Current Themes in Psychiatry 2

W0106243

Current Themes in Psychiatry 2

Raghu N. Gaind

Physician in Psychological Medicine,
Guy's Hospital, London

Barbara L. Hudson

Lecturer in Applied Social Studies,
University of Oxford

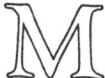

First published 1979 by
THE MACMILLAN PRESS LTD
London and Basingstoke
Associated companies in Delhi Dublin
Hong Kong Johannesbura Lagos Melbourne
New York Singapore and Tokyo

British Library Cataloguing in Publication Data

Current themes in psychiatry.
  Vol. 2
  1. Psychiatry
  I. Gaind, Raghu N II. Hudson, Barbara L
  616.8'9   RC454

  ISBN 978-1-349-04496-2   ISBN 978-1-349-04494-8 (eBook)
  DOI 10.1007/978-1-349-04494-8

Contents

List of Contributors

BANCROFT, John, M.A., M.D., F.R.C.P., F.R.C.Psych., D.P.M. (Lond)—Senior Scientific Officer, M.R.C. Unit for Reproductive Biology, Edinburgh.

BARNES, Thomas, M.B., B.S., M.R.C.Psych.—Research Fellow, Academic Unit of Clinical Psychopharmacology, Guy's Hospital Medical School, London.

BEAN, Philip, B.Sc. (Soc.), M.Sc. (Econ.)—Lecturer, Department of Applied Social Science, University of Nottingham.

BRYANT, Bridget, B.A.—Research Sociologist, Department of Educational Studies, University of Oxford.

CARSTAIRS, G. M., M.M., F.R.C.P., F.R.C.Psych.—Vice Chancellor, University of York.

CLARE, Anthony, M.B., M.Phil., M.R.C.P.I., M.R.C.Psych.—Senior Lecturer, Institute of Psychiatry, London.

CHRISTIE-BROWN, Jeremy, M.A., B.M., C.Ch., M.R.C.P., M.R.C.Psych., D.P.M.—Consultant Psychiatrist, The Maudsley Hospital, London.

EDWARDS, Guy, M.B., B.Ch., F.R.C.Psych., D.P.M.—Consultant Psychiatrist and Clinical Teacher in Psychiatry, University of Southampton Medical School.

FAULK, M., B.Sc., M.B., B.S., M.R.C.P., M.R.C.Psych., M.Phil.—Regional Consultant Forensic Psychiatrist, Wessex Regional Health Authority, Honorary Clinical Teacher, University of Southampton.

FREEMAN, Hugh, M.A., B.M., F.R.C.Psych., D.P.M.—Consultant Psychiatrist, Hope Hospital, Salford.

GELDER, Michael, D.M., F.R.C.P., F.R.C.Psych.—Handley Professor of Psychiatry, University of Oxford.

HIRSCH, Steven, B.A., M.D., M.Phil., M.R.C.P., M.R.C.Psych.—Professor of Psychiatry, Charing Cross Hospital Medical School, London.

KIDGER, Timothy, M.B., M.R.C.Psych.—Senior Registrar, Guy's Hospital, London.

LEFF, Julian, B.Sc., M.D., M.R.C.P., M.R.C.Psych.—Assistant Director M.R.C. Social Psychiatry Unit, Institute of Psychiatry, London.

LIPSEDGE, Maurice, M.B., M.R.C.P., M.R.C.Psych., D.P.M. (Lond)—Consultant Psychiatrist, St Bartholomew's Hospital, London.

MCAULEY, R., M.B., M.R.C.Psych.—Consultant Child Psychiatrist, Department of Child Psychiatry, Royal Belfast Hospital for Sick Children.

MILLARD, David W., Lecturer in Applied Social Studies, University of Oxford, Hon. Consultant Psychiatrist, The Warneford Hospital.

MORGAN, Gethin, M.A., F.R.C.P., F.R.C.Psych., D.P.M.—Consultant Senior Lecturer, Department of Health, University of Bristol.

PITT, Brice, M.D., M.R.C.Psych.—Consultant Psychiatrist, The London Hospital, London.

SHAW, Phyllis*, B.M., M.R.C.Psych.—Late Senior Research Psychiatrist, Department of Psychiatry, University of Oxford.

SILVERSTONE, Trevor, M.A., D.M., F.R.C.P., F.R.C.Psych., D.P.M. (Lond)— Reader in Human Psychopharmacology, Medical Colleges of St Bartholomew's and The London Hospitals.

SMITH, Selwyn M., B.S., M.D., F.R.C.P. (C), M.R.C.Psych., D.P.M.— Director, Department of Forensic Psychiatry, Royal Ottawa Hospital, Associate Professor of Psychiatry, University of Ottawa, Faculty of Medicine, Ottawa, Canada.

TRETHOWAN, W.H., C.B.E., M.B., F.R.C.P., F.R.C.Psych.—Professor of Psychiatry, University of Birmingham.

TROWER, Peter, M.Sc.—Senior Clinical Psychologist, Hollymoor Hospital, Northfield, Birmingham.

VAUGHN, Christine, Ph.D.—Former Research Worker, M.R.C. Social Psychiatry Unit, Institute of Psychiatry, London.

VENABLES, Peter H., Ph.D.—Professor of Psychology, Department of Psychology, University of York.

WATSON, J.P., M.D., M.R.C.P., F.R.C.Psych.—Professor of Psychiatry, Guy's Hospital Medical School, London.

YELLOLY, M. A., M.A., Ph.D.—Principal Lecturer, Goldsmiths' College, University of London.

*The death of Dr Phyllis Shaw is deeply regretted.

Preface

This, the second volume of *Current Themes in Psychiatry*, is based on a selection from the lectures delivered at Huntercombe Manor, Buckinghamshire in September 1977 at a course for senior psychiatrists arranged by the Senior Editor. We have tried to maintain the balance among the varied subject matter and approaches within psychiatry, selecting topics not included in Volume 1, and offering different perspectives. The first and largest section deals with issues of particular relevance to the contemporary psychiatrist who looks beyond his one-to-one treatment relationship to the inter-disciplinary team and the social systems to which both he and his patient are linked. However, alongside this broadening of perspectives, there is progress towards a sharpening of focus, a deepening of understanding, and a greater precision of treatment procedures. Chapters in the other sections demonstrate these developments.

Once again, we would like to thank the course participants, whose views have helped us in our selection of contents. We hope that this book, like its companion volume, will be of value to all those psychiatrists who seek to keep abreast of rapid increases in knowledge and innovative thinking in their speciality, and also to their colleagues, such as family practitioners and other mental health professionals.

B. L. H.
R. G.

University of Oxford,
January 1978

Foreword

John Pollitt
Physician in Charge
Department of Psychological Medicine
St Thomas' Hospital, London

It is a pleasure to be able to introduce and comment on this second series of articles based on original lectures organised by Dr Gaind in his capacity as clinical tutor. These lectures, like those in *Current Themes in Psychiatry*, Volume 1, were given in courses designed for senior psychiatrists to cover current research and development in modern psychiatry.

The fare in this volume is equally rich and varied, and the sections cater for all areas of the new broad spectrum in which psychiatric specialisation is developing. Early sections deal with interfaces ranging from the small group to cross-cultural studies. Moral and ethical issues are clearly to the fore and many of these articles emphasise the psychiatrist's evolving position in the community.

Not only did the original design cover the need for refreshment and stimulation which the sound discussion of growing areas can provide, but this book covers the further aim of enabling a much wider audience to enjoy these presentations. It will also allow those fortunate enough to have attended to digest at leisure the more compact areas. One hears often that outmoded ideas are 'layered' from one textbook to another and that traditional teaching dies hard, but this is an entirely different approach. Perhaps today's recent advances or contemporary views are the themes of membership teaching tomorrow. If so, we and our successors will have a much easier task. Dr Gaind's course has become very widely known. Its widespread positive appreciation is well deserved, and the reader is assured stimulation in this further series of distinguished contributions.

Acknowledgements

We are grateful to the Department of Postgraduate Education, Wyeth Laboratories, who helped to organise the 'Current Themes in Psychiatry' Conference at Huntercombe Manor in September 1977, to Miss Lilian Meekings, for first-class secretarial assistance, and to Mr Charles Fry, of the Macmillan Press Ltd, for helpful advice and endless patience.

In memory of the late Peter Duncan Scott, C.B.E.,
M.A., M.D., F.R.C.P., F.R.C.Psych., D.P.M.

SECTION 1
SOCIAL PERSPECTIVES

1 Community Psychiatry

Hugh Freeman

In all psychiatric literature, the word 'community' has appeared with increasing frequency for some years now, though this does not imply that there is any general agreement about its meaning in this connection. Very often, it is simply taken as equivalent to 'outside mental hospitals' and in the United States has commonly meant no more than providing psychotherapy under different financial arrangements from those of private practice. Sometimes it is used to refer to the whole of psychiatry and sometimes to a sub-speciality within it, though current British practice certainly assumes the former of these. A related concept is that of 'social psychiatry', which indicates the application of relevant scientific disciplines to the core of clinical psychiatry, or study of the interaction between social and clinical events; these disciplines include sociology, anthropology, statistics and economics. The result of this interchange is a practice of psychiatry greatly influenced by knowledge of social systems and of the epidemiological trends of disease.

Bennett (1977) has discussed the concept of community psychiatry and particularly commends Sabshin's definition (1966)—'the utilisation of the techniques, methods, theories of social psychiatry and other behavioural sciences to investigate and to meet the mental health needs of a functionally or geographically defined population over a significant period of time and the feeding back of information to modify the central body of social psychiatric and other behavioural science knowledge'. This refers therefore to the mental health needs of a defined population, rather than of individual patients, and not only those defined as sick, but also those whose health may be affected adversely by them. It takes account of the nature of the environment, as well as the clinical state of particular patients and does not assume any particular view as to where a patient should be treated or by whom. Another related aspect is 'community mental health', which has also suffered from a great excess of definitions. However, Schwartz (1972) sees this as a group of sub-systems (mental hospitals, private practitioners, welfare programmes, prisons, etc.) concerned with altering the ways in which society promotes the mental health of all of its citizens and responds to mental illness in some of them. Therefore, it involves many more people than the mental health professions—including the consumers of their services.

But in addition to any developments of theory or scientific knowledge, much has been added to community psychiatry through the everyday experience of psychiatrists and other professional staff in doing what they believed to be best. This is particularly relevant to circumstances in Britain, which has always favoured a pragmatic and dogma-free approach to the solution of problems—in A. J. Balfour's words, '. . . the principles of common sense, to do what seems to be the right thing in a given case'. British experience has, in fact, been influential on the ideas and practices of psychiatric services in many parts of the world during the past 25 years.

Among that experience, particularly full documentation has occurred of developments in the industrial city of Salford (Freeman and Mountney, 1967) resulting in the view of community psychiatry as a comprehensive arrangement of care for a defined population. It may also be described as 'district psychiatry' or 'psychiatrie du secteur'. This clearly includes facilities within hospitals and does not just refer to means of avoiding hospitalisation; within its defined area, the service must have continuous and final responsibility, whatever the clinical state of individual patients. It must offer, so far as resources allow, a continuous spectrum of integrated services from full-time, permanent care in an institution (for the relatively few people in any population who need it) to occasional support for a patient or family in their home. It must serve the whole community and not just those unable to afford private care; the more it is used by all social classes, the more likely are its standards to improve. As a general principle, it should be non-selective and non-rejecting in its activities, though clearly the extent to which it will be able to help different kinds of patients must vary greatly. It must particularly avoid the discontinuity which has existed between the internal activities of traditional mental hospitals and life outside, as well as their highly selective forms of intervention in psychiatric disorder (Freeman, 1977a). However, Wing (1977) has pointed out that discussions of organisation, management or staff training should not take place in such a way that the fundamental objectives of the service are forgotten, that is reduction of morbidity, distress and disability. Services should not become over-preoccupied with themselves. This model of community psychiatry has been particularly influential in the development of recent British policy for mental health services (D.H.S.S., 1971). It is basically an outward extension of the medical model of care.

There are a number of factors which have been important in influencing the development of community psychiatry (Freeman, 1968). The first of these is the progress made in psychiatric treatment; before the physical methods of treatment were discovered, it was very difficult to manage severe psychiatric illness outside a mental hospital, except for families with great private resources. However, the possibility of controlling fairly quickly most of the troublesome features of psychiatric disorder, particularly through medication and ECT, led slowly to general hospitals, family doctors, community nurses and social agencies all becoming able to play their part. Thus, the process of treatment and care can be distributed throughout a whole network of facilities in the population to be served, constituting a 'dispersed institution'. Compared with the type of service provided by the mental hospital alone, this should allow a greater variety of options of care for more kinds of psychiatric morbidity, yet preserving administrative integration of the service as a whole.

Secondly, the process has been affected by a broadening of the concept of psychiatric illness. At one time, psychiatric services dealt only with patients whose behaviour was severely disturbed through psychosis and who could not be managed by supporting relatives. More recently, the development of both physical and psychotherapeutic methods of treatment has allowed effective help to be given to patients with a wide range of psychotic and emotional disorders. At the same time, rising standards of living and of education in the general public have meant that the demand for such help has greatly increased. The result is likely to be the development of a system which is quite separate and additional to that of the mental hospital. Thus, in many countries, psychiatry has divided into an institutional kind, dealing with severe mental disorder, and an 'office' kind, dealing only with minor neurosis and personality problems. Such a split, which usually occurs mainly along the lines of social class, must have unfavourable consequences of many sorts, including the separation of both psychiatrists and patients into those of different levels of status. It is likely that only a comprehensive, community-based psychiatric service can avoid such a harmful division of resources, which in Holland for instance, results in three separate compartments of provision (Straathof, 1976). However, the fact that all services are publicly provided or financed certainly does not in itself guarantee integration; some countries which have no private practice also have an almost total separation between mental hospitals and extra-mural facilities.

Thirdly, there has been much greater awareness in recent years of the influence of social and psychological factors (which may be either therapeutic or anti-therapeutic) on psychiatric disorder and facilities. These factors include the institutionalism and authoritarian hierarchies of conventional mental hospitals, the harmful effects of intense emotion from relatives on schizophrenics (Vaughn and Leff, 1976) and the possible benefits to be gained from the introduction of therapeutic community principles into mental health facilities. As a result, intervention may be required in a variety of social situations, for example the visit of a psychiatrist or community nurse to a family with a member who is mentally ill, or the organisation of group activities in a day hospital. On the other hand, admission of a patient to hospital for physical treatment alone, without regard for the social circumstances of either the illness or the treatment process, will usually be of much more limited value. Awareness of the importance of these processes is likely to lead to a community-orientated, rather than an institutional system of care, though the series of comparative studies by Grad and Sainsbury (for example, 1968) suggested that a hospital-based service provided greater relief for the burdens imposed on families by psychiatric disorder. However, the 'community' service which was used as a comparison in this work seems to have been of only a limited nature—certainly in the earlier years.

Fourthly, but closely linked to the last factor, there are general social changes in the population. Mention has already been made of rising standards of demand and expectation, associated with an unwillingness of people to continue accepting the rigid and authoritarian practices of old mental hospitals. But there have also been great changes in age-distribution and in family structure; the average size of Western families has declined greatly, the number of unmarried adults has become much less, but the proportion of old people greatly increased. This means that it is much more difficult for cases of prolonged disability, such as severe mental illness, to be cared for within the family itself. At the same time, greater social mobility has caused the dispersal of extended families and of well-established social networks, such as exist in rural or older industrial communities. These patterns of kinship or neigh-bourhood could provide a great deal of support and practical assistance to families in trouble through illness, but many nuclear families now are quite isolated from any such source of help and must depend on the medical and social services of the community. Therefore, these services must be widely available and both comprehensive and flexible in their mode of operation; for instance, domestic help or babysitting might be more valuable in some cases than specifically psychiatric provision. Cooper and Sartorius (1977) have put forward some fascinating hypotheses on the possible relationship between industrialisation and the emergence of schizophrenia as a major public health problem in the nineteenth century; the view that these two may be linked is supported by findings from the *International Pilot Study of Schizophrenia* (W.H.O., 1975) showing that chronic disability from this disorder is less common in non-industrialised countries. Thus, the organisation of a com-munity psychiatric service must always be seen in social, as well as medical terms, though there is no evidence whatever that levels of psychiatric morbidity have any relationship to different political systems—something which would not be suspected from much non-medical writing and teaching on the subject. The relationship between mental health and environment is extremely complex (Freeman, 1978) and though deprived urban areas contain an excess of people affected by psychiatric disorder, this is likely to be due to drift, at least as much as to any influences of environmental conditions.

Another important influence in the development of community psychiatry is the fact that, with current treatment methods, a patient with a major psychiatric disorder will almost certainly spend much more time outside hospital than as an in-patient, in the long term. Therefore, we may expect that treatment will need to occur within a medical setting for a number of acute episodes, but that the main burden of continued care will be carried out elsewhere. This is because the patient will either be well enough to remain under the ordinary system of primary medical care, or else he will have chronic handicaps which require mainly social measures and facilities. For most of the time, medical and nursing interventions will be mainly of a monitoring nature and will only be intermittent.

For the episodes of illness which do require continuous medical and nursing management, there are strong social trends in most countries which favour this now taking place in a general hospital, rather than in a specialised institution. Both doctors and nurses in training generally favour a hospital in which all types of patients are treated and which is generally of higher status.

The isolated situation of many mental hospitals causes staffing difficulties because of the world-wide trend towards urbanisation and because staff wish to lead a normal life outside working hours. The use of the general hospital avoids the stigma or labelling effect of specifically psychiatric institutions, which can be personally very harmful to patients, and when given a choice, the consumer of psychiatric care will usually choose the general hospital. Finally, there is the fact that anti-therapeutic qualities and a peculiar internal culture have undoubtedly been prevalent in mental hospitals throughout the world, whereas the general hospital is usually a more open social situation and thus less vulnerable to manipulation by individuals. However, the general hospital psychiatric unit can only work successfully as part of a network of facilities, integrated with it, and these are missing to varying extents in nearly all parts of Britain at present.

Of course, not all the arguments are on one side. Where population density is relatively low, the psychiatric section of a district general hospital may be so small that it cannot provide a full variety of treatment methods or training for staff. Highly specialised facilities, which may serve a wider area can be difficult to accommodate on a general hospital site, particularly if they need plenty of space. Chronically handicapped patients may also find the large campuses of mental hospitals useful, particularly if they have peculiarities of behaviour, which are unwelcome to the public outside. There are some psychiatric hospitals that have developed a long tradition of excellence, which would be difficult to reproduce in a general hospital, though one must say frankly that these have always been a minority.

In fact, mental hospitals in most countries have tended, over the course of time, to develop into primarily long-stay institutions, to become over-crowded and to have low standards of care and staffing. It has become clear that it is generally wrong to deal with the chronically disabled by housing them in large institutions, which are separated and often remote from acute hospitals and from community-based medical and social services, as well as from their own families. The long-stay accommodation that is needed should be an integrated part of the comprehensive mental health service for that sector of population. It should therefore come within the responsibilities of a multi-disciplinary professional team, which is also concerned with acute care, home visiting, rehabilitation and all the other facilities which make up an integrated service. Unless the staff of residential institutions and those based in the community are made to feel part of the same organisation, it is inevitable that they will divide into two hostile camps and seek to pass the buck to each other. There is also the danger that staff in long-stay residential facilities may become as isolated and institutionalised as the patients. Wing (1977) has proposed as an objective that services should use the least degree of institutionalism that will cope with the needs of the family, for example bed-sitter, group home, hostel and hospital (in order of dependency)—'. . . it should be possible to provide appropriate accommodation within the area before families become unable to cope, so that the likelihood of handicapped people falling out of care altogether is minimised'. However, if this system is to work to any satisfactory extent, it does require co-ordination between agencies, as well as a reasonable provision of facilities—though what is satisfactory depends mainly on social expectations and 'illness' is a concept with many social determinants.

Hospital resources are now so expensive that it is logical to use them at maximum intensity and for the minimum length of time that will not produce undue hardship in the communities they serve. But in fact, a significant proportion of hospital beds nearly everywhere in developed countries are used primarily for social purposes—to house patients with chronic disabilities who cannot be cared for anywhere else at present. This situation is a very uneconomical one and it applies particularly to psychiatry and to geriatrics. In these specialities, curative medicine and nursing, along conventional lines, have very little to offer to a large proportion of the patients concerned. There is therefore a need to be much more flexible about the delivery of medico-social services; for instance, dispersing facilities for psychiatric consultation or maintenance treatment to primary medical care centres, which will be more accessible to most of the population served. Little is known yet about the cost – benefit aspects of most forms of medical and social service provision. However, since resources are limited and demands constantly increasing, there is an obvious need to examine the relative expense of all different kinds of provision and to seek for low-cost solutions where possible. For instance, supervision of patients with chronic psychiatric disorders living outside hospital has largely passed from the hands of social workers to those of community nurses—to the extent that it is undertaken at all. Yet the financial aspects of this change are unexplored, as are the actual transactions between nurses and patients to a large extent; we do not know what degree of further training should be provided for nurses who have previously worked inside hospitals, nor what this would cost. Similarly as far as accommodation is concerned, the 'purpose-built' hostel with a resident staff is now so expensive that very few more are likely to be provided. However, group homes are relatively cheap and are capable of dealing with a very large number of those who need a sheltered home because of psychiatric handicaps (Soni *et al.*, 1978). Early (1965) has developed the concept of the 'ladder' of rehabilitation facilities, concerned both with occupation and with social living, which should be available outside hospitals.

Every system of medical and social care, therefore, involves some process of rationing. If this is by money, the likely result—as in most parts of the United States—is that skilled psychiatric manpower will be concentrated on the fringes of psychiatric disorder, dealing with neurotic and personality problems in the urban middle class. However, community psychiatry must surely make an ideological choice (though not one between political ideologies) as to where its efforts are to be concentrated. If a genuine attempt is being made to meet the greatest human needs from psychiatric illness, then therapeutic goals are bound to be limited, because the numbers involved are large. Acute distress must be relieved and realistic attempts made to restore reasonable levels of functioning, but there can be little opportunity for remoulding personalities through intensive psychotherapy, nor for using resources on what has been described as 'primary prevention'. This concept owes much to the views of Caplan (1964) who made use of the public health model, and it would be very satisfactory if 'primary preventive' action could greatly reduce the demands made on services by the major psychiatric disorders. Unfortunately, as we have little real knowledge of their aetiology, there is no evidence at all that this desirable objective can actually be achieved. It would therefore be inhumane and unreasonable to direct our efforts in that way before an effective clinical service was available to every person in a community who might be affected by an acute psychiatric disorder.

Closely related is the concept of crisis intervention, which assumes that psychiatric illness may be prevented by intervening in crises of living, though these may have no definite clinical aspect at the time of occurrence. Certainly, many of the episodes which are presented to district psychiatric services, through either medical or social work channels, are primarily episodes of social disturbance (Mountney et al., 1969). Often, they could best be resolved by social action, for example obtaining a bed for the night in some non-clinical accommodation, though such action may currently be impossible for the service concerned. However, responding to a social crisis which has acquired a psychiatric label—perhaps through someone with a previous psychiatric history being involved in it—is a different matter from mental health staff actively seeking out those who are socially vulnerable, before any sort of clinical abnormality has appeared. The personal crises arising in the population of any community, for example marital, sexual, adolescent, bereavement, are so many that it would be quite impossible to have professional staff intervening in a high proportion of them, while at the same time providing a clinical service to those who are already ill. However, this is not to deny the importance of high-risk groups, such as the recently bereaved who may well develop clinical depression later, and the dilemma of how to offer help to them on a reasonable scale may be resolved to some extent by the use of trained volunteers. Similarly, it may be more practical and more honest to admit that a specialist psychotherapy service—particularly if undertaken by doctors—simply cannot be provided for all appropriate cases from a community's population. The alternative here is to place the responsibility firmly with the primary-care organisation, which may receive specialised help in the form of training and consultation from the community-based psychiatric service.

This raises, though, the question of how professional time should be divided between direct service to patients and indirect service through others, for example G.P.s, teachers, clergy, police, volunteers. It would be easy for the latter to swallow up almost the whole working time of a mental health service and to some extent American community mental health centres were founded on that basis. Brown (1977) points out that the emphasis on consultation and education in these centres assumes that there is a useful body of knowledge relating to 'mental health' which can be used to promote positive mental health, prevent mental illness and generally improve the quality of life. (Perhaps the optimism involved in these ambitious aims is typically American.) To qualify for federal support, a centre had to provide: in-patient services, out-patient services, partial hospitalisation (mainly day care), emergency services and consultation and education facilities. It was also recommended that there should be: diagnostic services, rehabilitation services, pre-care and after-care services in the community, staff training and research and evaluation. In practice, many difficulties have occurred in the development of this programme, not least financial; the centres have made relatively little contribution to the care of long-term disorders, their very ambitious objectives have not generally been met and their virtual abandonment of the medical model has led to wasteful controversies within their communities, far greater than those affecting conventional psychiatry. All in all, the more modest aims of the British model of community psychiatry seem more likely to be achieved, though the staggering cost of building new general hospital units has put the over-all replacement of mental hospitals far into the future.

Current British policy aims to relate community-based services to Health Districts, which have an average population of 250 000—300 000 though this figure may be much smaller in rural areas. Where a complete psychiatric unit does not exist in the district general hospital, the nearest mental hospital has to be divided functionally into clinical divisions, each of which serves one or more sectors of the population; a sector has a population of about 60 000 and is normally the responsibility of one consultant psychiatrist. The doctors and nurses of each division in the mental hospital are expected to develop close links with the G.P.s, social workers and community nurses operating in their district, so that a joint therapeutic team is formed. This situation is portrayed diagrammatically in figure 1.1.

In the long run, psychiatric facilities should be planned and developed to match the identified needs of the population of each community. However, we are still only at the beginning of this process and both thinking and practice still tend to be governed mainly by our familiarity with institutions, which were mostly built for circumstances that have now changed completely. Though services are still measured primarily by their number of hospital beds, this practice should be obsolete and probably the available time of skilled staff is the most important index available. However, day care places have become increasingly significant and sheltered housing, workshop places and transport should also be included; in fact, the day department could be seen as the central focus of the community psychiatry service, with some beds attached to it for those patients who currently need full-time hospitalisation. Though many people affected by psychiatric disorders need intensive care or rehabilitation over long periods, their actual place of residence may not be crucial and the fact that more psychiatric patients than previously are now

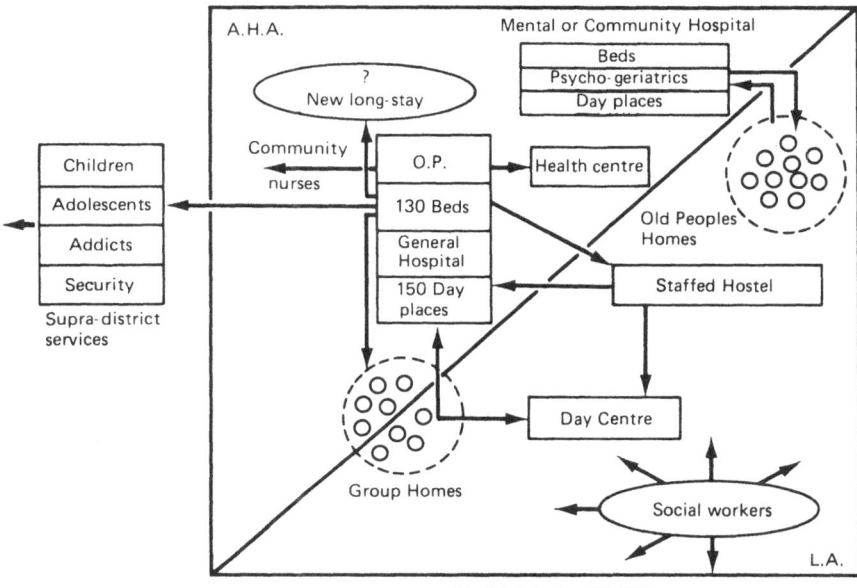

Figure 1.1

living outside hospital does not make the problem of caring for them any less. Measures of the case-loads of district services are provided by psychiatric case registers (for example Fryers *et al.*, 1970) but sophisticated instruments of this kind will not be generally available, nor necessary; accurate book-keeping, which does not demand expensive technology, is enough for most purposes.

Information about one important client-group of community psychiatry was obtained by Cheadle, Freeman and Korer (1977) who investigated all schizophrenics from a defined population of 124 000 who had been in contact with some psychiatric service during 1974 and were not long-stay hospital patients. The sample consisted of 190, with almost equal numbers of each sex, although the women tended to be older. Though many more of the women had been married, their marriages had often ended in divorce, whereas far more men were currently living with parents. Most said they were satisfied with relationships with their families and though 48 complained of social isolation, this was not necessarily related to living alone. Clinically, relatively few of the patients showed active features of psychosis, but many were troubled by neurotic symptoms, which were strongly associated with social handicaps. On the other hand, 49 were working and this was the social feature most strongly correlated with a favourable clinical state. Of the 190 patients, 156 were currently taking neuroleptics and of these, 137 were receiving them in the form of depot injections; it is very likely that the low level of overt psychotic illness in this group can be attributed to a large extent to the effective medication they were receiving. However, maintaining great numbers of people outside hospital on continuous pharmacological treatment for long periods requires management and information systems quite different from those used by hospitals or primary medical care in the past. A system of 'Continuous Care' is needed for patients who are vulnerable to further relapses of psychosis and only an integrated community psychiatric service is likely to be able to undertake this. A model of this system is presently being evaluated in Salford.

This discussion of community psychiatry has not referred to facilities provided by a community out of the personal resources of its individual members. Britain, however, has continuously followed the direction of creating a structure of public services, financed out of general taxation, of which community psychiatry is a part. But also, because of the social changes mentioned earlier (and others such as comprehensive urban redevelopment) there is no longer a 'community' in any real sense in many areas where the need for these services is greatest. It would clearly be wrong to look on the 'community' as a mythical society of healthy and well-adjusted people. In the United States, much emphasis has been placed on the idea of community self-help, including socially deprived areas, and the results have often been disastrous. Professional staff have strayed too far from their actual skills and body of knowledge, resulting in dissipation of effort into intractable social problems, for which they have no particular competence. The cobbler should stick to his last.

References

Bennett, D. H. (1977). Concepts of community psychiatry. Unpublished paper to *Symposium of Royal College of Psychiatrists*, London

Brown, A. C. (1977). The mental health centre. Unpublished paper to *Symposium of Royal College of Psychiatrists*, London

Caplan, G. (1964). *Principles of Preventive Psychiatry*. Tavistock, London

Cheadle, A. G., Freeman, H. L. and Korer, J. R. (1977). Chronic schizophrenic patients in the community. *Br. J. Psychiat.* **132**, 221–227

Cooper, J. and Sartorius, N. (1977). Cultural and temporal variations in schizophrenia. *Br. J. Psychiat.*, **130**, 50–55

D.H.S.S. (1971). *Hospital Services for the Mentally Ill*. H.M.S.O., London

Early, D. F. (1965). *Psychiatric Hospital Care*. (Ed. H. L. Freeman), Bailliere, London

Freeman, H. L. (1968). Community psychiatry. *Br. J. Psychiat.*, **114**, 481–484

Freeman, H. L. (1977). Continuity of care in the mental health service. *Int. J. ment. Hlth*, **5**, 3–13

Freeman, H. L. (1978). Mental health and the environment. *Br. J. Psychiat.* **132**, 113–124

Freeman, H. L. and Mountney, G. H. (1967). *New Aspects of the Mental Health Services*. (Ed. H. L. Freeman and W. A. J. Farndale), Pergamon Press, Oxford

Fryers, T., Freeman, H. L. and Mountney, G. H. (1970). A census of psychiatric patients in an urban community. *Social Psychiat.*, **5**, 187–195

Grad, J. and Sainsbury, P. (1968). The effects that patients have on their families in a community care and a control psychiatric service. *Br. J. Psychiat.*, **114**, 265–278

Mountney, G. H., Fryers, T. and Freeman, H. L. (1969). Psychiatric emergencies in an English Borough. *Br. med. J.*, **1**, 498–500

Sabshin, M. (1966). In *Community Psychiatry* (Ed. M. Roberts, S. L. Halleck and M. S. Loeb), University of Wisconsin Press, Madison

Schwartz, D. A. (1972). In *Progress in Community Health, II* (Ed. H. H. Barter and L. Bellak), Grune and Stratton, New York

Soni, S., Soni, S. D. and Freeman, H. L. (1978). Group homes for psychiatric patients. *Int. J. ment. Hlth.* (in press)

Straathof, L. J. A. (1976). General policies in the development of mental health services in the Netherlands. *Int. J. ment. Hlth*, **5**, 59–63

Vaughn, C. and Leff, J. P. (1976). The influence of family and social factors on the course of psychiatric illness. *Br. J. Psychiat.*, **129**, 125–137

World Health Organization (1975). *The International Pilot Study of Schizophrenia.* W.H.O., Geneva

Wing, J. K. (1977). Social and community psychiatry. Unpublished paper to *Symposium of Royal College of Psychiatrists*, London

2 Sociology and Psychiatry: Some Areas of Common Interest

Philip Bean

It is only recently that one could legitimately talk of a sociological contribution to psychiatry. To some extent this was caused by the different historical development of the two disciplines. Psychiatry had become a well-established branch of medicine by the mid-nineteenth century; sociology, by comparison, had its origins in the work of Auguste Comte in the first part of the nineteenth century, but did not become an extensive and established subject until after 1945. It was only in the 1960s that it achieved some form of general recognition.

Apart from the obvious differences in their historical antecedents sociological interest in psychiatry has never been profound, and even now remains largely divided between those sociologists interested in deviancy theory, who view ascriptions of mental illness as a deviant status, and those interested in the sociology of medicine who relate psychiatry to other forms of medical enterprise. There are others who specialise in studying psychiatry from a specific sociological position, such as through the sociology of organisations. There is, in addition, another group of sociologists who are primarily interested in the sociology of law and who concern themselves with developing theories about the psychiatrist's relationship with the Mental Health Act and its attendant legislation (Bean, 1975). Sociological interest is, therefore, fragmented and diffuse.

Sociology of Psychiatry and Sociology in Psychiatry

Although most sociologists have some knowledge about the role and functions of the psychiatrists, the reverse is not always the case. Psychiatrists often view social workers as sociologists (which may be true sometimes, but not usually when they are practising social work) and so confuse the nature of the sociological tradition. Social work could be seen as a form of applied sociology, although even then most sociologists would probably dispute this.

S. Kirson Weinberg makes the useful distinction between psychiatric sociology and social psychiatry (Weinberg, 1967). He defines psychiatric sociology as the study of mental disorders as social phenomena and identifies four features of psychiatric sociology. First, a study of social factors and social processes that contribute to mental disorders, for example family and social class; second, a study of the social definitions of mental disorders as forms of social deviance; third, the social facets in the treatment and care of disordered persons; and, last, the social aspects of the prevention of mental disorder. Weinberg argues that psychiatric sociology is derived from a sociological perspective where its theories and methods stem from a sociological base. 'Psychiatric sociology produces a social dimension (by) revising the object of study from an organism to a person in a social setting.'

In contrast, social psychiatry relates to social action and is seen by Weinberg as attempting to provide social patterns which facilitate the treatment and care of disordered persons. Social psychiatry is eclectic and is an applied discipline. Although clinical in orientation, it derives its perspective from the area of social relationships. Weinberg's definition of social psychiatry is heavily derived from the work of Jurgen Ruesch, who sees social psychiatry as a hybrid discipline which attempts to integrate the knowledge derived from the social sciences with the skills of the psychiatrists (Ruesch, 1965). Ruesch delineates seven major areas in the study of social psychiatry, most of which centre around epidemiological surveys and cultural and social factors such as the family, age, and sexual aspects that impinge on the mentally disordered persons.

To Weinberg and Ruesch, the differences between psychiatric sociology and social psychiatry can be seen in terms of aims and commitments. Psychiatric sociology is concerned with developing sociological theory whereas social psychiatry is concerned with assisting clinical practice. Another example would be the interpretation of social class. Psychiatric sociologists would be mainly concerned with the effects of social class on mentally disordered persons, social psychiatrists would be interested in the diagnostic conditions of the persons within the various social classes.

Weinberg and Ruesch provide a relatively clear distinction between psychiatric sociology and social psychiatry although, in practice, the two areas of study tend to overlap. A more certain view is provided by Leonard Schatzman and Anselm Strauss, who believe that it would be more fruitful for sociology if more research was done *about* psychiatry than *in* it or *for* it (Schatzman and Strauss, 1966). Their postion would, I think, be as follows. Criticisms of current sociological practices in the field of psychiatry tend to focus on the position that much of what goes by the name of sociological research contributes little towards developing theory essential to an exclusive sociological position. Sociologists tend to deal with problems of mental disorder by accepting the legitimacy of psychiatric practice and its supporting assumption, though not necessarily its underlying theories. Typically then, sociologists want to help psychiatrists understand how social events affect, or are related to psychiatric practice, but in so doing immediately accept the psychiatrist's stance. The shift, however slight, can be seen in the sociologist's use of psychiatric terminology. Whenever sociologists use terms such as 'mental illness', 'psychopath' or 'inadequate personality' or even 'schizophrenia', they have begun to accept the psychiatric stance. Unwittingly, say Schatzman and Strauss, sociologists have then committed themselves to the psychiatric position and their research is *in* psychiatry rather than *about* it.

Schatzman and Strauss could, of course, be accused of adopting a tribal position and be guilty of the same imperialistic stance of which they later accuse psychiatrists, that is of simply extending the boundaries of their academic discipline. In practical terms, however, their position is virtually unobtainable for as Stanley Plog and Richard Edgerton point out, there is really no way yet devised whereby psychiatric terms can be avoided in research in this area (Plog and Edgerton, 1969). Their own attempts to find a substitute for a term like 'mental illness' did not prove worthwhile, although they admitted feeling uneasy about the term for the same reason provided by Schatzman and Strauss. Yet in spite of the practical problems there are a number of advantages in adopting a sceptical position. First, an attempt to obtain a sociological perspective free from the inhibitions provided by psychiatric terminology has the advantage of forcing a much larger range of relevant questions into the field of study. Secondly, and linking this to the first point, a sceptical position affords protection against the assumptions that many psychiatrists take for granted. Finally, it stops the sociologist defining the psychiatrists' function in the psychiatrists' own terms. It is that very function of the psychiatrists that is to be questioned and placed under scrutiny. The disadvantages are clear also. The main one is that sociologists may be so concerned with their sociological perspective that they remove themselves from the subject matter and isolate themselves from the psychiatric realities.

From the standpoint of Schatzman and Strauss, and aided by the distinctions used by Weinberg, some differences between sociology and psychiatry can now be delineated. The sociologist is primarily concerned with developing the boundaries of the discipline, whereas those involved in social psychiatry have a commitment to the clinical requirements of the patient. The interesting question then becomes centred around the sociological *contribution* to psychiatry for with different aims the contribution must be of a qualitatively different nature.

Areas of Sociological Contribution

The first general and obvious point to make is that any sociological contribution must be within the methodology of sociology. The study of sociology involves lateral thinking, that is, sociological work involves making conceptual links between events over the same time period. In contrast, and by way of comparison, history involves making conceptual links between time periods and is, therefore, sequential thinking. Lateral thinking, which is specifically sociological, must also involve sequential thinking, for without it sociology would merely be the study of social forms divorced from any historical antecedents. Conversely, history would be reduced to describing events if it was never involved in lateral thinking. Inevitably the disciplines overlap, and the boundaries between the two are no less difficult to define than between sociology and psychiatry. However, the strengths (and weaknesses) of sociology make it ideally suited to ask a specific but limited set of questions which range from the macro level to the minutiae of the doctor/patient relationship. The types of questions considered below are not to be regarded as comprising an exhaustive list, but reflect the interests and views of one particular sociologist. They have been selected because they are considered to be the areas where sociological enquiry has been fruitful in the past and may continue to be so in the future.

Psychiatrists as Agents of Treatment

The term 'treatment' has now become sufficiently diffuse to encompass the specific features of the doctor/patient relationship and wide enough to include the area of 'society in general'—the latter involving arguments about 're-educating society' or 'societal perceptions of mental illness'. Nancy Waxler, for example (Waxler, 1974), relates treatment outcomes to differences in societal responses to mental disorder. Comparing Ceylon and Mauritius with Britain, Waxler notes that serious psychoses in peasant societies tend to be of short duration and have an excellent prognosis even though treatment facilities are considerably more limited. She argues that beliefs about mental illness in peasant societies centre around supernatural causation. This, she thinks, relieves the mentally disordered person of any sense of responsibility for his condition. In contrast, where psychiatric illness is seen to involve the total personality, and where treatment systems are both comprehensive and bureaucratic, the person may be engulfed in that system and find little reward or opportunity for improving his condition. Waxler's views must remain at the level of a tentative hypothesis, but are none the less interesting. In practical terms such a view has little value for the practising psychiatrist who must operate within the comprehensive and bureaucratic structure already established, except, of course, that large scale comparative studies act as a salutary reminder about some of the defects of our present system. These defects may one day be considered dysfunctional to the mentally ill.

At the same general level, arguments about 're-educating society' have been shown to have serious limitations. Attitudes about mental illness change slowly and in the thirty years since the Royal Commission, it is doubtful if 'public opinion in general is moving towards a more enlightened attitude (where) the mentally ill are sick people and that mental hospitals should be thought of as hospitals for the treatment of illness' (H.M.S.O.,1957). Mental illness and other forms of mental disorder are still, in Scheff's terms, forms of 'residual rule breaking' (Scheff, 1966), that is violate basic social norms of human conduct. Szasz, in a similar vein, says that although we may show more compassion and understanding than some of our forebears, the fact is that the person diagnosed as mentally ill is stigmatised. 'These stigmata cannot be removed by mental health "education" for the root of the matter is our intolerance of certain kinds of behaviour' (Szasz, 1974). Scheff and Szasz may be unduly pessimistic, but the research of Cumming and Cumming (1957) showed that mental health education programmes did not appear to change attitudes towards the mentally ill.

At a more specific level, and particularly at the level of the doctor/patient relationship, most sociological views of treatment rely heavily on Parsons' concept of the sick role (Parsons, 1951). Briefly, Parsons saw the sick role as involving two rights and two obligations. First, it exempts the sick person from normal social responsibilities; secondly, the sick person is not held responsible for his illness, and therefore needs care rather than punishment. Thirdly, the sick person is placed under an obligation to get well, and, finally, there is a moral obligation to seek competent help from a physician and co-operate with him in trying to get well. Parsons also emphasised that there is a fundamentally harmonious relationship between mental health and the broader social system. Adequate health for most group members is also a functional requirement of that social system, hence Parsons included the two obligations which were placed on the sick person.

Parsons' concept of the sick role is usually regarded as more appropriate to the area of physical sickness than to the psychiatric sphere, for the rights and obligations placed on the psychiatric patient may be of a different order. Even so, Parsons uses the sick role as a means of drawing attention to the subjective component in sickness, a factor which is rarely present in definitions provided by medical scientists. David Mechanic suggests that illness defined in medical terms is strictly organic phenomena occasioned by some disturbances of the normal functions of bodily processes marked by certain symptoms or syndromes (Mechanic, 1959). To the medical scientists, definitions of illness are operational definitions, and are non-theoretical. To the sociologist, illness is seen in terms of social action. In practice, a non-theoretical definition means that illness only exists when recognised by doctors—those persons not coming under medical scrutiny are not, therefore, regarded as ill. A theoretical definition related to social action considers the patient's view of his condition.

It must be recognised that for most of the time a pragmatic view works well. It is not without its limitations, the most obvious one being that it by-passes any consideration by the patient of his condition. Yet the subjective component cannot be easily ignored, for as Anthony Flew has recently pointed out, all definitions of illness should involve two distinct but related aspects; first that the illness must be recognised by the sufferer, and that, secondly, it must be regarded by him as being presumptively bad for him (Flew, 1974). Such a view stands in marked contrast to that stated by Sir Aubrey Lewis who saw illness as having a social context but not a social content (Lewis, 1953).

Sociological interest has been concerned with developing theory which accounts for the way in which illness can be related to the behaviour of the patient as well as that of the doctor. Mechanic and Volkart move some way towards this by introducing the concept of 'illness behaviour', which attempts to account for the way in which symptoms are perceived, elaborated and acted upon by a person who recognises some pain or discomfort or other signs of malfunction (Mechanic and Volkart, 1961). They emphasise the part played by social factors in illness behaviour, particularly that related to the way in which illness occurs within a complicated set of relationships, differential needs, and varied perceptions. These social factors begin at the point where the patient assesses his condition, for relatively few people consult a physician without first discussing their condition with a friend or next of kin. Initially, prospective patients rely heavily on non-medical explanations, which in turn help to provide them with some meaning about the illness and with some form of provisional validation. Most patients continue to define their condition, or at least assess it for themselves, after professional consultation has taken place, and decide whether to continue with their course of treatment. Geographical and social class factors operate too. In some areas of Britain, conditions such as bronchitis have different meanings for the sufferer: where bronchitis is common, it tends to be regarded more as a fact of life than an illness, whereas in other districts, or in higher social classes, bronchitis is seen to require immediate medical attention. Different interpretations of illness can also be related to roles. Where role expectations are high, entry into the sick role can be either immediate, as with someone holding high office who is important to the social group, or postponed as long as possible, as with the mother with small children who has different expectations placed upon her. Where role expectations are low, entry to the sick role varies accordingly. For example, those persons not working, or who are retired, may be encouraged to enter the sick role, even though the illness may be relatively slight. Seen in this way, illness behaviour is more than the physiological manifestations of the illness, but involves patterned networks and social relationships. Sociologists see their task as delineating these relationships.

In the field of psychiatry the arguments appear in a different but no less acute form. 'Mental illness' is first and foremost surrounded by an interesting and volatile debate as to whether 'mental illness' is an illness, and whether personality disorders can ever be regarded as a disease. Philosophers such as Anthony Flew regard 'mental illness' as a 'conceptual shambles' (Flew, 1974). Szasz regards it as a myth (Szasz, 1974) and Theodor Sarbin sees it as a myth born of metaphor (Sarbin, 1969). Conversely, David Ausabel says personality disorder *is* disease (Ausabel, 1961). Various British psychiatrists such as Sir Aubrey Lewis, would agree with Ausabel (Lewis, 1953). The debate, although interesting, lies slightly outside the sociologists' province, being more related to philosophy and psychiatry. It is relevant in that it adds a further element to the way in which the subjective component in mental illness has an altogether different flavour as far as the psychiatric patient is concerned. If Flew is right, that is that an illness must be regarded as such by the sufferer and also be presumptively bad for him, then it needs to be acknowledged that some mentally ill patients would not in those circumstances be ill. Neither would Flew's argument be weakened by adopting the stance of the 1954–57 Royal Commission who said that disorders of the mind are illnesses which need medical treatment, but added that mental disorders were special sorts of illness which affect the patient's power of judgement and appreciation of his own condition (H.M.S.O., 1957). That, Flew would say, was more a statement about intended policy than a debate about the nature of mental illness.

The debate about the nature of mental illness is also relevant for it leads to a basic weakness in Parsons' position. Parsons saw entry into the sick role as being ultimately regulated by the doctor so that entry into that role presumably shows the doctor and sick person to be in agreement. Yet in psychiatry there is often conflict between the psychiatrist and the sick person, concerning the existence of his sickness, hence the special powers created by the Mental Health Act. Michael Bloor and Gordon Horobin have refined Parsons' position by making a distinction between the sick role and the patient role (Bloor and Horobin, 1975); the distinction being based on the premise that not all people who are sick become patients, and not all patients are sick.

It is not always clear from Bloor and Horobin what they mean by 'sickness' in this context. None the less, the use of the 'patient role' helps to draw attention to the way in which psychiatrists have to negotiate entry into various roles and thus is another important area of sociological enquiry. Even if one accepts that the distinction between the sick and patient role is still in a crude form the potential is also apparent. As far as the individual person is concerned he may accept that he is sick in the psychiatric sense of the term and be willing to be a patient. Alternatively, he may accept that he is sick but not be willing to be a patient, or in some rare circumstances may not recognise he is sick but wish to be a patient (some people apply to be admitted to the patient role to escape other role demands such as those required by Courts, etc.). Finally, he may not recognise sickness nor be willing to be a patient. Conversely, as far as the psychiatrist is concerned, he may view the person as sick but is not willing to accept him as a patient (there are instances where the psychiatrist says he can do no more for this person, or that because of previous disruptive behaviour the person should not be allowed in the mental hospital), or he may view the person as not sick but needing to be a patient, or both sick and a patient, or not sick nor a patient. These points can be demonstrated diagrammatically as in figures 2.1 and 2.2. Figures 2.1 and 2.2 can be combined into a 16 × 4 table and this would show where the conflict is likely to occur. The psychiatrist still determines entry into the sick or patient role but conflict occurs where the psychiatrist wishes to ascribe roles not acceptable to the subject. In its most extreme form, the compulsory powers available under the Mental Health Act would be invoked where there was a dispute about entry into the patient role.

This type of presentation should be seen as a tentative step in an otherwise unchartered field. It could be used in other areas of medicine, but is at this

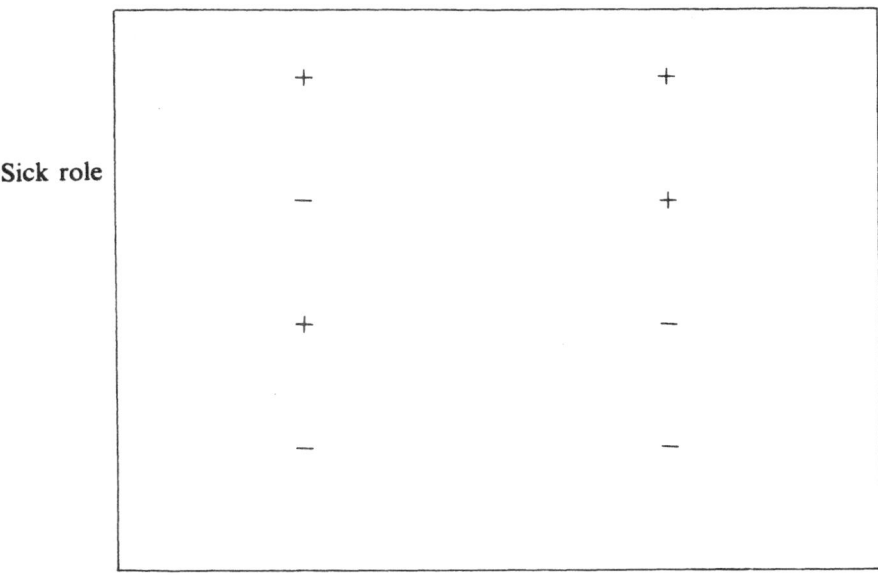

Figure 2.1   Subject's perception of sick and patient role

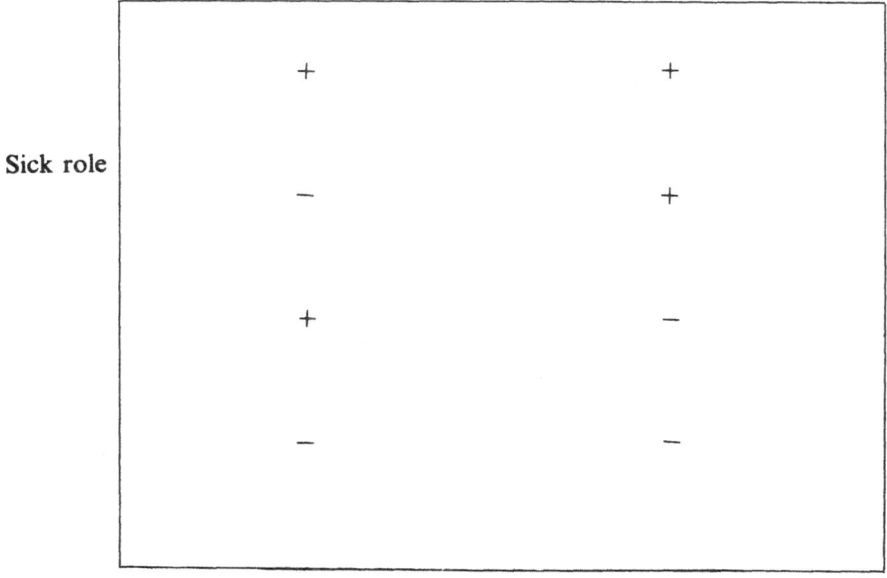

+ indicates acceptance, − indicates rejection

Figure 2.2   Psychiatrist's perception of sick and patient role

stage seen more apposite to the field of mental illness. To develop the analysis further we would need to know what features of the subject's condition determine entry into the sick or patient role and what features of psychiatric practice are key variables also. In short, a greater understanding is required of the interaction between psychiatrist (or any other doctor) and the person seen to be ill. Such an area of enquiry is still in its infancy.

Although the type of analysis presented above illustrates the possible area of future enquiry, studies relating to the mental hospital and the paths to the mental hospital show a more confident grasp of the subject matter. In their classic study of social class and mental illness, Hollingshead and Redlich showed how social class became a real factor in the prevalence of treated mental illness in the community, for the lower the class the greater the proportion of patients in the treated population (Hollingshead and Redlich, 1958). They also found that there was a direct relationship between class position and types of psychiatric disorders; again the lower the class the higher the rate for the psychoses. Finally, they found that there were real differences in where, how, and how long persons in various classes have been cared for by psychiatrists: those in the lower classes remained in hospital for a longer period. They concluded that 'treatment for mental illness depends not only on medical and psychological considerations, but also on powerful social variables to which psychiatrists have so far given little attention' (Hollingshead and Redlich, 1958, p. 300).

The importance of Hollingshead and Redlich's study is not confined to illustrating the basic structural inequalities in a class system which lead to differential diagnosis and differential treatment, but it also shows how language is used to present different aetiologies of similar conditions in varying classes. 'The class V neurotic behaves badly, the class IV neurotic aches physically, the class III defends himself and the class I and II is dissatisfied with himself. Thus we have a body language of pain and malfunction, social anxiety and verbal symbolic dislocation, all called neurosis' (Hollingshead and Redlich, 1958, p. 240). In a manner which preceded the labelling theorists by a decade, Hollingshead and Redlich pointed to the contingencies which determine whether abnormal behaviour is perceived as ill or merely idiosyncratic and indeed, whether it is perceived as ill or criminal. Mental hospitals may take mentally ill people, but so do other institutions, particularly in the penal system, and negotiation must take place between the members of the institutions to decide whether the person be regarded as 'ill' or 'criminal'. Hollingshead and Redlich argue that every person who follows a path that leads to a psychiatrist, and later perhaps to a mental hospital, must pass four milestones. First, the occurrence of 'abnormal' behaviour; second, the appraisal of that behaviour as disturbed in the psychiatric sense; third, the recommendation for treatment for acceptance into the patient role, and, last, the implementation of the decision to receive treatment (Hollingshead and Redlich, 1958, p. 171). At any point in that system the disturbed person can either drop out or enter another network, say the criminal one, or continue within the psychiatric network. Sociologists refer to the decision makers as social gatekeepers for social gates are opened or closed behind those who could enter the system. Once in the system, and once admitted for treatment then sociologists show how social pressures operate to neutralise or support psychiatric considerations. James Greenley, for example, shows how psychiatrists sometimes alter their evaluations of a patient's psychiatric condition in response to pressures from the patient's family (Greenley, 1972), whereas Goffman sees the psychiatrist as supplying traditional medical reasons for decisions which are rationales made on other grounds by other people (Goffman, 1961).

It has been left to labelling theorists such as Thomas Scheff to make a more distinctive sociological contribution, albeit a contentious one (Scheff, 1974). Labelling theory, or societal reaction theory shifts attention away from the individual attributes of the deviant and focuses on the societal reaction to those attributes. In this theory, deviance—or for our purposes, mental illness—is not seen as a physical defect of the so-called mentally ill patient, but as the outcome of a social process which involves conflicting values, labelling of the deviant and societal reactions or expectations. In Howard Becker's terms 'deviance is not a quality of the act a person commits, but rather the consequence of the application by others of rules and sanctions to an "offender" ' (Becker, 1963).

When the labelling theory is specifically applied to mental illness the mentally ill person is seen as someone who is not so much mentally ill, but who is forced by others to adopt that role. Scheff's formulation is that virtually everyone at some time commits acts or behaves in a way that could be seen as being mentally ill. However, if these acts are publicly made known, the person may, depending on certain chance events, become referred to appropriate officials. Routine processing of mental illness may then follow, with the result that the person labelled as mentally ill eventually accepts that role and internalises it into his life style. This is known as secondary deviance.

The importance of the labelling perspective is that it concentrates the activities of the control agents in those people who define and do something about a certain kind of activity. The labelling approach tends to ignore the motives and intentions of the deviant. It also emphasises the chance happenings where certain people are selected and defined as deviant members. As Goffman said, 'Society's official view is that inmates of mental hospitals are there primarily because they are suffering from mental illness. However, in the degree that the mentally ill outside hospitals numerically approach or surpass those inside hospitals, one could say that mental patients distinctively suffer not from mental illness but from contingencies' (Goffman, 1961, p. 126). Finally, it shows how the labels can be internalised and affect the person who is labelled.

Walter Gove takes issue with the labelling theorists (Gove, 1970). He sees the societal reaction approach as being incorrect, for hospitalisation occurs in most cases because the individual has a serious psychiatric disturbance, not simply because of societal reaction. He also argues that the societal reaction theorists overstate the amount of secondary deviance associated with hospitalisation. While this may be so, and my own research tends to support Gove's position, the labelling theorists are also correct in drawing attention to the often perfunctory and sometimes haphazard way in which labels relating to mental illness are applied. Labelling theorists are also correct in drawing attention to the way in which control agents become part of the problem. This is a refinement of the labelling viewpoint but sociologists have only recently begun to view the link between the patient and the psychiatrist as a relationship where each side shapes the behaviour of the other. Such a view can be seen in the development of social policy since 1945, for changes have rarely taken place unless professional interests have also benefitted. There is a trade in social problems and a lucrative one at that. Moreover, the view that social problems such as mental illness can be exacerbated by the control agents is a radical doctrine, because it enmeshes the helpers and the patients within the same problem area. Changes have not, to put it mildly, always been for the benefit of the patients, and as the labelling theorists continuously state, those changes have become part of the new problem.

No review of the contribution made by sociologists to treatment would be complete without some consideration of the sociological studies of organisations. There have been many such studies, particularly of mental institutions, but few aimed specifically at the types of care provided. Most studies have been concerned with providing a description and analytical account of the organisation, but the comparative study by Roy King, Norma Raynes and Jack Tizard has been selected for its methodology and the rigour used in conducting the enquiry (King et al., 1971). The authors were dealing with handicapped children and were concerned to explain the remarkable differences in child management practices between different types of institutions serving different types of children. They found that the differences could not be plausibly attributed to the characteristics of the children, nor to the personal characteristics of the staff. They sought their explanation in the social organisation of the regimes. They were able to divide the regimes into those adopting child-orientated practices and those adopting institutionally orientated practices, the latter associated with traditional hospital views of status divisions of staff and a low level of interaction with the children. The authors concluded that there were likely to be long-term benefits from child-orientated regimes as well as immediate future rewards. This type of enquiry is being continued within the Wessex Regional Hospital Board (Kushlick, 1968) and although it may lack the immediate impact of the labelling theorists, it may in the long run be more rewarding at an intellectual level and at the level of treatment.

Psychiatry as an Institution

To the sociologist psychiatry is more than a branch of medicine, it can be examined and analysed as an institution. The term 'institution' means an established form, or condition of procedure, characteristic of group activity. Institutions denote a mode or means of service. Analysis of institutions can be undertaken on a comparative basis, or in terms of the ways in which a particular institution is interrelated to other areas of society.

Psychiatry is clearly a medical specialism, but unlike many other such specialisms has close links with other professions and with other semi-professions such as social work. These links require additional sociological attention, and one could add, have implications for both psychiatrists and for their patients. Consider first the relationships with other areas of medicine. The links here seem tenuous and although the psychiatrist claims his medical expertise, this is not always reciprocated by his medical colleagues. In my own research the psychiatrists did not think that other doctors, and particularly those working in the general hospitals, understood the psychiatric position. Hospital doctors in turn, tended to regard psychiatrists as being 'not proper doctors', that is compared to their own expertise in high-technology medicine. Hospital doctors also reacted to psychiatrists in a way which reflected the traditional belief that psychiatry, alongside mental subnormality and possibly geriatrics, attracted low-quality personnel. This may of course not be true, but to many other medical personnel psychiatrists were still alienists. It is not clear how, and under what circumstances opinions from colleagues affect the psychiatric work. In one sense psychiatrists are dependent on G.P.s and hospital doctors for referral of patients, and from the study by Shepherd *et al.*, of general practice in London, only about 5 per cent of patients with psychiatric problems were referred to psychiatrists (Shepherd *et al.*, 1966). Who becomes referred and for what reasons are questions as relevant to the study of psychiatry as institutions are to the study of psychiatric treatment. One can only speculate that a moral hierarchy operates where psychiatrists and psychiatric patients are accorded low status on that hierarchy, and that the hierarchy develops within the wider institutions of medicine. If this is so, then a curious paradox exists, for the profession ostensibly devoted to the care, treatment, and social respect of the mentally ill has within it the structural requirements for producing the opposite effect.

The psychiatrist's relationships with social work are equally tenuous, although for different reasons. The ideological disputes between social work and psychiatry are now being rehearsed in the press and in the literature. Social workers no longer see themselves as compliant semi-professionals eager to learn from their psychiatric superiors, but as members of a strident group intent on expanding their influence and domain. That these claims may be exaggerated is not the point; the claims are being listened to and reflect an important shift in the political stance of government. It would, I think be possible to speak of a watershed for psychiatry in the late 1960s and to suggest that the psychiatrists' political influence is beginning to decline. From 1959 to the late 1960s psychiatry accepted the confidence given to it by the Royal Commission and became the institutionalised means to achieve solutions to social problems. Psychiatric influence was paramount and was reflected in the way in which psychiatrists became key personnel who advised on matters far beyond their boundaries of medical training. Since 1970, psychiatry has begun to lose that political confidence and social work has replaced it as the dominant occupational group which is to provide the solution to modern social problems. The shift is partially political but also reflects a belief that social problems cannot be solved on an individual basis but require an element of social action. I would suggest that this view is likely to be temporary, but the manner in which it has affected psychiatry is likely to be permanent. It is doubtful if we shall again see the expansion of psychiatric influence as a pervasive social movement.

Even so, psychiatry as an institution still retains high status and still has relative power commensurate with that status. It holds positions of influence, it has control of key resources. It also retains that level of expertise which befits a professional group. What is uncertain is the future direction of psychiatry. Will it attempt to foster stronger relationships with other branches of medicine, or attempt to compete in the social field? The next decade may provide the answers.

Psychiatry's relationship with law is equally tenuous. Szasz, in his usual pungent way has said that psychiatric testimony in the Courts is up for sale; meaning more than that psychiatrists sell their views to the highest bidder, but that psychiatric judgement is moral and partisan, or in a word, strategic (Szasz, 1965, p. 34). The problem is, however, wider than this and is related to the perennial question about the nature of treatment, control and liberty. Psychiatrists and psychiatry are at the centre of that debate, their presence in the Courts merely provides the public arena for that debate to be rehearsed. Under the demands for treatment, the 1959 Mental Health Act provided psychiatrists with power to recommend that a person be detained in an institution without a trial, and without any rights of appeal prior to that commitment. The requirement that psychiatric treatment ought to be obtained as rapidly as possible for those requiring psychiatric attention fits in with the tradition of humanism, which runs throughout our society. Yet it conflicts with other values such as liberty and the right not to be detained without due process of law. The conflict has a timeless quality about it but needs to be resolved if psychiatry is not to be forever tarnished with the label of being against the individual's civil rights. Institutional psychiatry has, for laudable reasons, come to be regarded as part of the soft machine of social control. It is seen as an agent of the therapeutic state, which, for therapeutic reasons puts people in therapeutic jails (Bean, 1976). Sociologists such as Goffman have drawn attention to this and psychiatrists must face this issue soon, for it is likely to be another key issue in psychiatric practice over the next decade.

References

Ausabel, D. (1961). Personality disorder *is* disease. *Am. Psychol.*, **16**, 69–74

Bean, P. T. (1975). The Mental Health Act. 1959: some issues concerning rule enforcement. *Br. J. Law Soc.*, **2** (2), 228–238

Bean, P. T. (1976). *Rehabilitation and Deviance*. Routledge and Kegan Paul, London

Becker, H. (1963). *Outsiders*. Free Press, Chicago

Bloor, M. J. and Horobin, G. (1975). Conflict and conflict resolution in the doctor/patient relationship. In *A Sociology of Medical Practice* (Ed. G. Cox and A. Mead), Collier Macmillan, London, pp. 271–281

Cumming, E and Cumming, J. (1957). *Closed Ranks*. Harvard University Press

Flew, A. (1974). *Crime or Disease*. Macmillan, London

Goffman, E. (1961). *Asylums*. Pelican, London

Gove, W. R. (1970). Who is hospitalized: a critical review of some sociological studies of mental illness. *J. Hlth soc. Behav.* **11**, 294–303

Greenley, J. R. (1972). Alternative views of the psychiatrists' role. *Soc. Problems*, **20** (2), 1–11

H.M.S.O. (1957). Royal Commission on the law relating to mental illness and mental deficiency, 1954–1957. *Cmnd 169* (Percy Commission), H.M.S.O., London

Hollingshead, A. B. and Redlich, F. C. (1958). *Social Class and Mental Illness*. Wiley, New York

King, R. D., Raynes, N. and Tizard, J. (1971). *Patterns of Residential Care*. Routledge and Kegan Paul, London

Kushlick, A. (1968). The Wessex Plan for evaluating the effectiveness of residential care for the severely subnormal, 650. In *Proceedings of the First International Congress for the Scientific Study of Mental Deficiency*. Montpellier

Lewis, Sir. A. (1953). Health as a social concept. *Br. J. Sociol.*, **4**, 109–124

Mechanic, D. (1959). Illness and social disability. some problems in analysis. *Pacif. Sociol. Rev.*, **2**, 37–41

Mechanic, D. and Volkart, E. H. (1961). Stress, illness behaviour and the sick role. *Am. sociol. Rev.*, **26**, 51–58

Parsons, T. (1951). *The Social System*. Free Press, Chicago

Plog, S. G. and Edgerton, R. B. (1969). *Changing Perspectives In Mental Illness*. Holt, Rinehart and Winston, Eastbourne

Ruesch, J. (1965). Social psychiatry: an overview. *Archs gen. Psychiat.*, **12**, 501–509

Sarbin, T. (1969). The scientific status of the mental illness metaphor. *Changing Perspectives In Mental Illness* (Ed. S. G. Plog and R. B. Edgerton), Holt, Rinehart and Winston, Eastbourne, pp. 9–30

Schatzman, L. and Strauss, A. (1966). A sociology of psychiatry: a perspective and some organizing foci. *Soc. Problems*, **14**, (1), 3–16

Scheff, T. (1966). *Being Mentally Ill*. Aldine, Chicago

Scheff, T. (1974). The labelling theory of mental illness. *Am. sociol. Rev.*, **39**, 444–452

Shepherd, M. Brown, A. C. and Kalton, G. W. (1966). *Psychiatric Illness In General Practice*. Oxford University Press, Oxford

Szasz, T. (1965). *Psychiatric Justice*. Collier Books, London

Szasz, T. (1973). Mental illness as a metaphor. *Nature*, **242**, (5396), 305–307

Szasz, T. (1974). What psychiatry can and cannot do. In *Ideology and Insanity* (Ed. T. Szasz), Pelican, London, pp. 78–85

Waxler, N. (1974). Culture and mental illness. *J. Nerv. Ment. Dis.*, **159** (6), 379–395

Weinberg, S. K. (1967). *The Sociology of Mental Disorders*. Staples Press, London, Chapter I

3 Social Work in Psychiatric Rehabilitation

David W. Millard

The potential contribution of social work to the rehabilitation of patients is such a broad topic that it is first necessary to locate within it those aspects which are discussed in the present paper. As will become clear, rehabilitation provides a particularly convenient focus for considering the relationship between psychiatrists and social workers as occupational groups, and our chief purpose is to discuss this relationship—which is currently vexing all concerned. We shall place ourselves in context by recalling at once that social work forms but a part of a wide range of welfare and personal social services. Even those local government departments which, in England and Wales, we rightly call Social *Services* Departments (less correctly known in Scotland as Social *Work* Departments) have functions wider than simply that of the delivery of social work. It is surely arguable that a perfectly imaginable change in public provision, such as a quadrupling of the financial benefits available to chronically handicapped patients and their families, might at a stroke do more for psychiatric rehabilitation than all the social work—or, for that matter, all the psychiatry—in the world.

Social work, then, is a more limited matter than social service. However, we must include within its definition not only that combination of personal and social adjustments that constitutes individual and family *casework*, but also *groupwork*, certain examples of *community work* and, most importantly from the point of view of psychiatric rehabilitation, the professional elements in *residential work* and in *day care*.

All these elements will normally be represented in the curriculum of courses leading to basic professional qualifications. Since the way members collectively of any occupation see themselves is both reflected and to some extent defined by their arrangements for professional education, we may take this to be an indication of the scope of contemporary social work (C.C.E.T.S.W., 1975).

After some hesitation, social work seems to have settled for a pattern which is general at the qualifying level and provides for specialisation in terms of methods of working or of client groups at post-qualifying level. There is a fairly rapid development at present of such opportunities either through in-service training or, increasingly, in university and college-based courses. Some psychiatrists have regretted the loss of the specialist mental health social worker but in this chapter it will be argued that the broader general background is itself of considerable relevance to psychiatric rehabilitation;

moreover it is certainly possible that the eventual quality of social workers specialising in mental health work will be the better for such a grounding once appropriate post-qualifying training is established. The point here, however, is to claim real value for that broad survey of social structures and processes, psychological development and behaviour, the complex interplay of facts and values, and of those policies, techniques and skills that are required in order to meet a wide range of social problems, all of which constitutes basic social work education today.

Hospital-based doctors still tend to hold a rather partial view of the nature of social work, and to judge it accordingly; although, to give them their due, psychiatrists are perhaps less blinkered in this respect than colleagues in other specialities. It remains the case that individual and family casework, which is what the doctors usually have in mind and which we will chiefly consider in this paper, is probably still the 'centre of gravity' of social work, but that profession as a whole would also see itself as concerned with, for example, not only the administrative access to a hostel or a day centre, but the expertise required to run such places. All this is part of the contribution of social work to psychiatric rehabilitation.

We may summarise in the words of the White Paper *Better Services for the Mentally Ill* (H.M.S.O.1975)—in which social work has the invidious distinction among the professions of being thought to require several paragraphs of description and justification:

> Successful rehabilitation entails the deployment of a whole range of services of which the health and personal social services are only a part; housing, employment and education and the voluntary services, can be particularly important. It is the concern of the social services department to see that all services are mobilised in helping the mentally ill and in supporting their families. The relationship between the social services and the other agencies concerned is thus of crucial importance; in some instances social service staff may need to undertake a liaison function in exploring the needs of mentally ill people and the nature of the help they need from other services. The unifying element in these activities is the professional skill of the social worker, whether deployed in the fieldwork in primary care, in residential or day care, or in hospital. (Paras. 3.15 and 3.16.)

Addressing the American Psychiatric Association in 1973 on *Community Mental Health Services in Britain*, Dr Douglas Bennett remarked:

> So much has been said and written about continuity of care, cooperation, coordination and team work that the words have all but lost their meaning. They do not tell us how to work or what to do. They provide no basis for teaching psychiatrists.

The platitudes of *Better Services for the Mentally Ill*, or, indeed of official formularies such as the Royal College of Psychiatrists' recently published report on *The Responsibilities of Consultants in Psychiatry within the National Health Service* (1977) seem to get us very little further. Can we do better? Yes; it may be that we can.We should observe that the question 'What is the place of social work in psychiatric rehabilitation?' might be answered descriptively or prescriptively. Both approaches are important, but the data which would allow the present paper to be descriptive simply do not appear to exist. We would need empirical investigations studying in a controlled way the particular inputs of members of a specified professional group to the rehabilitation of a specified group of patients. And the precise behaviours of the professionals concerned would presumably differ somewhat according to whether we are considering the rehabilitation of a psychiatrically disturbed adolescent, an acutely disordered adult patient, a chronically handicapped and perhaps institutionalised patient, or an elderly person; with or without, in each case, the complication of mental subnormality. It is easy to specify in theory the requirements of such an investigation; very difficult in practice to isolate as a particular variable the social worker's contribution. The available literature makes it quite clear that very detailed distinctions appear as soon as the processes or experiences of rehabilitation are examined critically.

A couple of recent examples taken more or less at random will serve to make the point. In a carefully conducted study, Pryce (1977) has shown in a group of long-term schizophrenics resettled from hospital into accommodation in a residential home that whereas the female patients improved on the whole, the men did not; this, however, may have less to do with sex and with gender-related behaviour such as the patient's occupation and more to do with the severity of their illness in relation to the degree of social stimulation. In a quite different study Byrne *et al.* (1974) demonstrated that the various disabilities shown by a group of discharged chronic psychotics when observed by their families at home bore little relation to the behaviours observed by the nurses in a day centre which they attended; home behaviour therefore could not be inferred from that displayed at the day centre. Such examples could be multiplied, but distinctions of this degree of detail clearly imply that statements about rehabilitation need to be made with some precision.

It so happens that these are investigations by psychiatrists, but some important studies of psychiatric rehabilitation have also been written by social workers. They would include, for example, the definitive account of the well-known boarding-out scheme for long-stay psychiatric patients from the North Wales Hospital, Denbigh, which appears in a collection of papers highly recommended to psychiatrists, and published by the British Association of Social Workers in 1976, *Differential Approaches in Social Work with the Mentally Disordered*. This account is written, and the collection edited, by a senior social work teacher Dr Rolf Olsen (1976). The social work literature in this area is, however, generally disappointing; a rapid survey of the leading British publications since the beginning of the decade yielded, in the main, statements which, although broadly covering individual, residential, group and community work, are generally anecdotal, judgemental, theoretical or prescriptive. There is nothing which helps us in any empirical way to answer the question concerning the place of social work in psychiatric rehabilitation.

We have therefore, to turn to a theoretical discussion in our attempt to define this contribution more precisely; and we shall start by considering in general the relationship between social workers and psychiatrists as part of the wider problem of teamwork in psychiatric care, and afterwards focus more particularly on rehabilitation.

The theory concerned is that of organisations. This aims to proceed by a clear definition of its questions followed by systematic attempts to collect the information which would help to answer them.

We may as an example take the coherent conceptual framework for discussing the relationships between professional groups which has been provided by the Health Services Organisation Research Unit of Brunel University (1976a, b). These workers distinguish, for instance, between *network* and *team* and the concepts are accurately characterised. Both are situations in which practitioners work together; but in the team they are necessarily known personally to each other, and work face to face together with the whole group or some part of it (while in a network this may or may not be the case.) They have to be mutually acceptable as co-members; and they have to intend to work together over an extended period of time. Networks and teams each imply a rather different set of rights and duties of membership, and these also are specified. The College of Psychiatrists' report on the Responsibilities of Consultants within the National Health Service found it necessary ' . . . to outline the College's policy with regard to the multi-disciplinary team concept and to relate consultant responsibility within that framework'—a laudable objective, if ungrammatically expressed—but the discussion is rather muddled, and it seems a pity that a statement of official policy should not make use of the conceptual clarifications which are in fact available.

This would be especially useful in considering the relationship between the individual roles within the team. Here the Brunel workers define *managerial, prescribing, co-ordinative* and *monitoring* relationships, together with concepts which are also useful in this discussion such as *independent practice, primacy of responsibility,* and the *encompassing profession.* We do not need to reproduce the definitions attaching to the whole of this vocabulary; the work needs careful study, and psychiatry, being at present much troubled by its relationships with other professions, might benefit from looking at it more closely. For the purpose of the present chapter, it will suffice to say that the question whether the relationships between psychiatrists and social workers are managerial, prescribing, co-ordinative or monitoring (as defined) hinges on two factors: the knowledge bases of the two professions, and the nature of psychiatric disorders. The contention is that these two factors are such that, irrespective of whatever distinction of status there may be between the professions, the authority of the psychiatrist *vis-à-vis* the social worker is co-ordinative or monitoring but *not* prescribing or managerial. (We should recall that in sociology, status and authority are not necessarily directly related.)

There is not much debate about two out of these four possibilities. Few of those involved would disagree with the view that the psychiatrist's authority is not managerial. Most would be happy to accept a relationship which includes co-ordinative aspects; indeed this function is claimed for the consultant in the College's report. Some social workers would be doubtful about monitoring, which the Brunel terminology suggests is a relationship '. . . in which the monitor is expected to keep himself aware of certain specifically defined areas or aspects of activity, to discuss deviation from acceptable standards in these areas and to report continual or serious deviation to higher authority'— although others might accept this. The chief dissension surrounds the question whether or not the psychiatrist has, or should have, prescribing authority in respect to social workers. A prescribing relationship, according to the Brunel workers, '. . . arises where a member of one occupational group has by virtue of his membership of that group the right to determine the objectives to be pursued and the contexts to be observed in specific cases by members of certain other occupational groups whose knowledge base is encompassed by that of his own' (1976a, p. 27). It is this matter of the encompassing profession that is at the heart of the problem. Where two disciplines are quite distinct, the problem does not arise but (rather like the phenomenon of *cognitive dissonance* within individual psychology) the closer two occupational groups become without actually coinciding, the greater the discomfort seems to be. This, surely, is the present situation of psychiatry and social work. The Brunel work, which is based on a wide range of field studies, is intended to apply to the health services in general, but their report itself stresses the particular difficulties which arise here in relation to mental health.

However, these are not only matters of theory: they are also open to empirical research. Unhappily, there is rather little of it available at present, at least in Britain (and national cultural characteristics are likely to be important in such studies). But Agnes Miles (1977) has published a study from three psychiatric hospitals which investigated the judgements made about occupational competence (among other matters) by doctors, nurses, social workers and occupational therapists. An important distinction was made between an occupation's 'area of competence' and its 'area of exclusive competence'—the former possessed by that group in common with other groups; the latter possessed by that occupation alone. The doctors, without exception, denied the possibility of exclusive competence for any of the other health professions in any part of the treatment process; that is, they claimed the role of an encompassing profession. The other health professionals, all of whom had been employed in the hospitals for at least three years, and notably the social workers, dissented from this view. Now that may seem a commonplace conclusion in the light of most psychiatrists' impressions of contemporary practice; but the point is surely that a careful analysis of the situation such as that provided by the Brunel research clears a great deal of the ground and enables us to isolate the remaining problems.

We turn next to use the nature and processes of rehabilitation in support of the contention that the knowledge base of social work and the nature of psychiatric disorders are such that psychiatry is not an encompassing profession *vis-à-vis* social work and therefore the relationship between psychiatrist and social worker does not include prescribing authority. For this purpose we must first consider a social sciences view of rehabilitation.

It generally helps to clarify a concept if it can be set over against other related concepts. This was usefully done nearly twenty years ago in the juxtaposition of 'rehabilitation' and 'treatment' by Rapoport (1960) in *Community as Doctor*. Although written with particular reference to the Henderson Hospital, the discussion of these concepts is of much wider application to psychiatric care. Rapoport traces their historical development, pointing particularly to the initial separation between treatment as directed towards the care of the disease and rehabilitation as a residual activity, 'taking up what was left of the patient when treatment was over' and having to do with the transition 'between the technical medical measures and the private matter of making a life outside the hospital'. Such a view came to particular prominence during the 1939–45 war, 'reflecting' (as *Black's Medical Dictionary* has it) 'the growing awareness of the medical profession . . . that a man with a fractured limb or spine has to recover the full use *not only of the injured parts* but of his whole body' (present author's italic). Rapoport describes the way in which in psychiatry the two concepts gradually became blurred with the growth in the last 30 years of that concatenation of interests which we might broadly call 'social psychiatry' until we reach the view that 'all psychiatric treatment is rehabilitation'. (As a matter of fact towards the end of the book Rapoport makes a plea for retaining the distinction between these concepts, with specific reference to the work of therapeutic communities; but that need not detain us here.) He also quotes from Charlotte Schwartz (1953) the observation that in psychiatry the word rehabilitation has confusingly been taken to include '*what is done* to the patients, the *processes* that stem from this, the *goals* of the activity or the measures taken at a particular *phase* in the patient's career'.

Recently, one of my social work students and I worked out another conceptual distinction which belongs to the recovery phase in the patient's experience, namely that between 'convalescence' and 'rehabilitation' (Beckingham, 1976). We may start by quoting again *Black's Medical Dictionary*: *Convalescence*, the conditions through which a person passes after having suffered from some acute disease, and before complete health and strength are regained; and *Rehabilitation*, the restoration to health and working capacity of a person incapacitated by disease, mental or physical, or by injury. And, from the *Oxford English Dictionary: Convalescence*, to recover from sickness, or get better. (This word derives ultimately from the Latin verb *Valere*, which is also the root of words such as valid and invalid. Indeed there is a Roman Law meaning of the word convalescence 'to become Valid' so perhaps our usage of the word *invalid* to describe a person who is weakened by sickness properly conveys overtones of defective social competence in the same sense that a legal contract might be held to be invalid.) The *Oxford English Dictionary* gives for *rehabilitation*: to restore by formal act or declaration (a person degraded or attainted) to former privileges, rank and possessions; to re-establish a person's good name or memory by authoritative pronouncement; to restore to a previous or proper condition; to re-establish the character or reputation (of a person or thing.) In the writer's own copy of the dictionary, the medical usage has not yet been added to these essentially political definitions.

The point here is that the word convalescence is patient-centred and the word rehabilitation is other-centred. Convalescence refers to the inner experiences of healing; rehabilitation refers to a series of activities done to or on behalf of the patient by others. Convalescence belongs to the vocabulary of Being; rehabilitation belongs to the vocabulary of Doing. Convalescence has to do with the first of that pair of concepts indispensible to social psychology— the *self* and *social roles*—and rehabilitation has to do with the other.

We may have a simple mental picture of the individual as a cartwheel; the hub at the centre represents the 'self', the spaces between the spokes surrounding it being the various roles—occupational, family, economic, political, leisure roles and so forth, in which the energies of the self are from time to time invested. '*And one man in his time plays many parts.*' A person in psychotherapy (whether this is being undertaken by psychiatrist or social worker) is being invited to consider the two-way traffic between the self and his social roles; we speak of material learned in the patient role as being 'internalised', and use terms like 'acting out' or 'working through' to describe the manifestations, undesirable or otherwise, of such material in the variety of role performances.

During illness, many of these roles are surrendered—even obliterated— and one, the *sick role*, whose characteristics were classically described by Talcott Parsons (1972), becomes salient. (There are, incidentally, some modifications of the classical description of the sick role which obtain in chronic illness, and these are also described in the sociological literature (Kassebaum and Baumann, 1972).) Indeed, it is part of the Parsonian definition that the sick role takes precedence over other social obligations. Rehabilitation is the replacing of the sick role as salient by a selection of role performances which most closely match those of people in society who are like the patient in all respects save that they are not, or have not recently, been particularly sick; that is, it aims to minimise the differences between the individual patient and other members of his 'reference group'. This process is needful for any patient. The examples of empirical studies of rehabilitation quoted earlier were all to do with the chronically handicapped and institutionalised, but, within this definition, rehabilitation is required for patients in any clinical group. It is, of course, always to be hoped that the experiences of rehabilitation will be internalised in forms that enhance the self and enrich the performance of each one of the patient's ordinary social roles. Convalescence is ideally an experience of growth and maturation of the personality. The particular contribution of social workers to the processes of minimising the differences between the patient and other members of his reference group follows from their broad acquaintance with the variety of social roles within British culture. This is, in part, a consequence of the range of social and psychological studies which, as indicated earlier, is an important feature of the general professional education for social work at the qualifying level. The professional education of members of most other helping professions, on the other hand, ordinarily has different preoccupations, and leaves these matters to general knowledge and to common sense—or, regrettably, to prejudice. Examples abound; a recent one from the author's own experience occurred in the case of an immigrant patient whose psychiatrist was giving her the benefit of the doubt concerning a particular child-rearing practice until told firmly by the social worker that such behaviour would be abnormal in *any* culture. This reference to 'the variety of social roles in British culture' is, of course, a more general statement of the social worker's competence than is generally offered. It represents that 'life outside the hospital' of the quotation from Rapoport; it is really what is implied by the claim advanced by the social workers in Miles' study to a 'knowledge of the patient's family and home environment', and it covers a wider range of social behaviour than is represented by those familiar 'ladders' of housing and occupation which have traditionally guided the thinking of psychiatrists about rehabilitation.

But this claim concerning the independent knowledge base of social work is only one of the two factors underlying its problematic relationship with psychiatry. The other is the familiar question of the precise status of psychiatric disorder. We do not need to discuss this here at any length; the question, of course, is how far it is possible in psychiatry to separate the symptomatology and the sick role behaviour.

This distinction works well for physical illness; we have little difficulty in conceptualising separately the phenomena of illness in, say, rheumatoid arthritis, and the behavioural consequences for a patient crippled by this condition. In the case of many of the problems confronting the psychiatrist, however, the concepts are harder to separate. Take all the sick role behaviour away from one's clinical description of an hysterical patient, for example, and remarkably little seems to be left. Is not the same true of any one of a number of functional disorders? The sick role behaviour *is* the illness. Moreover, do not the really taxing clinical problems of even unequivocally organic disorders such as dementia reside in their effect on the patient's performance in his or her ordinary social roles rather than in the physiological side of the problem?

There is a problem here which seems insoluble in the present state of our understanding. It leads to the periodic discussion on both sides of the Atlantic concerning psychiatry 'moving away from' or 'towards' medicine, and also to the currently fashionable practice of carving up the subject-matter of psychiatry for redistribution among the disciplines.

A notable proponent of the latter is Eysenck (1975) whose well-known proposal is that the part which is unequivocally 'medical' should remain the province of the psychiatrist, the remainder becoming the province of the clinical psychologist. Eysenck's own view of the professional preparation required is worth quoting:

This training would embody a realistic training in psychology particularly those aspects of it concerned with learning, with conditioning, with personality and with psychometrics, as well as the principles of abnormal psychology; social psychology would also figure strongly. A limited amount of sociology (of the factual rather than the ideological and political variety) might also be useful, together with some information on anthropology.

Apart from the references to psychometrics, this sounds at least as much like a social work curriculum as it does a psychology course.

To the extent that symptoms and role performance are indistinguishable, much of the sociologists' critique of the 'medicalising' of psychiatry is justified, as is Rapoport's aphorism 'all psychiatric treatment is rehabilitation'. If to this be added the assertion of the independent knowledge base of social workers we might ultimately find ourselves redefining psychiatry as a branch of social work! This perhaps would not do. However, were we willing to entertain that kind of professional territorialism (which the present author is not) the claim of social work to be the professional group equipped to take over does seem to be rather stronger than that of the psychologists. Social workers are much more numerous; their responsibilities in the task— particularly in relation to after care and rehabilitation—are already great (some of them, indeed, are statutory), and the processes of their professional socialisation fit them for it rather explicitly.

Meanwhile, we persist in our rather uneasy dualism—a word which, with its overtones of Cartesian philosophy, is chosen deliberately. At the level at which it would be useful to the clinical management of the individual psychiatric patient, we do not in fact know quite how to handle the relationship between body and mind.

The College of Psychiatrists' report itself tends to make this dualistic assumption. It appears in the medical emphasis within such statements as: 'The Consultant has, by virtue of professional qualification, Acts of Parliament and contract, the authority and responsibility to diagnose and prescribe medical treatment, and this responsibility cannot be wholly devolved elsewhere'. We can agree with that; but it does not solve any problem, it merely relocates it. The problem is that we do not know how far psychiatric disorder is of the same ontological status as rheumatoid arthritis; how far, that is, it calls for 'the diagnosis and prescription of medical treatment', as opposed to the consideration of a variety of role performances. The points of transition, the induction into the sick role and rehabilitation from it, present this dilemma most acutely—and this is why rehabilitation is so convenient a focus for discussing the relations between psychiatry and social work.

The wise answer is surely to accept for the present the uncertainties of professional relationship which are forced upon us in large part by the real nature of the problems which our patients bring to us. The difficulties in teamwork are generated not so much by the aspirations to status and power of competing occupational groups as by the difficulties in deciding what kind of event is a psychiatric disorder. It is, after all, only during the past 200 years that such disorders have been assimilated to the model of diseases. Social history suggests both that the changing understanding of human problems alters the provision to meet them, and also that new patterns of provision change the social definition of the nature of the problems. This being so, we would be well advised to regard as provisional the claims of any occupational group in relation to the care of the psychiatrically disordered.

If we choose to adopt this stance, what can we say of the relations between individual team members of different disciplines? Experience in therapeutic communities' regimes emphasises that staff members have essentially a common task, and this indeed seems frequently to be the case across a broad field of psychiatric care. But they come to it by different routes, from the separate starting points of their different professional trainings. Perhaps what they have had to discard from their separate backgrounds is at least as important as any residual differences in the contributions which they bring to clinical care. There is an old tag of the psychologists: no perception without contrast. We might borrow the Gestalt idea, and suggest that individuals of the various disciplines perceive the same figure but against differing backgrounds—the need and the task are the same; the context within which they are seen is not. To the psychiatrist the mental disorder is not precisely like the diseases of medicine, to the social worker it is not precisely like other deviations from social norms with which he will be familiar. Yet both may function very similarly in working with a particular patient. A recently published report of a quite successful rehabilitation programme for chronic psychotic patients at Long Grove Hospital notes without differentiation that the 'primary therapists' were 'nurses, social workers or chaplains' and it has as co-authors two social workers and one consultant psychiatrist (Barker *et al.*, 1977). This seems a perfectly proper state of affairs. It may be that the task of isolating a specific contribution to psychiatric rehabilitation of social work or of any other discipline is in some ways misguided.

Perhaps it is a partial response to Bennett's observation that the words co-ordination and teamwork 'do not tell us how to work or what to do' that we should make better use of what is known of the nature and problems of multi-disciplinary practice, and understand more clearly their relationship to the content of professional education and to the intractable difficulties of conceptualising psychiatric disorders; and that we should be well-content to leave our inter-professional relationships to a process of quiet evolution.

References

Barker, G. H. B., Woods, T. J. and Anderson, J. A. (1977). Rehabilitation of the institutionalized patient. *Br. J. Psychiat.* **130,** 484–488

Beckingham, C. R. (1976). *Relinquishment of the Sick Role: Convalescence and Rehabilitation.* M.Sc. Dissertation. Department of Social and Administrative Studies, University of Oxford

Bennett, D. (1973). Community mental health services in Britain. *Am. J. Psychiat.,* **130,** 1065–1070

B.I.O.S.S. (1976a). *Professionals in Health and Social Service Organisations.* Health Service Organisation Research Unit, Brunel University

B.I.O.S.S. (1976b). *Collaboration between Health and Social Services.* Health Service Organisation Research Unit, Brunel University

Byrne, L., O'Connor, T. and Fay, T. J. (1974). The home behaviour of schizophrenic patients living in the community and attending a day centre. *Br. J. Psychiat.,* **125,** 20–24

C.C.E.T.S.W. (1975). *Education and Training for Social Work.* Central Council for Education and Training in Social Work, Paper 10

Eysenck, H. J. (1975). *The Future of Psychiatry.* Methuen, London

H.M.S.O. (1975). *Better Services for the Mentally Ill.* Cmnd 6233, H.M.S.O., London

Kassebaum, G. G. and Baumann, B. O. (1972). Dimensions of the sick role in chronic illness. In *Patients, Physicians and Illness* (Ed. E. C. Jago), Free Press, Chicago

Miles, A. (1977). Staff relations in psychiatric hospitals. *Br. J. Psychiat.,* **130,** 84–88

Olsen, M. R. (1976). Boarding out the long-stay psychiatric patient. In *Differential Approaches in Social Work with the Mentally Disordered* (Ed. M. R. Olsen), British Association of Social Workers

Parsons, T. (1972). Definitions of health and illness in the light of American values and social structure. In *Patients, Physicians and Illness* (Ed. E. C. Jago), Free Press, Chicago

Pryce, I. G. (1967). The effects of social changes in chronic schizophrenia: a study of forty patients transferred from hospital to residential home. *Psychol. Med.,* 7, 127–139

Rapoport, R. (1960). *Community as Doctor.* Tavistock, London

Royal College of Psychiatrists (1977). The responsibilities of consultants in psychiatry within the National Health Service. *Bull. R. Coll. Psychiat.,* September 1977, 4–7

Schwartz, C. (1953). *Rehabilitation of Mental Hospital Patients.* U.S.P.H.S. Monograph No. 17

4 Cross-cultural Psychiatry

G. M. Carstairs

Instances of socially unacceptable behaviour occur in every society, and every society has developed explanations to account for them, and procedures for dealing with such deviant persons. The commonest explanation —inspired no doubt by the subject's change of personality and his often incomprehensible speech—is that of spirit possession; indeed Ackerknecht (1968, p. 1) has suggested that this mode of explaining mental derangement became, by extension, the explanation for all other forms of illness also. Rosen (1968) has drawn attention to recognisable descriptions of psychotic behaviour in ancient Hebrew literature as long ago as 1020 B.C. He also refers to the distinction made in early Greek medicine between madness due to natural causes (such as abuse of alcohol) and *enthusiasmos* or divine madness, which was seen as a mark of election, so that its victims were treated with some awe, as people who had enjoyed direct communication with supernatural powers— a concept which we saw temporarily revived by R. D. Laing, in some of his apocalyptic utterances, some eight years ago.

During the period of colonialism, the Western powers found it necessary to make provision, in their own way, for socially unacceptable deviants: they created prisons and asylums, frequently built to the same design, for this purpose. Early in the present century Kraepelin visited a number of mental hospitals in Malaya and in Java and found that he could recognise familiar patterns of behaviour among their inmates. His conclusion that both organic and functional psychoses occur, perhaps with differing rates of incidence, in industrially under-developed countries, has since been confirmed by several epidemiological surveys since Lin (1953) carried out his pioneer study in Formosa. He was able to demonstrate, as later on Dube (1970) showed in his North Indian survey, that prevalence rates for the major forms of mental disorder were not greatly different, in their respective populations, from those found in Europe or America.

Until these studies were reported, most publications on 'Cross-Cultural Psychiatry' contained accounts of peculiar syndromes such as *Windigo* (a form of psychotic depression, leading to cannibalism found among isolated Eskimo tribes in northern Canada) or *Amok* (an excess of indiscriminate murderous frenzy, usually ending with the death of the patient, found in Malaysia) or the other typically Malaysian phenomenon of *Latah* (a state of dissociation with compulsive imitation of another person's words, gestures or acts) or *Koro*, a panic state occurring among males from the southern provinces of China in which they believe that the penis is shrinking and being retracted inside the abdomen with fatal results.

The early examples of psychiatric epidemiology, which were so ably reviewed by Strømgren (1950) at the first World Congress of Psychiatry, understandably focused their attention on the psychoses and on severe forms of subnormality because only for these cases could ascertainment and enumeration be carried out with an acceptable level of reliability. At the same time, however, psychiatrists were aware, as some general physicians have been aware over the centuries, of the much larger amount of minor pathology which finds expression in the symptoms of the neuroses and the psychosomatic disorders. Already in 1951 Bremer had shown that a psychiatrically-orientated physician living in prolonged contact with his patients could perceive a much higher prevalence of these minor forms of psychiatric morbidity than had been noted in any previous epidemiological surveys. Subsequently, many research workers have addressed themselves to the difficult task of developing valid and reliable criteria for the identification of these conditions in cross-sectional or in longitudinal surveys. Among them have been Michael Shepherd and his team (1966) who showed that 14 per cent of adult patients in a large sample of general practices consulted their doctors because of psychiatric or 'psychiatric-related' symptoms during the survey year. In North America, Alexander and Dorothea Leighton (1963) and their co-workers carried out painstaking studies of the prevalence of psychiatric disorders in a small town and in a rural community. Their methods were also deployed in a large-scale sample survey of citizens in a district of New York (Srole et al., 1962). The findings of both these studies were greeted with some incredulity and a good deal of hostility, simply because they revealed such high rates of symptoms, and of disability caused by these symptoms.

The possibility that there might also be high rates of minor, but still disabling, neurotic and psychosomatic symptoms in peoples of the developing countries was not explored until quite recent years—partly, no doubt, because they seemed to have other, and more pressing health problems due to the high prevalence of very serious illnesses caused by infection and malnutrition. I myself, during the course of two years' residence in villages of northern India, while engaged on studies of culture and personality, came to recognise that neurotic and psychosomatic symptoms were often presented by my rustic patients, and that psychotherapy appeared to play a large part in the ministrations of their traditional healers (Carstairs, 1955, 1956).

Westerners have tended to regard witch doctors and spiritual healers with a degree of condescension, as survivals from the pre-scientific Dark Ages. Recently, however, anthropologists have begun to explore the roles which these healers play in their respective societies: and they prove to be key roles for both individual health and social cohesion. If the anthropologist is himself medically trained, he is soon compelled to realise that part of his own training has consisted of learning to conform to the role-expectations of doctor and patient in his own society, and that the expectations of the people he is studying are quite different.

This confrontation occurred in my own experience on the very first night of my stay in a village in Rajasthan, over twenty years ago. My tent was full to overflowing with men and boys from the village which I had planned to study, and a concert of drumming, sitar-playing and singing was under way when a distracted villager appeared, asking me to come to the aid of his wife, who was possessed by a devil. Carrying my stethoscope as a talisman, I followed him through the darkness to his hut where, to my relief, I was able to diagnose a well-advanced normal labour: my talisman even reassured me that the infant's heart was beating regularly. I told the father that this was a healthy little devil whom he would soon see face to face; and indeed the child was born before our sing-song had ended.

During the ensuing months I saw many patients and gradually learned how to live up to their expectations as a healer. At first, all seemed rather familiar: my clients would squat patiently until I was free to attend to them, and then would extend their right hand, apparently expecting me to feel their pulse, because they seemed pleased when I did so. After this, however, I would ask what was troubling them, and this caused them to look at me with dismay: 'You are a wise, learned man' they would say: 'It is for *you* to tell *us* what is the matter'.

During these few months I had many opportunities of watching their own folk-healers at work. They were of two kinds, the *Bhopas* and the *Mantar-janne-walas*; the former were attendants at a shrine whose deity, summoned by drumming and chanting, would take possession of the *bhopa's* body and speak directly to the supplicants, while the *mantar-janne-wala* was the possessor of secret powerful charms which could exorcise ghosts, witches and evil spirits. One rather celebrated exorcist consulted me for treatment, and having benefitted from a course of sulphathiazole he was kind enough to teach me the basic elements of his expertise. In order to do so, he reached for my right hand, laid a finger across my wrist and explained that flickering movements of the tendons betrayed the presence of a witch or demon. For some months my village patients had assumed that this was what I was doing, when I took their pulse.

There was plenty of sickness in that area, especially chest and bowel diseases, malnutrition and anaemia; but it was only during the course of my second year of fieldwork that I began to feel sufficiently familiar with the prevailing culture to recognise that some of my clients were suffering from anxiety, depression or hysteria. This was a casual observation, but one which came back to mind in subsequent years when further studies carried out by T. Y. Lin in Taiwan, by Leighton and Lambo in Nigeria, and by Robert Giel in Ethiopia all reported quite a high prevalence of disabling psychiatric symptoms in these populations.

The qualification 'disabling' is an important one. All of us suffer or have suffered at some time from depression, anxiety, sleeplessness or bodily discomfort which disappeared when a recognised cause for such feelings ceased to operate. In assessing the prevalence of such symptoms of psychic disturbance, we need to know whether or to what extent they have interfered with a person's normal activities: only then can we begin to assess the contribution of emotionally-determined symptoms to total morbidity in a given population.

The Leightons (1963) had again been pioneers, by carrying out, with the collaboration of T. A. Lambo and other Nigerian colleagues, a replication of their North American survey of psychiatric symptoms in a population sample drawn from Nigerian town and country dwellers. In order to do this the original screening questionnaires had to be translated into Yoruba, and some additional items had to be included, to cater for some local concepts of pathology which had no American counterpart. The survey revealed a very high prevalence of psychiatric symptoms in this West African population, especially in the category of 'psychophysiological disorders'. This was not surprising, because all skin conditions, all musculoskeletal, respiratory, cardiovascular, gastrointestinal, genito-urinary or endocrine reactions, all headaches and all cases where the respondent appeared to be conspicuously over- or under-weight were included under the category of psychophysiological disorders. The authors realised that by so doing they would include an undetermined number whose symptoms were due to physical rather than emotional causes: but they believed that it was not possible to make this distinction under the conditions of a field survey. When they compared the findings from Nigeria with those of the Stirling County survey, they found that the former sample yielded more symptoms, but fewer cases of clearly evident psychiatric disorder than did the latter. They also found an interesting reversal of the respective prevalence rates in men and women: in the North American sample, women showed higher rates of neurotic symptoms than the men, while in the Nigerian sample the men showed higher rates than the women. This was ascribed to the greater and more stressful impact of recent social change on the role and status of the Yoruba men, as compared with their womenfolk.

Leighton and his collaborators were well aware of the difficulties inherent in trying to make cross-cultural comparisons of neurotic symptoms. In a chapter of their monograph, entitled 'The Problem of Cultural Distortion' and at several points in the discussion of their methodology and their findings, they drew attention to likely sources of error, and presented their study as a first step towards obtaining data which would make more valid comparisons possible. In contrast, Kessel (1965) speaking at a conference on international comparisons of morbidity argued that rates of psychiatric symptoms found in one culture could not be compared with those found in another culture, because the perception and reporting of such symptoms must inevitably be influenced by their respective cultural values: hence, we cannot compare like with like. Instead of trying to carry out cross-cultural comparisons, he advocated comparisons between sub-cultures whose members shared many cultural attributes and differed only in a few, definable respects.

Kessel also drew attention to the difficulty of translating the terms in which psychiatric symptoms are described: all too often, the other language is found to contain only words which convey a slightly different meaning. This has been the experience of many Western-trained psychiatrists who have to practice in a non-Western culture. For example, Ebie (1972) on returning to psychiatric practice in Nigeria after completing his training in Edinburgh, found that depressed West Africans described numerous physical complaints, but would acknowledge psychological symptoms such as depressed mood, only on questioning. This was partly attributable to the fact that these patients regarded the hospital doctor (perhaps correctly) as being only interested in the treatment of physical complaints; and partly to the fact that most Nigerian languages do not have a term precisely equivalent to 'depression', nor any expression which conveys the meaning of 'sadness of mood'. Depressed patients in India are also selective in their 'choice' of symptoms (Neki, 1973).

Can the members of any culture suffer from a complaint which their language cannot put into words? The anthropologically-minded linguist Benjamin Whorf (1956) was an early exponent of the school of thought which holds that every people's perception of the self and of the external world finds expression in, and in turn is limited by, the formal structure as well as the vocabulary of its language. Even sub-groups within a single language area may develop styles of speech which constrain the range of their perceptions, as Basil Bernstein (1961) has shown in his analyses of British working-class and middle-class utterances.

It is evident that to use a questionnaire, or a structured interview in a culture other than that in which it was developed must entail some degree of error, no matter how carefully it has been translated. In spite of this, the attempt has been made, for example in Ethiopia (Giel and Van Luijk, 1969) in Uganda (Assael and German, 1970) and in northern India (Wig and Verma, 1973 *a, b, c*; Verma and Wig, 1974; Verma *et al.*, 1974 *a, b*) and in each case has shown both the high prevalence of neurotic symptoms in sample populations, and some interesting variations in the type of symptoms reported.

Wig and his colleagues began by using the Cornell Medical Index with their English-speaking patients and comparing their scores with those reported from England and America. Soon, however, they decided to develop a symptom checklist in the local vernacular. This abbreviated instrument, the 'Postgraduate Institute Health Questionnaire N-1' is based on the translation of items in the CMI 'suitably modified to be as near to patients' own description of symptoms as possible'. A study of this Hindi version of the CMI reveals some interesting transmutations. For example, where the English item is phrased in the active voice (for example 'I feel sick', or 'I don't sleep well', or 'I don't have a good appetite') the Hindi equivalent takes a passive form (for example 'Ulti ati hai'—vomiting comes over me, or 'Nind thik se nahin ati'— sleepiness doesn't come properly, or 'Bhuk thik se nahin lagti hai'—hunger doesn't affect me as it ought to do). The translated questionnaire is pervaded by common Hindi usages, 'ata hai'—it comes; 'lagta hai'—it touches, or affects; 'rahta hai'—it keeps on. Clearly, one of the biases built into the language is the Hindi speaker's expectation that this world is a place where things happen to him, without his own volition, rather than one on which he imposes his own will.

In spite of these limitations, instruments adapted and translated from originals developed in Britain or America have been used to good effect in India and in many other countries; but their users have always been troubled by doubts as to just how appropriate such instruments are in a different culture, and particularly as to whether some important elements have been left out, because they are not perceived as important in the English-speaking world. These considerations prompted my Indian colleague, Dr R. L. Kapur, and myself, in planning a survey of psychiatric symptoms and their social correlates in a rural population in southern India, to begin by studying the terms in which members of this language-area describe their symptoms, and the comparative frequency with which different symptoms are mentioned by patients and by their nearest relatives, respectively. This preliminary task kept Dr Kapur and his co-workers occupied for some two and a half years during which he developed and tested for reliability two related instruments, the Indian Psychiatric Interview Schedule (IPIS) and the Indian Psychiatric Survey Schedule (IPSS). The development, pilot trials and final employment of these instruments in a population survey have been reported in a series of articles (Kapur et al., 1974a, b; Carstairs, 1975) and in a book (Carstairs and Kapur, 1976).

We chose to carry out our survey in Kota, a cluster of villages near the coast of the Arabian Sea, in southern India. Here we could study three communities who had lived side by side, for several centuries, sharing a common language, and a common adherence to Hinduism but differing in a number of other respects. These were the priestly, privileged *Brahmins*, the formerly rather prosperous *Bants*, who are farmers, and the underprivileged *Mogers* or fishermen. During recent years the Brahmins' status has been challenged, but they remain firmly on top, the Bants find themselves in economic and social decline, while the Mogers are rapidly coming up in the world. Another important social change has been the progressive (but still incomplete) abandonment on the part of the Bants and the Mogers of their former matriarchal system of inheritance and of family location, in favour of the patriarchal system which prevails in most Indian communities. We were interested to see whether these social changes would be reflected in differences in the prevalence of symptoms, in the three castes.

First of all, the general prevalence of symptoms: of our 1233 respondents, 37 per cent presented one or more psychiatric symptoms (32 per cent of the men, and 40 per cent of the women). Of course, to have one symptom did not necessarily mean that the respondent felt ill, or was disabled. We therefore carried out a number of other analyses—for example, we noted that of the whole sample 63 per cent had no symptoms; 12 per cent had one symptom only; 15 per cent had two or three symptoms and 10 per cent had more than three symptoms. We also ascertained whether their symptoms were such as to render them unable to cope with their normal activities, and also whether they had actually consulted a doctor or a healer of any kind because of these symptoms. Finally, we constructed a 'Need Scale' (table 4.1), combining numbers of symptoms, 'inability to cope', and whether they had sought a consultation. In terms of this Need Scale, we found that 6 per cent of the whole sample had four or more symptoms, complained of inability to cope, and were currently consulting a healer. Clearly, this gave us an indication of the number in the wider population who shared a similar degree of 'psychiatric need'.

Table 4.1
Distribution of the sample on the Need Scale

Need score	N	%
0	778	63
1	70	6
2	81	7
3	117	9
4	112	9
5	75	6

We found that case rates differed between the three castes (table 4.2). Among the males, the Bants had clearly the highest rates, while among both males and females the Brahmins showed the lowest rates.

Table 4.2
Caste and 'case' rates

	Brahmins (%)	Bants (%)	Mogers (%)
'Case' rate – males	29	39	32
'Case' rate – females	33	43	42

When we looked to see whether case rates were any higher among spouses who had 'changed over' from a matrilineal to a patrilineal life-style, we found that among those who had made the change, 'case' rates were higher—significantly so, for the wives (table 4.3). Evidently, the transition to a mode of life which was unfamiliar to both partners but particularly stressful for the wives (who had formerly enjoyed the support of their brothers and other kinsfolk) took its toll in the form of neurotic complaints.

During the course of the study we also carried out sample surveys to ascertain, among other things, the degree of 'modernisation' of attitudes in members of the three castes; Brahmins were clearly the most 'modernised', and Mogers the least; but the women of all three castes lagged well behind the men in this respect. We were, therefore, rather surprised to find, in another

Table 4.3
Residence patterns and 'case' rates among formerly matrilineal spouses

	Pattern of residence	
	Traditional	Changed over
Males: (N)	(113)	(93)
'Case' rate	32%	38%
Females: (N)	(222)	(115)
'Case' rate	36%	55%

sample survey, that women were significantly more likely than men to consult the village's sole Western-trained doctor first rather than either of the two types of traditional healers who enlisted supernatural powers as the agents of their therapy. At first this seemed to indicate a realistic grasp of the efficacy of modern medicines; but on further inquiry we found that these women shared a common belief that the traditional healers were also endowed with super-naturally enhanced sexual potency, and therefore judged it safer to consult the doctor first.

In this Indian population, as in many developing countries, the pheno-menon of 'possession', in which the subject goes into a state of dissociation and appears to assume an altered personality, is far from rare. Western observers have tended to regard this as a manifestation of hysteria, a condition notoriously liable to be influenced by surrounding cultural expectations. Here, however, we found that there were two quite distinct forms of possession, which we categorised as 'voluntary' and 'involuntary' respec-tively. Subjects who reported the former state were in no way inconvenienced by it; instead, their visitations, like that of the ancient Greek *enthusiasmos*, enhanced their prestige and frequently gave them a form of livelihood. In contrast, those whose episodes of possession were unbidden and unwelcome tended to exhibit numerous other symptoms, and to consult local healers frequently for their relief.

It would be unwarranted to extrapolate from this small sample to the six hundred millions of India, 85 per cent of whom are still village dwellers; but at least our survey does convey an inkling of the enormous size of the problem of mental morbidity in that sub-continent. On the one hand there are perhaps 2 per cent suffering from epilepsy or psychosis, many of whom could experience alleviation of their symptoms if modern drugs were made available to them; and on the other hand there are the tens of millions who suffer from, and are in varying degrees disabled by neurotic or psychosomatic disorders. The latter almost invariably resort to their traditional healers (Neki, 1973). Clearly, in terms of public health the former patients are the ones who need priority. The military term 'triage', which means concentrating on those cases where one is most confident of being able to intervene effectively, has recently acquired undesirable connotations when whole populations have been deemed beyond help, but it remains a valid guide in planning the deployment of limited resources. As to the much larger numbers of persons with neurotic symptoms, they will, in the majority of cases, either recover or learn to live with their symptoms and in both cases they will continue to receive moral support from the same traditional healers who have brought solace to their ancestors for countless generations. That, at any rate, is what one would wish for them; but my experience of the development of 'general hospital psychiatry' and of private practice in Indian cities, during the past twenty-five years compels me to recognise that other forces will almost certainly come into play. In India, just as in the West, there is a ready market for tranquillisers and other psychotropic drugs, a market which the pharmaceutical industry and their not unwilling salesmen, the General Practitioners, exploit all too indiscriminately. As yet, the masses of the Indian population have been spared from the excesses of iatrogenic illness, whose prevalence in North America has been so eloquently documented by Ivan Illich (1974); they have been protected by two factors, first by the high cost of the psychotropic drugs, and secondly by the persistence of a world view in which pain and suffering are accepted as aspects of normal experience, to be contended with and mastered or, should this prove impossible, to be lived with. This philosophy has served India well for centuries and will continue to underlie the ministrations of her traditional healers for many years to come.

References

Ackerknecht, E. (1968). *A Short History of Psychiatry* (2nd edn). Hafner, London and New York

Assael, M. and German, G. A. (1970). Changing society and mental health in Eastern Africa. *Israel Ann. Psych. Rel. Discip.*, **8**, 52–74

Bernstein, B. (1961). Social class and linguistic development: a theory of social learning. In *Education, Economy and Society* (Ed. A. H. Halsey, J. Floud and A. Anderson), Free Press, Chicago

Bremer, J. (1951). A social psychiatric investigation of a small community in northern Norway. *Acta Psychiat. neurol.*, Supplement 62

Carstairs, G. M. (1955). Magic and faith in rural Rajasthan. In *Health, Culture and Community* (Ed. B. D. Paul), Russell Sage, New York

Carstairs, G. M. (1956). Hinjra and Jiryan: two derivatives of Hindu attitudes to sexuality. *Br. J. Med. Psychol.*, **29**, 5

Carstairs, G. M. (1975). Measuring psychiatric morbidity in a South Indian population. *Bull. Br. Psychol. Soc.*, **28**, 95–101

Carstairs, G. M. and Kapur, R. L. (1976). *The Great Universe of Kota: Stress change and Mental Disorders in an Indian Village*. Hogarth Press, London; California University Press, Berkeley

Dube, K. C. (1970). A study of prevalence of mental illness in Uttar Pradesh, India. *Acta psychiat. scand.*, **46**, 327

Ebie, J. C. (1972). Some observations on depressive illness in Nigerians attending a psychiatric outpatients clinic. *Afr. J. Med. Sci.*, **3**, 149–155

Freud, S. (1930). *Civilisation and its Discontents*. Hogarth, London

Giel, R. and Van Luijk, J. N. (1969). Psychiatric morbidity in a small Ethiopian town. *Br. J. Psychiat.*, **115**, 149

Illich, I. (1974). *Medical Nemesis: the Expropriation of Health*. Calder and Boyars, London

Kapur, R. L., Kapur, M. and Carstairs, G. M. (1974a). Indian Psychiatric Interview Schedule (IPIS). *Social Psychiat.*, **9**, 61–69

Kapur, R. L., Kapur, M. and Carstairs, G. M. (1974b). Indian Psychiatric Survey Schedule (IPSS). *Social Psychiat.*, **9**, 71–76

Kessel, W. I. N. (1965). 'Are international comparisons timely?' In *Comparability in International Epidemiology* (Ed. R. M. Acheson), Milbank Memorial Fund, New York

Leff, J. P. (1973). Culture and the differentiation of emotional states. *Br. J. Psychiat.*, **123**, 299–306

Leighton, A. H., Lambo, T. A., Hughes, C. C., Leighton, Dorothea C., Murphy, Jane M. and Macklin, D. B. (1963). *Psychiatric Disorder among the Yoruba*. Cornell University Press, Ithaca, New York

Leighton, Dorothea C., Harding, J. S., Macklin, D. S., Macmillan, A. M. and Leighton, A. H. (1963). *The Character of Danger: Psychiatric Symptoms in Selected Communities*. Basic Books, New York

Lin, T. Y. (1953). A study of the incidence of mental disorder in Chinese and other cultures. *Psychiatry*, **16**, 313

Lin, T. Y., Rin Hsien, Yeh, E. K., Hsu, C. C. and Chu, H. M. (1969). Mental disorders in Taiwan, fifteen years later. In *Mental Health Research in Asia and the Pacific* (Ed. W. Caudill and T. Y. Lin), East-West Center Press, Honolulu, pp. 66–91

Neki, J. S. (1973). Psychiatry in South-East Asia. *Br. J. Psychiat.*, **123**, 257–69

Rosen, G. (1968). *Madness in Society*. Routledge & Kegan Paul, London

Shepherd, M., Cooper, B., Brown, A. C. and Kalton, G. (1966). *Psychiatric Illness in General Practice*. Oxford University Press, London

Srole, L., Langner, T. S., Michael, S. T., Opler, M. K. and Rennie, T. A. C. (1962). *Mental Health in the Metropolis: The Mid-town Manhattan Study*. McGraw-Hill, New York

Strømgren, E. (1950). Statistical and genetical population studies within psychiatry: methods and principal results. In *Report of the International Congress of Psychiatry*, Vol. VI, Herman et Cie, Paris, pp. 155–190

Verma, S. K. and Wig, N. N. (1974). A cross-cultural comparison of psychiatric patients on some of the parameters of Cornell Medical Index. *Manas*, **21**, 17–25

Verma, S. K., Wig, N. N. and Pershad, D. (1974a). A comparative study of medical and psychiatric patients in India on Cornell Medical Index. *Indian J. Clin. Psycholog.*, **1**, 104–8

Verma, S. K., Wig, N. N. and Pershad, D. (1974b). A comparative study of rural and urban population in India on Cornell Medical Index. *Indian J. Clin. Psycholog.*, **1**, 109–113

Whorf, B. (1956). Science and linguistics. In *Language, Thought and Reality* (Ed. J. B. Carroll), Cambridge, Mass.

Wig, N. N. and Verma, S. K. (1973a). PGI Health Questionnaire N–1: a simple Neuroticism Scale in India. *Indian J. Psychiat.*, **15**, 80–88

Wig, N. N. and Verma, S. K. (1973b). PGI-HQ-N1: further data on the patient population. *Psychol. Studies*, **18**, 10–13

Wig, N. N. and Verma, S. K. (1973c). A cross-cultural study of psychiatric patients on Cornell Medical Index. *Indian J. Psychiat.*, **15**, 363–6

Yap, P. M. (1951). Mental diseases peculiar to certain cultures: a survey. *J. Ment. Sci.*, **97**, 313–27

Yap, P. M. (1967). Classification of the culture-bound reactive syndromes. *Austral. N. Z. J. Psychiat.*, **1**, 172–79

5 The Small Group as a Therapeutic Medium

M. A. Yelloly

Interest in the therapeutic effects of experience in small groups is by no means confined to psychiatry; social workers, occupational therapists, marriage guidance counsellors, and many others in the helping professions are equipping themselves with the skills and knowledge to conduct small groups, in the belief that this is a powerful medium for beneficial change. In this chapter the term 'therapeutic' will be used in a broad way to denote any group deliberately established with the aim of producing psychological change or growth in its members. Defined in this way, the kinds of groups under consideration will include not only formally constituted psychotherapy groups and those aimed at psychodynamic change, but counselling groups, activity groups for disturbed children, groups for bereaved people and those with a variety of physical and social handicaps, as well as for those with interpersonal problems. On the whole, such groups are regarded as being particularly valuable in overcoming isolation and increasing social effectiveness and social functioning. Research which has implications for the group conductor comes from a number of sources: from the field of group psychotherapy, from the encounter movement, and from social psychologists with an interest in small group phenomena in relation to problem-solving, morale, decision-making and the like in the work situation. This chapter draws mainly on the first two of these sources—group psychotherapy and the encounter group movement.

In recent years there has been a burgeoning of interest in the small group. Within psychiatry it is regarded as a flexible and economic mode of treatment with considerable potential; outside psychiatry there has been an immense proliferation of intensive group experiences of various kinds — encounter groups, sensitivity groups, sensory awareness groups, consciousness raising groups, Gestalt and many others. Some of these groups are not overtly 'therapeutic' in that they set out to provide a therapeutic experience for psychologically distressed individuals, but they do generally claim to lead to personal growth and change through fostering greater openness and honesty in interpersonal relationships, by enabling people to get rid of hang-ups and relate to others with greater freedom and lessened defensiveness. Rogers (1970) has identified some of the characteristics of encounter groups as follows:

A facilitator can develop, in a group which meets intensively, a psychological climate of safety in which freedom of expression and reduction of defensiveness gradually occur.

In such a psychological climate many of the immediate feeling reactions of each member towards others, and of each member towards himself, tend to be expressed.

A climate of mutual trust develops out of this mutual freedom to express real feelings, positive and negative. Each member moves towards greater acceptance of his total being — emotional, intellectual, and psychical — as it is, including its potential.

With individuals less inhibited by defensive rigidity, the possibility of change in personal attitudes and behaviour, in professional methods, in administrative procedures and relationships, becomes less threatening.

With the reduction of defensive rigidity, individuals can hear each other, can learn from each other, to a greater extent.

There is a development of feedback from one person to another, such that each individual learns how he appears to others and what impact he has in interpersonal relationships.

With this greater freedom and improved communication, new ideas, new concepts, new directions emerge. Innovation can become a desirable rather than a threatening possibility.

These learnings in the group experience tend to carry over, temporarily or more permanently, into the relationship with spouse, children, students, subordinates, peers, and even superiors following the group experience.

These characteristics are very similar to the kinds of formulations made by group therapists and demonstrate the impossibility of drawing hard and fast distinctions between what is or is not a therapeutic group.

With this intense interest in the small group as a medium of growth and change, and the very ambitious claims which are often advanced as to its effectiveness — often by those espousing very different ideologies and styles — we must look to research for guidelines to assist us in establishing and conducting counselling or therapeutic groups.

Three Models

One of the difficulties in discussing the effectiveness of group methods is that there is little homogeneity of method, approach, theoretical assumption or therapeutic style; as little as within psychiatry itself. Indeed, what evidence there is suggests that theoretical orientation is only very loosely related to actual therapist behaviour. It is thus not always easy to know what is being measured, or to what aspects of the very complex group process change is to be attributed. It is useful, however, to identify at this stage three main orientations reflected in the literature — the psychodynamic, the Rogerian, and the behavioural.

1. The Psychodynamic

This term usually includes a number of theoretical orientations which are derived ultimately from the work of Freud, and whatever differences they may have, share a fundamental interest in the unconscious mind, and in the phenomena of transference and resistance. Therapists with a psychodynamic orientation will in general tend to avoid personal disclosure, and will focus especially on the unconscious (by which is meant dynamically unconscious and not merely covert) processes going on within the group; their interventions will be primarily of an interpretive nature designed to increase the insight and cognitive mastery of group members. Interpretations may be primarily directed to individuals, or to unconscious group processes (Bion, 1961).

2. Rogerian

This refers to the client-centred therapy of Carl Rogers. The client-centred school has been particularly influential, partly because of the sheer numbers of participants through the encounter group movement, and partly because of the great volume of research it has stimulated. In this approach, the main task of the conductor is to foster a warm, supportive, facilitative climate in which honest self-disclosure and expression of feelings can take place. All group members are seen as sharing in the therapeutic tasks, but the therapist's role is central; although non-directive (in the traditional sense of leading or charting a course) the therapist is nevertheless highly influential in creating a group climate which is facilitative — he is referred to as a facilitator rather than leader or conductor. The warmth, empathy and genuineness of the facilitator are assumed to be as important to the development of the group as in the one-to-one counselling situation (Truax and Carkhuff, 1967). Rogerian groups are like those of a more psychodynamic orientation in their non-directiveness, but differ from them in two important respects: interpretations are eschewed, the facilitator being more likely to call attention to covert aspects of group process or personal feeling than to interpret them; and there is a greater openness and transparency on the part of the conductor, the expression of whose own feelings is regarded as valid and helpful. There is a deliberate attempt to lessen rather than accentuate the psychological distance between therapist and group members. The degree to which therapist transparency is a facilitating or restrictive condition is a matter of considerable debate, and the reader is referred to Dies (1977) for a recent review.

3. Behavioural

Behavioural group therapists assume that dysfunctional behaviour is learned, and that both troublesome and adaptive behaviour come about as the result of identifiable learning processes. Eradication, and the learning of new skills or the making up of behavioural deficits can therefore most effectively be induced through known and well-proven procedures of behaviour modification, such as response shaping, modelling, systematic desensitisation, and (increasingly) cognitive restructuring. The therapist is both an expert in these procedures and a teacher of them, and (initially at least) takes an active role in structuring, controlling and directing the activities of the group to facilitate the achievement of clearly defined and mutually agreed treatment objectives. Later such leadership tasks may be undertaken by group members (Rose, 1977). On the whole the group is seen as advantageous in offering the opportunity for learning and testing out new behaviours with clear feedback in a situation which closely approximates to the everyday world; in powerfully controlling and reinforcing members' behaviour — far more influentially than in the therapist–patient dyad; and in providing a variety of models. The group process is only of interest in so far as it facilitates or obstructs the achievement of individual goals.

In practice it may be difficult to relate specific therapist styles to particular orientations; for instance, a psychodynamic group will permit re-learning and testing-out of new social skills as well as the acquisition of insight, and the therapist may influence members by acting as a model as well as through his interpretations. Nor is there marked difference in objective, though there may be considerable differences of view as to the means whereby this is to be achieved. Although Bednar and Lawlis (1971) note a variety of specific goals, these resolve themselves into two broad objectives: (1) enhanced social functioning (particularly characteristic of behavioural groups), and (2) personal growth and discovery of identity (particularly characteristic of Rogerian, Gestalt and other existentialist groups). Both objectives may be present, but they are separated here because they may conflict with each other, in which case one or other will be paramount.

Some Questions about Groups

This chapter addresses itself to three groups of questions most significant for the practitioner:

(i) What do groups offer? What is the evidence that they lead to patient improvement? What kinds of changes occur, in what patients in what kinds of groups, and with what degree of permanency?

(ii) Can there be change not only for the better, but for the worse, as the result of group experiences, and if so, is it possible to identify either participants who are particularly at risk, or high-risk styles of leadership?

(iii) With the variety of models there now are in the group field, can we identify group or therapist variables which seem to be commonly associated with therapeutic outcomes — the 'curative factors'?

What do groups offer?

Walton (1971) maintains that the evidence supports the contention that (a) desired behavioural changes occur more readily in group psychotherapy than with other psychological treatments; (b) such changes are more enduring; (c) people treated in groups improve their social functioning. It is reasonable to suggest that in contrast to one-to-one treatment, the group offers at the very least the following conditions:

(1) A closer approximation to the real world in which behavioural difficulties become readily apparent. Within the group situation, a range of interpersonal and peer relationships quickly confront the member with his characteristic difficulties in a vivid and inescapable way. Thus there is the opportunity for testing out and modifying perceptual distortions and for corrective emotional experiences.

(2) From the therapist's point of view, there are diagnostic advantages. He can observe his patient in action, and does not have to rely on reported accounts. This provides a unique opportunity for on the spot diagnosis, and for monitoring change over time and in a developmental way (Feldman and Wodarski, 1975).

(3) There is the possibility of therapeutic interventions from other group members as well as the therapist; feedback from peers may be more acceptable than from the 'expert' and hence more readily utilised.

(4) It is well-established that group influences on behaviour are very strong, and while this can have negative effects in inducing undesirable conformity, it can also be utilised very positively, for example, in encouraging a withdrawn person to become more self-assertive.

(5) A cohesive group provides a safe climate within which new behaviours that may involve risk for individuals can be tried out.

(6) The group can become an important reference point for its members, outside the specific boundaries of group meetings, that is, it can be internalised. Thus a group member, faced with a difficult situation, may ask himself, 'I wonder what the group would say about this?'.

What evidence is there that groups do actually benefit patients in the way that these conditions might lead us to expect? Varied criteria for the assessment of outcome have been used. Kelman and Parloff (1957) discuss comfort (relief of distress or symptoms), effectiveness (in social role performance and management of transactions with others), and self-awareness (insight, correction of perceptual distortions, and the release of repressions) and these seem to be fairly typical of the kinds of changes expected. A thorough survey of outcome studies can be found in Lieberman (1976). But there are many problems in assessing the results of empirical research: one is the variety of outcome measures used; another, that 'group therapy' covers a variety of theoretical and stylistic differences; a third, that dynamic changes may occur independently of behavioural changes, and vice versa (Malan *et al.*, 1976). Despite all this, Bednar and Lawlis (1971) in a review of some 38 studies found a clear convergence of evidence consistent with the view that group therapy is an effective tool. In terms of more specific changes, their review suggested that patients suffering from mood disorders, anxiety states and somatic complaints experience relief from distress, depression being the symptom most frequently reported as improved. Thought disorders and severe interpersonal withdrawal do not seem to be readily influenced by group therapy.

In sum the results of group psychotherapy are encouraging, but we need to know far more about what kinds of group benefit what patients; in general it is likely that therapists have been far more optimistic about the beneficial effects than have patients. In a very careful follow-up study undertaken by staff of the Tavistock Clinic (Malan *et al.*, 1976), which involved 42 randomly selected patients interviewed after 2–14 years and was concerned with identifying dynamic changes, it was found that the majority of patients were highly dissatisfied with their group experiences. Further, a comparison of those who stayed less than 6 months with those who stayed more than 2 years showed no significant differences. But there was a strong correlation between positive outcome and previous individual psychotherapy.

Encounter groups are an important source of information about intensive group experiences, partly because of the number of those who participate in such events; these have produced very useful data about what kinds of changes occur. One large study concerned 17 groups totalling 206 participants (Lieberman *et al.*, 1973). Viewed from the perspective of the participant, at the termination of the groups, rather over 60 per cent saw themselves as having benefited. Six months later, 10–20 per cent of this group were less enthusiastic and rated the groups in more negative terms — a change which suggests that the results are not necessarily lasting. Leaders tended to be more optimistic about outcome than did participants, seeing some change in about 90 per cent of the participants, and substantial gain in about one-third. Over all, one-third of those who participated in the groups benefited from them, a little over a third remained unchanged and the remainder experienced some form of negative outcome. Types of change related to values, attitudes and the Self. Participants were more likely to shift their value structure towards being more change-oriented and growth-oriented. Their self-images moved towards being more lenient and towards increased congruence between their ideal image and their self. Behavioural changes were much less stable than changes in values and attitudes.

The Hazards of Therapy

In sum, encounter groups show 'a modest positive impact'. But of greater interest is that very significant differences *between* the groups emerged on detailed study (Lieberman *et al.*, 1973). Some proved to be highly productive learning experiences; others were on balance destructive, leaving participants more harmed than helped. This is in line with the findings of Bergin (1963) and Truax and Carkhuff (1967) that patients in psychotherapy show greater variability in personality change at the conclusion of therapy than do controls; in other words, they show greater improvement or greater deterioration. In a controlled study of 209 encounter group participants (Yalom and Lieberman, 1971) 16 members (around 8 per cent of the total) were identified as casualties in that they had had a destructive experience when the damage had sometimes to be repaired through psychotherapy. A casualty was defined as one demonstrating an enduring, significant, negative outcome. These mainly occurred in groups with a leader whose style was characterised by high aggressive stimulation, high charisma, high individual focus, and high confrontation. The risk factor was then considerable and particularly in groups where individuals were put in the 'hot seat' or were 'worked on'. Negative outcome was associated with attack, rejection, failure to achieve unrealistic goals, and coercive expectations on the part of the group or its leader. (This finding contradicts that of Gibb (1971) who claims that in one follow-up study of 1200 participants, only one rated his experience as 'negative'.)

Some Variables Associated with Positive Outcome

I turn now to the third question, and attempt to identify some variables which research suggests are critical to the success of a group, and to relate these to therapist tasks. Of especial importance are *group cohesiveness* and *group culture*.

(1) There is strong evidence that *group cohesiveness* is a key variable (Yalom, 1970). Though as Yalom observes, it is 'a widely researched, poorly understood, basic property of groups', cohesiveness is generally defined as the attractiveness of the group to its members. It is a *sine qua non* for therapeutic change, and feelings of personal involvement, a sense of warmth and unity and of being accepted are important antecedent conditions for corrective experience and interpersonal learning. Correspondingly, an atmosphere of distrust and non-involvement is unlikely to provide these conditions.

Cohesiveness may be deliberately increased in a number of ways. First, *selection* of group members provides a degree of homogeneity and compatibility. There are, however, examples of non-selected groups (for example in day centres for offenders) where nonetheless a high degree of cohesiveness may develop. Similarly homogeneity is not desirable in all circumstances and heterogeneous groups (that is containing patients with dissimilar problems) may have certain advantages. Thus in adult treatment groups in a psychiatric ward, patients in heterogeneously composed groups were more productive and problem-centred than were those in homogeneous groups (Rose, 1977). This may be because a heterogeneous group provides greater stimulation and more variety and richness of experience. Second, the *size* of the group also relates to cohesiveness. Eight is usually considered a desirable number for the therapy group, though the potentialities of larger groups (particularly for the treatment of paranoid individuals) is still being explored (Kreeger, 1975).

Third, beneficial outcome is significantly increased by *pre-training* (Bednar *et al.*, 1974), which ensures that patients have a reasonably clear expectation about therapist and patient roles and about the purpose of the group; clear mutually agreed goals obviously contribute also to the establishment of a cohesive group. Pre-training is often done by using videos or tapes of groups thought to be functioning in a therapeutic way. Fourth, the therapist can contribute to the development of cohesiveness through reinforcing and prompting verbal expressions of solidarity and affection, and he is a potent influence in shaping the behaviour of the group (Liberman, 1971).

(2) *Group culture.* All groups develop a characteristic culture based upon certain common ideas, beliefs and norms. One group may differ very greatly from another in the degree of commitment to the group, the importance attached to the task and the work achieved, the level of hostility which is regarded as acceptable, and the openness and freedom of communication. In therapeutic groups high value is placed on the development of a climate of trust which allows frank discussion of problems to take place and encourages an honesty which the patient may never have experienced in his ordinary social relationships. It is an important part of the therapist's task to foster a climate which encourages free interaction among group members, high levels of involvement and self-disclosure, mutual acceptance, and expression of both conflict and affection. This may be achieved by reinforcing such expressions, or by modelling; it can also be furthered by dealing with restrictive conditions such as scapegoating, and the discouragement of destructive personal attacks. It should be added that although these have been referred to as 'therapist tasks' they are not necessarily dependent on the presence of a formally designated therapist, and self help groups such as Alcoholics Anonymous in which members act as models and therapists to each other can be very effective (Hurvitz, 1970; Madison, 1972). Another example is Mowrer's 'integrity groups', in which all members share in these therapeutic tasks; each group contains some new members and a core of those already experienced in such groups; new groups are seeded from the membership of those already in existence (Mowrer, 1964).

Whatever the theoretical position of the therapist, one of the main tasks is to help the group define its work and keep it productive and task-focused. This means an alertness for when work is being done and when it is being avoided. It is not always easy to identify when work is going on. At the manifest level, discussion about apparently irrelevant or trivial matters may also be an indirect way of expressing concern about the here-and-now situation of the group (Whitaker and Lieberman, 1964). For instance, a group of adolescents on probation met with a probation officer. At the first meeting discussion centred on the police, and whether or not they were to be trusted. This could be seen as an indirect questioning of the good intentions of authority in general, and the probation officer in this group in particular. The group has, as it were, a hidden agenda which it may be necessary to make explicit if it is to surmount the difficulty and move on. In psychodynamic groups a great deal of the therapist's activity will be concerned with interpreting the latent content of such communications, particularly as they relate to the transference between group members and therapist (Bion, 1961; Ezriel, 1950).

Conditions for Effective Work

Groups can be a medium for significant therapeutic gain. Conversely,.they can be a source of disappointment, boredom, frustration, or even negative learning for their members. There is, sadly, no way in which success can be guaranteed; the process and outcome of any group depends on many conditions only some of which can be known by or are within the control of the conductors. Nevertheless there are identifiable and well researched conditions which are likely to maximise the chances of a successful group, and others which are likely to stack the cards against it, and these can act as guidelines for the group conductor. Stock Whitaker (1975) has identified four sets of conditions for effective work:

(1) *The institutional or organisational environment within which the group is conducted.* Careful preparatory work with colleagues may remove some resistance and distrust among those in a position to affect the group; but the chances of success in an unfavourable or distrustful environment may be so low as to make the group non-viable.

(2) *The state of consensus within the group with respect to its aims and procedures.* This has been discussed under cohesiveness.

(3) *Structures which facilitate or undermine the group's work*; that is, size, composition, duration, constancy of membership, proportion of leaders to members and the like.

(4) *The maintenance or loss of impact and productivity.* Some groups seem to have the capacity to retain their impact and significance for members over periods of years, and members continue to use the group productively. Others become sterile or repetitive, and though they survive, little useful work seems to be being done. A frank stock-taking of the progress of the group may indicate some reorganisation, or even termination.

In conclusion, it must be said that the nature of the expertise required of group conductors is still inadequately defined. Lieberman (1976) notes that the influence of the therapist and his actions and skills has been emphasised in the group therapy literature; he is assumed to be central and indispensable to any changes which take place, much as in the dyadic situation. Lieberman suggests, however, that 'the behaviour, personality and skill level of the leader may have taken on mythic proportions as a basic force for successful personal change in groups'. More important may be the relationships members have with each other and opportunities for feedback, heightened emotional experience, and self expression, which may only peripherally relate to the leader; support for this view comes from studies of consciousness-raising and similar peer-led groups which have like goals to therapy groups, and appear to work very effectively without designated leadership. The small group is a complex social system, and the influences which lead to change are equally complex, and as yet very imperfectly understood (Lieberman, 1975). The group is a dynamic, changing entity, in which events, thoughts and feelings chase each other with bewildering rapidity. No-one can hope to have more than a limited awareness and understanding of a process of such complexity, or even of his own part in it. Experienced conductors, however, whatever their orientation, regard as crucial the capacity of the leader to distance himself sufficiently from the emotionally charged events of the group to enable him to maintain a perspective on what is happening—and on what is happening to himself. By so doing he is more likely to be able to recognise how he and others are being affected, to recognise and deal with potentially destructive activities such as scapegoating, and so influence the process in more therapeutic directions.

References

Bednar, R. L. and Lawlis, G. (1971). Empirical research in group psychotherapy. In *Handbook of Psychiatry & Behaviour Change* (Ed. A. E. Bergin, and S. L. Garfield) Wiley, New York

Bednar, R. L., Weet, C., Evensen, P., Lanier, D., and Melnick, J. (1974). Empirical guidelines for group therapy: Pre-training, cohesion and modelling. *J. appl. behav. Sci.*, **10**, 149–65

Bergin, A. E. (1963). The effects of psychotherapy: negative results revisited. *J. Counsel. Psychol.*, **10**, 244–250

Bion, W. R. (1961). *Experiences in Groups*. Tavistock, London

Cooper, C. L. (1974). Psychological disturbance following T-groups: Relationship between the Eysenck Personality Inventory and family/friends perceptions. *Br. J. soc. Work*, **4**, 39–49

Dies, R. R. (1977). Group therapist transparency: a critique of theory and research. *Int. J. Group Psychother.*, **27**, 177–200

Ezriel, H. (1950). A psychoanalytic approach to group treatment. *Br. J. med. Psychol.*, **23**, 59–74

Feldman, R. A. and Wodarski, J. S. (1975). *Contemporary Approaches to Group Treatment*. Jossey-Bass, San Fransisco

Gibb, J. (1971). The effects of human relations training. In *Handbook of Psychotherapy and Behaviour Change* (Ed. A. E. Bergin and J. L. Garfield) Wiley, New York

Hurvitz, N. (1970). Peer self-help psychotherapy groups and their implications for psychotherapy. *Psychotherapy: Theory, Research and Practice*, **7**, 41–49

Kelman, H. C. and Parloff, M. B. (1957). Interrelationships among three criteria of improvement in group therapy: comfort, effectiveness and self-awareness. *J. abnorm. soc. Psychol.*, **54**, 281–288

Kreeger, L. (1975). *The Large Group: Dynamics and Therapy*. Constable, London

Liberman, R. (1971). Reinforcement of cohesiveness in group therapy: behavioural and personal change. *Archs gen. Psychiat.*, **25**, 168–177

Lieberman, M. A. (1975). Group methods. In *Helping People Change* (Ed. F. H. Kanfer and A. P. Goldstein), Pergamon Press, New York

Lieberman, M. A. (1976). Change induction in small groups. In *Annual Review of Psychology*. Palo Alto, pp. 217–249

Lieberman, M. A., Yalom, I. D. and Miles, M. (1973). *Encounter Groups: First Facts*. Basic Books, New York

Madison, P. (1972). Have grouped, will travel. *Psychother. Theory, Res. Pract.*, **95**, 324

Malan, D. H., Balfour, F. H., Hood, V. G. and Shooter, A. M. (1976). Group psychotherapy: a long-term follow-up study. *Archs gen. Psychiat.*, **33** (ii), 1305–1315

Mowrer, O. H. (1964). *The New Group Therapy*. Van Nostrand, Princeton, New Jersey

O'Donnell, C. (1972). Group behaviour modification with chronic in-patients: a case study. *Psychotherapy: Theory, Research and Practice*, **9**, 120

Rogers, C. R. (1970). *Encounter Groups*. Penguin Books, London

Rose, S. D. (1977). *Group Therapy: a Behavioral Approach*. Prentice-Hall, Englewood-Cliffs, N.J.

Truax, C. B. and Carkhuff, R. R. (1967). *Towards Effective Counselling and Psychotherapy*. Aldine, Chicago

Walton, H. (1971). *Small Group Psychotherapy*. Penguin Books, London

Whitaker, D. S. (1975). Some conditions for effective work with groups. *Br. J. soc. Work*, **5** (4), 423–439

Whitaker, D. S. and Lieberman, M. A. (1964). *Psychotherapy Through the Group Process*. Tavistock, London

Yalom, I. D. (1970). *The Theory and Practice of Group Psychotherapy*. Basic Books, New York

Yalom, I. D. and Lieberman, M. A., (1971). A study of encounter group casualties. *Archs gen. Psychiat.*, **25**, 16–30

6 Psychiatric Ideologies

J. P. Watson

'Ideology' is a sub-set of 'Attitude', a term which is used in many different ways to cover a wide range of phenomena. It is sometimes hard to distinguish 'attitudes' from other concepts such as values, beliefs, ideas, opinions, or feelings. 'Ideology' is also an ambiguous term. Hence, we begin with matters of definition. We can then consider psychiatric ideologies and their importance in psychiatric practice.

Definitions

Attitude

Scott (1968) has drawn attention to the large number of definitions of attitude to be found in the literature. His own definition makes sense; he states that an attitude is 'an enduring organisation of motivational, emotional, perceptual and cognitive processes with respect to some aspect of the individual's world'. An attitude is enduring, not a mere whim; it has something to do with action, affects—some say predisposes to—behaviour, is 'motivational'; and is affect-laden, not simply a more or less coherent conceptual system, important though its cognitive aspect is.

Scott also culled from the literature eleven empirical derivatives of the hypothetical construct 'attitude'. Four seem particularly important. 'Direction' is the psychological distance of a person from an object, and refers to his tendencies to approach and avoid it. 'Magnitude' refers to the degree of (un)favourableness (or, positive or negative movement) with which a person responds to an object, and is the most frequently measured aspect of attitude. The other two empirical derivatives are 'intensity', reflecting the strength of feeling associated with attitude, and 'salience', the importance of the object of attitude in the person's view of the world.

Ideology

According to the *Oxford English Dictionary*, 'ideology' is a 'manner of thinking characteristic of a class or individual'. A social psychological view of ideology is as a 'set of values determined by material or quasi-rational considerations' (Allport, 1968). In explication of this general statement, Allport defines Marxist 'ideology' as including the belief that there are 'elaborate beliefs promulgated by the capitalist class to justify its favoured position in society'.

Clearly, ideologies have to do with ideas, and action, but are also accompanied by semantic uncertainty. This could be advantageous to those working to advance certain ideologies but is counterproductive in psychiatry. It seems to me to accord with common usage to regard ideology as a sub-set of attitude and thereby an 'enduring organisation', as defined previously. We talk of ideologies in relation to principles, classes of objects, or broad abstractions of reality, as opposed to attitudes towards individual persons, objects or things. I might then have attitudes to persons A, B and C (enduring organisations of motivational, etc., processes with respect to them) individually. And, I might have attitudes toward the class or group of persons which included A, B and C; I would call my attitude to this group my ideology about it. My over-all view of A or B or C might be a product of my ideologies about the groups of which they are members *and* also of individual attitudes to them derived from other sources.

This chapter is concerned with the possible importance of ideology in determining views of psychiatric patients. We will restrict ourselves to the view of psychiatric staff towards patients.

Psychiatric Staff Ideology

Varieties of Ideology

Three ideological types of psychiatrist were identified using a questionnaire method in an extensive study in the United States by Strauss *et al.* (1964). The types were called 'somatotherapeutic', 'psychotherapeutic' and 'sociotherapeutic' to refer respectively to contrasting emphases upon biological, individual psychological and environmental factors in the aetiology, formulation and treatment of psychiatric disorder. Almost a decade previously a distinction between 'custodial' and 'humanistic' ideologies had been drawn by Gilbert and Levinson (1957a) in the United States and in Britain by Carstairs and Heron (1957). There are substantial similarities between the descriptions given of custodial and somatotherapeutic ideologies, while the humanistic ideology has much in common with both psychotherapeutic and sociotherapeutic ideologies. The three ideological types of Strauss *et al.* seem essentially the same as those obtained in Britain a little later by Caine and Smail (1969).

It is not difficult to think of giants in the post-war psychiatric scene who could be regarded as exemplars of these three ideological types. However, it may occur to the reader that these varieties of psychiatrist are rarely found in pure culture in Britain (Freudenberg, 1966). Some may think that many psychiatrists today espouse an eclectic view, the central feature of this ideology being its emphasis upon the need to accommodate biological, psychological and social factors in a single coherent view.

Two points are important here. The first is that a 1970s investigation along the lines of Strauss *et al.* has not been done and would be needed to show if ideologies have changed since the early 1960s. Secondly, it is reasonable to enquire if the 'ideologies' of all these above workers are mere artefacts, derived from the methods used by the investigators. This proposition requires some comments upon the methods in question.

Methodology

Psychiatric ideologies have emerged from questionnaire studies and the method is exemplified by that of Caine and Smail (1969). It is helpful to review the stages involved in this kind of work.

(a) Caine and Smail interviewed a considerable number of the sort of people they were interested in (psychiatric staff of various professional affiliations), asking them to talk freely about the subject matter of the investigation (psychiatric practice, hospitals, and treatment). The conversations were recorded.

(b) Statements of view about the different parts of the subject matter were culled from the recordings and listed so that respondents could indicate degrees of (dis)agreement to them.

(c) The list was pruned of redundant and relatively unintelligible items following a pilot study.

(d) The resulting list (of 75 items in Caine and Smail's case) was given to a suitably obtained sample of psychiatrists (and subsequently to other relevant groups of people).

(e) The results were subjected to multivariate analysis.

(f) Measures derived from this analysis were used in studies with further groups of psychiatric personnel.

One of the most important things about any psychological measure is the set of rules governing the interpretation of data derived from it. That is to say, in what circumstances is it legitimate to make which inferences from test results? These approaches are sometimes more helpful than traditional concerns about reliability and validity, which cover some of the same ground.

In clarifying 'interpretation rules', two questions can be usefully asked. These are: what was the experimental task? And what constraints did the task place upon the test subjects? It is important to note that psychological test constraints may be positive (subjects are prevented from doing misleading or inappropriate things) or negative (subjects are not able to do meaningful things relevant to the test subject matter). In assessing the task set before the respondent in a psychological test, it is important to note test items, and test instructions.

Consider Item 48 in Caine and Smail's questionnaire. The subject is here invited to express (dis)agreement with the proposition, 'Patients should not call nurses by their Christian names'. (It should be remembered that, for the most part, persons perform psychological tests however absurd if asked nicely to do so and if they do not take exception to the matter presented to them. Test compliance *per se* does not indicate cogency, relevence or meaning, although it may imply intelligibility.)

What is made of a 'mildly agree' response to Item 48? It could be a composite of 'some patients should certainly call some nurses on some wards by their Christian names' and 'some patients should certainly not call some nurses on some wards by their Christian names'. This is because the test form gives no opportunity for the registration of a qualified 'yes sometimes', 'it all depends' view of the matter, whether strongly felt or not. Alternatively, 'mildly agree' to Item 48 could indicate 'yes but I don't feel very strongly about this issue'. And other possible detailed meanings of such responses can be devised without difficulty. The point to be made here is that the test t isk entails a constraint which prevents certain responses of prima facie importance. It is possible in principle that constrained responses and the analyses to which they are subjected generate artefacts. In this instance, one might conclude that the ideological types inferred by Caine and Smail from principal component analyses of arrays of questionnaire responses are nothing but products of data manipulation, without empirical referents. (After all, principal components arise from matrices of numbers, not from anyone's mind. Tables of random numbers have principal components.)

Are then Caine and Smail's ideological types spurious? The answer to this is to be found by reference to the data source. The investigators interviewed many staff under conditions of minimal constraint and included their statements in their questionnaire. They put into their instrument the views of the people they were interested in, suitably summarised, and were at pains not to impose their own views in their test. This is substantial evidence for meaning in the results they obtained.

(In contrast, we may note that some workers, mostly of sociological origin, have asked various repondents, including psychiatrists, to rate 'mental illness' as a single class (see Rabkin (1972) for a review). Anyone who has day to day contact with the whole range of psychiatric disorders would immediately note the importance of the heterogeneity of this class when asked to talk about it. Similarly, any psychiatric staff person would emphasise that 'mental patients' are not all the same if asked about this class. Much work assuming the homogeneity of 'mental illness' and 'mental patients' has been misleading or at best valueless because of the constraints entailed by the use of such imposed categories, a mistake readily preventable by adequate conversation with relevant persons at the outset.)

In any field in which individual persons are the objects of experience, generalisations must be interpreted with caution. Yet, people who work in 'mental hospitals' with 'mental patients' and have experience of giving 'mental treatment' tend to derive general views from repeated particular experiences.

We know that persons 'anticipate events by construing their replications' (Kelly, 1955, p. 50) and hence understand that a person who infers a general principle from experiences of individuals will tend to make predictive deductions from that principle about subsequent similar individuals. In the sense of general principles about classes, everyone has ideologies and all psychiatric staff persons have psychiatric ideologies. Problems arise if people have 'nothing but' ideologies which hinder registration of the humanity of the individual. Without an ideology, on the other hand, personal phenomena cannot be related to other experience, and thereby lack personal meaning.

The Effects of Psychiatric Ideologies

Work in this field has indicated some of the associations between psychiatric ideology and other factors.

(a) In the first place, staff ideology does relate to (reflect, and predict) staff behaviour. Custodial ideology is linked to custodial role performance (Gilbert and Levinson, 1957b). (People who said they were custodial were custodial.) It is reassuring as well as banal to know that, generally, somatotherapeutic psychiatrists actually give drugs, psychotherapeutic psychiatrists actually espouse psychotherapy and so on. Similarly with ward or hospital clinical policies. But the importance of this is to draw attention to problems which may arise because people do not actually do what they think they do, their ideology having become divorced from practice. The determinants of this interesting state of affairs warrant discussion elsewhere.

(b) Other effects of staff ideology on patients have been reported. An admixture of ideologies among a ward or hospital's staff can evoke inter-staff conflict and tension (Strauss et al., 1964) and hence issue in disturbed patient behaviour (Stanton and Schwarz, 1954). Also, ideologies of nurses and other staff affect interactions and relationships with patients. For instance, 'custodial' staff tend to interact with patients less and value interaction less than 'humanistic' staff (Altschul, 1972). Evidence that patients suffer or benefit from more or less interaction with staff is, however, sparse, as Altschul points out.

(c) This leads to the question of the relationship between staff ideology and treatment outcome. This most interesting and important matter is complex and it is not possible to deal with it fully here. It is worth reiterating the obvious but still often forgotten clinical truism that statements about treatment outcome are meaningless (or at worst pernicious) unless outcome criteria are clearly defined and clinically relevant. Different ideologies may affect different outcome criteria differently. Outcome criteria may be administrative (length of hospital stay, for example), social (for example a measure of occupational adaptation), clinical (for example severity of depression), or 'personal' (relative's satisfaction with services). There was a time when administrative outcome paralleled clinical outcome, hospital discharge indicating recovery. Now, however, leaving hospital has as little to do with recovery from illness as entering hospital has to do with onset of illness, and statements about outcome which refer only to such criteria are of 'little value', if not misleading.

(Unhappily, official sources continue to claim that discharge from psychiatric hospital is good *per se*.)

It is also worth reiterating the obvious clinical fact that treatment outcome varies between psychiatric disorders. Ideologies may be expected to have different effects on people with different illnesses. For instance, an ECT-responsive psychotic depression is likely to respond to ECT given on a sociotherapeutic, psychotherapeutic or somatotherapeutic ward, for the effects of ECT override those of any other influence. Again, the outcome of a single episode of mania is likely to be subsidence of the episode within a relatively short time whatever the treatment—this course being a function of the natural history of the illness. Schizophrenics in contrast may respond specifically to any aspects of ideology which issue in actions impinging upon illness-related susceptibilities. Thus an ideology which encouraged affect-laden contact with relatives might induce symptomatic worsening, or an ideology which allowed 'institutionalism' might permit symptomatic deterioration thereby (Wing and Brown, 1970).

The possible effects of ideology upon outcome are of particular interest with patients with neurotic and personality disorders. This is because these patients are particularly responsive to environmental characteristics affected by ideology such as quantity and quality of staff–patient interaction, and also because the very definition of disorder is a function of staff and patient ideology. Staff ideology may be such as to preclude acceptance of the patient for treatment; and failure of the patient, once accepted for treatment, to accept the ideology made manifest to him, may indicate a poor outcome (Rapoport, 1960). It would seem that a staff ideology which allows a person to be exposed to 'treatment' may *thereby* tend to help persons of the kind in question.

Morale

It is difficult to separate the possible effects of ideology from those of enthusiasm. Staff morale tends to be improved by any innovation approved by the organisation's policy makers, such as nurses ceasing to wear uniform (Walker *et al.*, 1971) or introducing unrestricted visiting (Barton *et al.*, 1961). Levels of staff morale have demonstrable effects upon the hospital career of non-psychiatric patients (Revans, 1962, 1964). Enthusiasm has been implicated in many psychiatric activities, including the effects of psychotropic drugs (Rickels, 1968), industrial and occupational rehabilitation programmes (Morgan *et al.*, 1965; Miles, 1971), group treatment (Astrachan *et al.*, 1968) and individual psychotherapy (Goldstein, 1962). The wide range of these effects suggests the possibility that the therapeutic potential of an ideology depends less on its content than on its association with charismatic leadership (Clark, 1964, p. 124), for charismatic leaders tend to enthuse those around them and thereby to raise morale. The possible value of this kind of leadership as a function of its capacity for innovation, is reminiscent of the industrial phenomenon of increased productivity following organisational change of more or less any kind (Hawthorne effect). It seems possible that it is precisely the more charismatic varieties of leadership which the administrative arrangements of the British National Health Service are designed to stifle.

Every psychiatric staff person has a psychiatric ideology. Psychiatric ideologies differ, are of three main kinds and have demonstrable effects on ward life and staff behaviour. They may also affect patient progress. However, little specific information is available about the kinds of patient affected in different ways by particular ideologies.

References

Allport, G. W. (1968). The historical background of modern social psychology. In *The Handbook of Social Psychology*, Vol. 1, 2nd ed. (Ed. G. Lindsey and E. Aronson) Addison-Wesley, Reading, Mass.

Altschul, A. T. (1972). *Patient-Nurse Interaction: A Study of Interaction Patterns in Acute Psychiatric Wards*. Churchill Livingstone, Edinburgh and London

Astrachan, B. M., Harrow, M. and Flynn, H. R. (1968). Influence of the value-system of a psychiatric setting on behaviour in group therapy meetings. *Soc. Psychiat.*, 3, 165–172

Barton, R., Elkes, A. and Glen, F. (1961). Unrestricted visiting in a mental hospital. *Lancet*, i, 1220–1222

Caine, T. M. and Smail, D. J. (1969). *The Treatment of Mental Illness*. London University Press, London

Carstairs, G. M. and Heron, A. (1957). The social environment of mental hospital patients: a measure of staff attitudes. In *The Patient and the Mental Hospital* (Ed. M. Greenblatt, *et al.*) Free Press, New York

Clark, D. H. (1964). *Administrative Therapy*. Tavistock, London

Freudenberg, R. K. (1966). The function and attitudes of professional staff in psychiatric hospitals. *Proc. R. Soc. Med.* 59, 591–594

Gilbert, D. C. and Levinson, D. J. (1957a). 'Custodialism' and 'humanism' in mental hospital structure and in staff ideology. In *The Patient and the Mental Hospital* (Ed. M. Greenblatt, *et al.*) Free Press, New York

Gilbert, D. C. and Levinson, D. J. (1957b). Role performance, ideology and personality in mental hospital aides. In *The Patient and the Mental Hospital* (Ed. M. Greenblatt, *et al.*) Free Press, New York

Goldstein, A. P. (1962). *Therapist-Patient Expectancies in Psychotherapy*. Pergamon Press, Oxford

Kelly, G. A. (1955). *The Psychology of Personal Constructs*. Norton, New York

Miles, A. (1971). Long-stay schizophrenic patients in hospital workshops. *Br. J. Psychiat.*, 119, 611–620

Morgan, R., Cushing, D. and Manton, N. S. (1965). A regional psychiatric rehabilitation hospital. *Br. J. Psychiat.*, 111, 955–963

Rabkin, J. G. (1972). Opinions about mental illness: a review of the literature. *Psychol. Bull.*, 77, 153–171

Rapoport, R. N. (1960). *Community as Doctor*. Tavistock, London

Revans, R. W. (1962). Hospital attitudes and communication. In *Sociological Review Monographs* No. 5 (Ed. P. Halmos) University Press, Keele

Revans, R. W. (1964). *Standards for Morale. Cause and Effect in Hospitals*. Nuffield Provincial Hospitals Trust and Oxford University Press, London

Rickels, K. (1968). *Non-specific Factors in Drug Therapy*. Thomas, Springfield, Ill.

Scott, W. A. (1968). Attitude measurement. In *Handbook of Social Psychology*, Vol. 2, 2nd ed., (Ed. G. Londzey and E. Aronson) Addison-Wesley, Reading, Mass. Chapter 11, p. 204–274

Stanton, A. H. and Schwartz, M. S. (1954). *The Mental Hospital. A Study of Institutional Participation in Psychiatric Illness and Treatment.* Tavistock, London

Strauss, A., Shatzman, L., Buckner, R., Ehrlich, D. and Sabshin, M. (1964). *Psychiatric Ideologies and Institutions.* Free Press, New York

Walker, V. J., Vorneskos, G. and Dunleavy, D. L. F. (1971). The effects of psychiatric nurses ceasing to wear uniform. *Br. J. Psychiat.*, **118**, 581–2

Wing, J. K. and Brown, G. W. (1970). *Institutionalism and Schizophrenia.* Cambridge University Press

7 Ethics in Psychiatry

A. Clare

My justification for having the temerity to discuss matters of ethics in the absence of any formal training in moral or philosophical enquiry derives from two sources. There is Hippocrates who insists that 'every physician should be a philosopher' in the sense that every doctor should not shirk from the ever-present necessity to assess and reappraise the values and attitudes on which his practice of medicine is founded. There is also the more contemporary view, expounded by, among others, Paul Ramsey, to the effect that in order to become an ethicist the physician has only to quit resisting being one. Neither of these positions should be taken as suggesting that ethical questions are easily defined and mastered. But both lend substance to the conviction that ethics are concerned with the actual moral judgements of practical men and with the formulation of relevant general principles, values and criteria to support the value judgements and moral decisions made daily in the clinical practice of medicine.

I draw considerable comfort too from the observations recently made on the subject of medical ethics by a philosopher engaged in a research project involving nurses, doctors and medical students. To start in medical ethics with the actual moral judgements of doctors, nurses and other health care professionals, Thompson (1976) argues, 'has the advantage of empirical veracity and immediate relevance'. It also ensures that no alien methodology or preconceived schemata will be imposed from outside.

Ethics in psychiatry are but a specialised variation of medical ethics which in turn reflect the application of ethical judgements in the wider human community. The moral requirements governing the relationship between psychiatrists and their patients are only a particular example of the moral requirements or covenants among men. The nature of the contemporary issues and crises which confront physicians demands critical scrutiny by the professionals involved but such issues and crises cannot be resolved, or at least not satisfactorily, without the involvement of informed lay opinion. Thus, for example, the ethical problems posed within psychiatry by such issues as consent to treatment and compulsory certification cannot be resolved solely by psychiatrists. Indeed, the medical profession must shun being tempted to draw the complacent conclusion that the personal integrity of physicians alone is enough.

In the interests of clarity, it seems best to outline a number of areas within psychiatry wherein ethical issues tend to converge. The basic level is where individual professionals sense there is a conflict between their personal and private moral convictions and what appears to be demanded of them in their public and professional roles. The most publicised example of conflict between individual conscience and legal policy in the wider field of medicine is, of course, the issue of abortion but the intense interest focused on that controversial subject has tended to obscure the fact that issues of personal conscience do occur in other areas too. They may be less dramatic—the dilemmas experienced by some social workers attempting to implement aspects of the 1959 Mental Health Act are but an example of such an issue within psychiatry—but they are no less complex.

The next level of problems relates to dilemmas which arise when different professionals encounter one another in areas which require inter-professional co-operation but where there is often no firm foundation of shared attitudes, values or goals. Issues such as clinical responsibility and confidentiality assume gargantuan proportions and individuals, who at other times can be counted upon to manifest a lethargic disinterest in such questions of principle become possessed by a spirit of moral righteousness which would not be out of place in a revivalist preacher.

Finally, there is that level of problems seen where there is a conflict between the ethic of psychiatric practice and conventional social morality or declared political and public policy. The abuse of psychiatry in relation to dissidents in the Soviet Union is a case in point but again the ethical principles involved can be found in less publicised situations closer to home. The latter examples, it is true, do appear to be more isolated and less systematised than the Russian abuses but moral issues are moral issues whether they relate to the Gulag Archipelago or the Home Counties.

Each of these levels of problems demands an approach which is informed by the relevant psychiatric expertise, is based upon practical considerations, is sensitive to differences of ideology and training between professional groups within the specialty and is open to the need to provide effective yet realistic representation of conflicting groups, interests and opinions in the formulation of crucial ethical decisions. Clearly it is not going to be possible within the confines of this paper to discuss all the many and varied ethical issues arising at these different levels in the course of psychiatric practice. What can be attempted, none the less, is a consideration of the more pressing areas of professional concern.

Consent

One vital element in any answer to the fundamental question concerning the nature of right action in psychiatric practice is the requirement of reasonably free and adequately informed consent. In Ramsey's view (Ramsey, 1970), it is the chief covenant or canon of loyalty between the person who is patient/subject and the person who is doctor/investigator. While it is true that there is a considerable degree of lip-service paid to the idea of 'informed consent', how it operates in actual clinical practice remains elusive. The attempts to qualify the word 'consent' with terms implying that the subject has to have a full and proper understanding of the nature, procedure and risks of a proposed treatment first appeared in profusion in 1946 with the appearance of the Nuremberg Code on medical experimentation. One of the eminently sensible principles enshrined in that code declares that a subject in a medical experiment 'should have sufficient knowledge and comprehension of the elements of the subject matter involved as to enable him to make an understanding and enlightened decision'. It has been argued (Garnham, 1975), with some justification in my opinion, that only medically qualified people can judge with any degree of competence the therapeutic efficacy and necessity of a given therapeutic procedure. Yet there are those who appear to believe that consent can only be truly informed if the individual concerned is made aware of all the details, possible hazards and actual difficulties attendant on any proposed clinical intervention. I have commented elsewhere (Clare, 1976) on how a truthful and exhaustive account of what is actually involved in the average appendicectomy is hardly conducive to persuading patients suffering from acute appendicitis to undergo surgery. Not surprisingly, given the nature of many medical interventions, such information as is provided by doctors to patients about proposed treatment is emotionally biased. The doctor has a massive personal investment in his proposed treatment. That is part of the nature of being a doctor. Indeed, this aspect of being a doctor is one of the reasons for the misunderstanding, in my view, which many non-medical critics manifest concerning the clinical situation.

If we consider for a moment the issue of non-compliance then this point becomes clearer. A typical ethical analysis of non-compliance revolves around the issue of a patient's right to refuse treatment, the question of self-determination and the idea of mutual contractual obligations between doctors and patients. However, doctors can see other issues and indeed these same issues but from a different perspective. In Churchill's words (Churchill, 1977), 'non-compliance is viewed not only as a threat to a patient's life or health but as an abridgement of the physician's authority and as a threat to his identity as a healer'. The doctor who declares that as long as such-and-such an individual is his patient he is going to do what he is told may be seen as coercive or abusive—by others. By the doctor, it may merely be seen as a legitimate professional response brought about by the doctor's anxiety to push ahead with the care of his patient. In the majority of cases, the patient can of course absolutely refuse to consider any further treatment and that is that. But the point which merits emphasis is that throughout all this the doctor and the patient are not participating in a moral dispute as between one autonomous individual and another but as doctor and patient with all the particular assumptions and qualifications that this relationship embodies in our culture. Churchill's striking conclusion to this particular analysis is worth quoting: 'Because the conventional ethical analysis of such a situation does not probe into the value components of professional training and practice, clinicians rarely get an adequate hearing for their mode of decision making'.

If this is true of those situations in which the patient is assumed to be able to make a responsible and voluntary choice, then it is doubly so when it comes to the question, crucial to psychiatric practice, of compulsory treatment. At the present time, the atmosphere is charged with a feeling that medical power with regard to compulsory detention and treatment is largely unfettered and often abused. The discussion is polarised by the views of Thomas Szasz on the question, views which, while largely ignored within the psychiatric profession, are strikingly influential in certain areas of social work training. For Szasz, arguments on how best to implement legislation on compulsory treatment are irrelevant. The problem is not how to improve commitment but how to abolish it:

> ... In the final analysis, what makes a medical intervention morally permissible is not that it is therapeutic but that it is something the patient wants. Similarly what makes a quasi-medical intervention of involuntary psychiatric hospitalisation morally impermissible is not that it is harmful but that it is something the so-called patient does not want.
>
> (Szasz, 1974).

Quite the opposite view has been expressed by Birley (1973) in his unequivocal contention that compulsory psychiatric care is not a threat but in fact a right. 'Every citizen should have the right to be admitted against his will to the care of a first-class psychiatric service.' In practice, the ethical issue revolves itself around the issues of personal responsibility and harm. That an individual's judgement can be impaired, that the balance of his mind can be affected by disturbances within various mental part-functions, is recognised not merely by psychiatrists but it is built into the criminal and civil law of every civilised community. In practice, it is the difficulty of predicting harm or dangerousness which poses much greater difficulties and raises a number of ethical issues. That is to say, the more frequent situation is one in which the individual is indeed unarguably mentally ill and insistently refusing treatment. The doctor is faced with deciding whether treatment is to be enforced on the grounds that the individual's safety is threatened or that he represents a danger to the safety of others. Such a decision is both a professional one (deciding the likely risk) and an ethical one (deciding whose rights are to be jeopardised, the individual's or the community's). While psychiatrists are clearly unhappy that they have been cast in the role of arbiters of such situations, it is difficult to see how such a role could have been avoided. Nor, at present, can they rely on much assistance, either of a practical or a moral nature, from outside their professional ranks. Recent publications and statements by MIND (the National Association for Mental Health), among others, reflect the low opinion held of the ability of psychiatrists to make accurate predictions concerning dangerousness and, in the circumstances, the preoccupation with curtailing and confining the powers to commit, currently held by psychiatrists, to a minimum is understandable.

Interestingly enough, there has been no evidence that psychiatrists are anxious, in public at any rate, to extend the harm principle to include not merely the risk of physical violence and death but economic hardship, social deprivation and public nuisance considerations. It is worth noting in this regard that a recent paper on non-compliance, discussing a patient who had refused an operation for cancer, wondered whether compulsory intervention could be justified 'in terms of a public harm principle by appealing to the costs to health and welfare institutions resulting from the patient's failure to accept treatment'. Such an extension strikes this observer as fraught with danger but my clinical experience of working in a busy emergency clinic attached to a major psychiatric clinic in London supports the impression that doctors do have a wider concept of harm than merely physical harm. The MIND Report (Gostin, 1975) argues that 'only grave and genuinely probable future harm to others should form the basis of compulsory admission and this prediction should be based upon recent overt acts'. That it means by harm, physical harm, is illustrated by an annotation provided on the same page which, drawing on the experience of the Graham Young case, supports compulsory treatment in the case of individuals who have behaved violently in the past. 'But it is not acceptable', the statement continues, 'that a person who is mentally disordered and has not behaved violently should be detained because two doctors have said that he may act violently at some time in the future'.

A short case-history may illustrate how practice challenges theory. One of the first cases in which I was involved which raised the question of certification involved a middle-aged businessman who, while on a trip abroad, became quite suddenly hypomanic. He became preoccupied by an extraordinary scheme to turn a disused airfield into a rock concert arena and proceeded to run up enormous bills telephoning a dazzling assortment of world figures for their support in his venture. Eventually he was ejected from his hotel (not for running up telephone bills but for interrupting a dance by his insistence on playing the drums) and somehow persuaded to return home by a distraught colleague. His family were immensely distressed by the financial impact of his illness—his job in jeopardy, bills coming in for all manner of crazy purchases, his public name at risk—but he himself insisted that he was well and interpreted attempts to admit him to hospital as cunning ploys by his business rivals to prevent him reaping the benefit of his brilliant scheme.

Now, in this case-history, the question of violence never arose as indeed it rarely if ever arises in so many cases which provoke doctors to consider compulsory intervention. What is striking is the 'harm' in a more general but in a no less dramatic sense which it involved. The fact that there is effective treatment for mania is irrelevant to the ethical issue of curtailing a patient's rights. Or is it?

For this brings us to another aspect of the question of compulsion which has ethical implications. Birley speaks of a person's right to compulsory treatment in 'a first-class psychiatric service'. That there are such services goes without saying but that there are others which might not merit such a Michelin-style grading is likewise difficult to deny in this era of the public enquiry. Much of the reluctance to include psychopathy within the mental illness rubric is derived from the fact that at present we lack any truly effective medical treatment for those so classified. Theoretically, it should not greatly affect the issue whether we had such a treatment or not but in practice it does.

Much of the reluctance to leave current legislation on compulsory admission and treatment alone also stems from a belief that much that passes for psychiatric treatment is in actual fact scarcely distinguishable from incarceration and, on some occasions, from punishment. Indeed, much of the vigour in the movement to diminish psychiatric powers in this area does stem from a disenchantment with many psychiatric therapies, such as ECT and drugs. It is fair to wonder whether quite so much time and effort would be devoted to ensuring that as many people as possible are kept out of our psychiatric facilities if these facilities enjoyed a higher level of confidence among the members of the general public than they currently do.

I have concentrated more on the issue of harm than on the issue of the existence or otherwise of mental illness in the individual for whom compulsory detention is being considered because in practice the issue of harm is usually the critical one. However, the dispute over Russian practice has served to focus attention on ways in which psychiatrists can be ethically compromised as a consequence of pressure exerted by their political masters. This issue is raised again when the related problem of psychiatrists working within the prison system is briefly discussed.

ECT

The question of consent arises once again when we come to consider some particularly controversial treatments within contemporary psychiatry. The Royal College of Psychiatrists has just published a memorandum on the use of ECT (Royal College of Psychiatrists, 1977a) which, in addition to reviewing the evidence in favour of its efficacy, the associated morbidity and mortality and the various methods of its administration, considers the question of consent. However, the memorandum is not especially expansive on the subject. It advises psychiatrists that consent for ECT should be written using the standard forms suggested by the Department of Health and Social Security and the Medical Defence societies. It continues:

> Consent is a matter between the patient and doctor and it is a medical responsibility to ensure that the patient has been given an explanation of the procedure, benefits and dangers of ECT.
>
> (Royal College of Psychiatrists, 1977).

Given what we have already discussed concerning the difficulties of establishing what constitutes 'informed' consent, the memorandum seems wise to refrain from being more explicit in its advice. It emphasises that if ECT has to be given to compulsorily detained patients, this can only be done under Section 26. (Current legal advice is that Section 25 does not entitle psychiatrists to use such a treatment.) The memorandum also recommends that the nearest relative should always be consulted and again the procedure should be explained and approval in writing obtained. Consultation should take place with staff who are to assist or give the patient ECT. In practice, it suggests, patients unable to understand the nature and purpose of the treatment proposed and therefore 'unable to give consent' should be treated as 'unwilling' and the procedure adopted in the case of compulsorily detained patients applied. 'Compulsory treatment under the Mental Health Act', it emphasises, 'can only be applied to treatments directed to the alleviation of psychiatric conditions, and cannot be used for the compulsory treatment of physical conditions'.

It is interesting to note that the memorandum steers clear of any suggestion of an independent adviser or tribunal with powers to oversee the administration and prescription of ECT. This is one example of how the situation with regard to ECT differs from that pertaining to psychosurgery. With regard to the latter, most authorities support the idea of an independent medical 'referee' or panel whose assessment of the indications for intervention and agreement to it has to be registered before treatment can proceed. For ECT, however, as is clear from the memorandum, no such special provision is judged necessary. It is a treatment like any other treatment involving an anaesthetic. It falls within the doctor's competence to decide how and when it should be used and the normal professional restrictions governing his performance apply. I have no reason to doubt that this is the view of ECT held by the vast majority of British psychiatrists at the present time.

Psychosurgery

As befits a controversial subject, there is some disagreement concerning its exact definition. The World Health Organization (1976) has suggested 'the selective surgical removal or destruction . . . of nerve pathways . . . with a view to influencing behaviour'. Bridges and Bartlett (1977) are not happy with such a definition since to them most modern psychosurgery 'is concerned with the treatment of severe and intractable affective illnesses without any intended effect on behaviour at all' and they suggest that psychosurgery should instead be defined as 'the surgical treatment of certain psychiatric illnesses by means of localised lesions placed in specific cerebral sites'. However, as they concede, attempts have been made to correct 'abnormal sexuality' by placing lesions in the hypothalamus (Reeder et al., 1972), 'abnormal aggressiveness' by means of amygdalotomy (Narabayashi et al., 1963; Hitchcock and Cairns, 1973; Kiloh et al., 1974) and sociopathy by attacking multiple limbic targets (Hunter Brown and Nighthill, 1968). Given this state of affairs, it is difficult to agree that the W.H.O. definition is seriously misleading. It is worth noting that two recent reviews of the subject, namely the New South Wales Committee of Inquiry into Psychosurgery (1977) and the Report on Psychosurgery prepared by the U.S. National Commission for the Protection of Human Subjects of Biomedical and Behavioural Research (1977), both employ definitions which allow for alterations in both emotions *and* behaviour as the intended end-result of surgical intervention.

There is at least one State in the United States in which psychosurgery has been banned. Such has been the situation in the Soviet Union for many years. Psychosurgery has been the subject of two lengthy and hostile entries into the Congressional Record. In this country, attempts to mount a controlled study of psychosurgical procedures have met with considerable opposition from amongst a number of politicians and lay critics of psychiatry.

Such opposition, much of it shrill and a great deal of it misinformed, has not been without its positive aspects. One of these is that it has served to provoke a number of careful evaluations of the evidence now available concerning the efficacy of the many technical procedures subsumed under the general term, psychosurgery.

Perhaps the most extensive of these has been the American report already referred to. The report is based on evidence accumulated over the decade 1965-75 and from a number of studies performed under contract to the National Commission involved. Its recommendations, though lengthy and detailed in the original report, merit summarising:

Psychosurgery should only be performed at an institution with an approved review board (IRB) by a competent surgeon on a properly assessed, informed and consenting patient.

It should not be used for any purpose other than to provide treatment to individual patients.

A National Psychosurgical Advisory Board should provide guidelines concerning the demonstrable efficacy of specific psychosurgical procedures. Psychosurgery should not be performed on (1) a prisoner, (2) a patient who is involuntarily committed to a mental hospital, (3) a person with a legal guardian or (4) a patient believed by the IRB to be incapable of giving informed consent to such a procedure *unless* (among other qualifications) the patient has given informed consent or, where there is doubt that he is in a position to do so, his guardian or a court in which the patient had legal representation has approved the operation.

The New South Wales Report, like the American one, was precipitated by massive adverse publicity. (It is interesting to note that the U.S. study estimated that approximately 400 psychosurgical operations are performed annually in the United States compared with approximately 200–250 in the United Kingdom and approximately 80 in Australia.) This report recommends that psychosurgical treatment should only be given to patients who are able to give informed consent. All intended cases should be assessed by a Psychosurgery Review Board composed of seven members including a lawyer, a psychologist, two psychiatrists, a neurosurgeon and a representative of the public. No member of the board shall be directly engaged in practising psychosurgery. Where there is doubt about the quality of a patient's consent, the case shall be referred to a Justice of the Supreme Court for a ruling on the matter.

The N.S.W. Report has already provoked a critical response from Kiloh (1977) who argues that in the case of those patients capable of giving informed consent the decision concerning whether or not to operate should be left to the group of clinicians concerned with psychosurgery employed by the approved institution. Kiloh is particularly incensed by the N.S.W. Committee's insistence that 'the decision to perform any psychosurgical operation . . . cannot be left to the medical advisor or advisors proposing the performance of the operation'. Given that earlier in its report, the Committee expresses the view that psychosurgery is 'a safe, effective, simple and worthwhile procedure', Kiloh regards the demand for a Board to decide whether to operate or not as 'a near-libellous slur upon the medical profession with its implications of irresponsibility, coercion of patients, inadequate selection of cases and the use of ineffective and dangerous operative procedures.'

It is interesting to note that the U.S. Report argued that individuals should not be denied access to potentially beneficial therapy simply because they are involuntarily confined or unable to give informed consent. In such instances, where surgery appears indicated, it recommended access to a court review in addition to the assessment by the various boards. It totally opposed, however, using involuntarily committed individuals as subjects in psychosurgical experiments.

Ethical Aspects of Forensic Psychiatry

Ethical considerations of the appropriateness of psychosurgical procedures applied to prisoners mainly revolve around the difficulty of teasing out informed consent from consent acquired through coercion. This in turn reflects the more basic problem faced by the forensic psychiatrist, namely the question of accountability. Bowden (1976) has argued that a doctor cannot serve two masters and that the dual allegiance of the prison medical officer to the state and to those individuals under his care results in activities which largely favour the former. Whereas the World Health Organization prescribes a system of health ethics which qualitatively indicates the responsibility of each state for health provisions, the World Medical Association acts as both promulgator and guardian of a code of medical ethics which determines the responsibilities of the doctor to his patient. A number of other codes, including the 'Standard Minimum Rules for the Treatment of Prisoners' adopted by the first U.N. Congress on the Prevention of Crime and the

Treatment of Offenders in 1958, have attempted to clarify this issue without obvious success. The role of the doctor in caring for prisoners under his care and his role in certifying the fitness of a prisoner to undergo some form of punishment or discipline are often described in the same list of regulations and ethical prescriptions although it is not always easy to see how they can be reconciled successfully. A practical example of the tension involved was shown in the investigation of interrogation procedures used in Ulster. Two of the three members of the Parker Committee, set up to examine the whole question of interrogation, concluded that the methods employed could continue to be used if they were subject to more stringent controls, one of which was that a doctor trained in psychiatry should be present to see that the prisoner was not being pressed too far. Fortunately, the third member, Lord Gardiner, produced a minority report of such uncompromising hostility to the whole idea that the methods of interrogation were subsequently forbidden (Gardiner, 1972).

There does appear to be a conflict between medical ethics and health ethics in the forensic situation which cannot be resolved by the appointment of an individual as guardian to both. Bowden (1976) suggests the provision of a separate and independent health service to prisoners 'which should be intimately linked with extrapenal facilities'. However, as he himself points out, others (e.g. Prewer 1974) see no real conflict and argue that 'treatment and control are merely two sides of the same coin'. Yet Bowden's view is neither a lonely nor an original one. The first congress of the British Commission on Human Rights (London, November 1972) considered conditions for convicted prisoners, for those awaiting trial or sentence, and for those held under emergency regulations. One recommendation was that all procedures under emergency regulations should be monitored by regular and frequent inspection, especially medical inspection and that the internee should have the right to choose his doctor.

Confidentiality

One of the few sections of the Hippocratic Oath which has remained intact over almost 3000 years is that relating to confidentiality:

> And whatsoever I shall see or hear in the course of my profession, as well as outside my profession in my intercourse with men, if it be what should not be published abroad, I will never divulge, holding such things to be holy secrets.

This undertaking is repeated in the Declaration of Geneva:

> I will respect the secrets which are confided in me even after the patient has died.

Now, with the development of such technological advances in the recording, storage and reproduction of material, advances such as photocopying, computer storage, videotaping and microfilm, the situation has become extremely complicated. With the increase in documentation goes an increase in the amount of sensitive, personal information recorded. Professionals, including medical practitioners, do not hoard information quite as assiduously as they did.

A major problem concerns the availability of hospital case notes. While in some hospitals, these are handled only by doctors and their secretaries, in others they are readily available to all members of the therapeutic team, including social workers, nurses, clinical psychologists, occupational therapists and students of all these disciplines. In some hospitals, patients are encouraged to read their own case notes which may include confidential letters from external agencies. A report on confidentiality to the Council of the Royal College of Psychiatrists (1977b) noted that 'Quite apart from what is supposed to happen, in some hospitals security is so lax that patients and casual visitors can easily pick up and read 'confidential' case notes'.

The fact that it is no longer practicable to look upon the single physician as the patient's sole therapeutic agent in any serious illness implies the widening of the notion of confidentiality to some degree. The concept of 'extended confidentiality' has developed and is assumed to cover the exchange of confidential information about patients between the immediate members of the clinical team. However, given the numbers involved in the treatment of the individual psychiatric patient, the easy accessibility of the case records and the haphazard nature of much record storage, it is hardly surprising that in some countries, particularly the United States, there has been something of a counter-reaction to the practice of widely disseminating sensitive information. In some States of America, doctors are accorded the same privilege as priests—of being allowed to refuse disclosure in Court of information they have received in confidence. There is no such privilege for anyone except a lawyer in Britain.

The Royal College of Psychiatrists' Ethical Working Party has made a number of recommendations to the Council of the College on the subject of confidentiality. The following represent the more important:

(1) The College should continue to press for privilege in Court to be extended in the public interest beyond lawyers to other groups who require confidentiality to carry out their tasks, especially registered medical practitioners.

(2) The College should press the Department of Health and Social Security to make a public statement about the legal position with regard to access to hospital case notes so that the public may know where they stand.

(3) The College should press for an immediate interdisciplinary Working Party to inquire into the problems of security, access to and confidentiality of psychiatric case records.

(4) Every hospital should have a Psychiatric Records Committee which should include doctors, nurses and a Records Officer and which should have as its major responsibility the security and confidentiality of the medical records of the hospital.

(5) The rules of each hospital and its constituent units with regard to the question of access to notes must be clarified and kept up to date. If all members of the staff and many patients have access to case notes, then less information should be recorded in them.

(6) The Psychiatric Records Committee should clarify and codify the practice of the hospital with regard to sending letters of information, summaries or case notes to other institutions and persons. The decision should be a medical one and should not be left to the discretion of the unsupported Records Officer. Information gathered for one purpose (e.g. treatment) should not be used for another purpose (e.g. litigation) without the consent of the person who gave the information. The hospital policy should take account of photocopying: if something should not be photocopied, it should not be sent out of the hospital.

This Working Party was sufficiently worried about the situation to suggest guidance on the subject for the College's members. In particular it noted that since the case records are the property of the D.H.S.S. and can be available to many other N.H.S. staff, doctors should be very careful what they include in them. 'If intimate, shameful or legally damaging facts about a person are elicited', the Working Party declares, 'very careful consideration should be given to what is recorded in the records'. It suggests that if such details have to be recorded, it might be better to place them in a separate filing system with a much higher degree of security. 'Psychiatrists', it is pointed out, 'would do well to remember that they may be questioned in Court about anything they have written in the hospital records. The only justification for writing is that the record was true and that it was necessary for the effective medical treatment of the patient and in his best interest.'

Clinical Responsibility

A problem circumscribed with as many ethical problems as confidentiality is the problem of responsibility. Again, the development of the so-called multi-disciplinary team has altered the doctor–patient relationship and has affected the traditional position of authority exercised by doctors in the clinical setting. Within the N.H.S., however, the consultant psychiatrist is still the person who has the ultimate responsibility and the over-all authority to diagnose illness and prescribe treatment. In the uncompromisingly forthright opinion of the Royal College of Psychiatrists (1977c), 'this authority may be delegated but the responsibility cannot be abrogated'. The concept of the multi-disciplinary team, while attractive and currently influential, is lacking in clarity and it is unclear from the writings of those who greatly favour it as a method of delivering patient care and treatment whether decisions reached through its deliberations are thought to override the decisions of individual clinicians. However, the current ethical position does suggest that certain medical responsibilities, such as the legal and diagnostic ones, cannot be delegated to a team. Multi-disciplinary in this context, from the medical viewpoint, is a process of consultation, the final decision resting with the Consultant on matters where the Consultant has the final responsibility. 'Similar considerations may apply to other professions', observes the College report 'when the central responsibilities germane to these disciplines are involved.'

One such discipline, recently the subject of a Sub-committee of Enquiry set up by the D.H.S.S. under the Chairmanship of Professor William Trethowan, is clinical psychology. Developments in the theoretical and practical basis of the subject have led to psychologists playing a more forceful role in the diagnosis and management of many psychiatric conditions. Not surprisingly, there have been those who have argued that there are circumstances in which a psychologist might reasonably exercise clinical responsibility in relation to patients referred to him for treatment by a doctor. The British Psychological Society, in its submission to the Sub-committee, declared:

It is the responsibility of a referring medical practitioner . . . to assure himself that the clinical psychologist is qualified. Thereafter the psychologist is responsible for whatever acts he carries out in treatment . . .The clinical psychologist's responsibility covers all acts which are within his competence. As is the case with all independent professionals, it is part of his competence not to exceed the boundaries of his skill. Where a clinical psychologist and a medical practitioner are jointly engaged in the care of an individual, they should establish by agreement their specific areas of responsibility.

Many medical witnesses to the Sub-committee, however, strongly expressed the view that there were no circumstances under which a psychologist should take clinical responsibility for patients. The General Medical Council commented,

Within the N.H.S., the practice of psychology as a therapeutic procedure by persons other than registered medical practitioners is ultimately the responsibility of the referring general practitioner or consultant. In extreme cases, improper delegation of medical duties to unregistered persons may render a doctor liable to charges of serious professional misconduct.

The Trethowan Sub-committee, in its discussion of the concepts of legal and medical responsibility, raised a number of questions concerning the independant status of psychologists (and by implication of other professional groups engaged in the diagnosis and treatment of the mentally ill). While recognising that there is a continuing medical responsibility which cannot be handed over to any other profession, the report wondered whether there are not also spheres of competence special to other professional groups. The members of each group can be seen as responsible for their decisions within their sphere. The report continues:

> They are also individually responsible for recognising the limits of their own competence and enlisting the involvement of their colleagues when necessary. The decisions which involve the team as a whole are those concerning the patient's care as a whole which involve a choice between different forms of professional intervention.

This report distinguishes therefore between independent professional status and full clinical responsibility within the N.H.S., the latter to be exercised only by certain medical practitioners (consultants or general practitioners, depending on whether or not the patient is receiving hospital treatment). Such a view does appear to envisage a situation wherein all patients attending psychologists are first referred by doctors. Whether psychologists consider such an arrangement acceptable remains to be seen.

Much of the difficulty encountered in clinical practice involving many professional disciplines may well be derived from professional rivalry, jealousy, insecurity and ignorance. Much of it too may derive from insufficient consideration of the ethical bases and professional traditions and ethos underpinning the various groups involved. If multi-disciplinary teamwork is to become more than a fashionable trend and catchword, then it will do so through the various professional interests examining the issues involved with as the guiding mainstay the fundamental interest of the patient.

If medical responsibility appears to be under threat of curtailment as a consequence of multi-professional expansionism, it appears itself to be enlarging in another area altogether. Psychiatrists are playing an increasing role as advisors to the police in the management of sieges and of crimes involving the taking of hostages, in selection procedures in industry and in the military area. New ethical issues and old ones in new guises constantly appear and lend support to Thompson's (1976) appeal to professionals to involve themselves not merely in the construction of codes of conduct or rules of etiquette but in the more demanding task of clarifying the nature of the fundamental ethical principles which form the moral base of clinical action.

The World Psychiatric Association, mainly as a response to the growing concern over the political abuse of psychiatry in the Soviet Union, has recently laid down a series of broad ethical guidelines, the so-called 'Declaration of Hawaii' (Appendix A). Perhaps the best that can be hoped from such a broad exhortatory document is that it may help to stimulate a greater awareness of, and sensitivity to ethical issues in psychiatry and the constant danger of abuse and misuse of psychiatric power.

References

Birley, J. L. T. (1973). *Coercion and Care*. Lecture delivered to the London Medical Group

Bowden, P. (1976). Medical practice: defendants and prisoners. *J. med. Ethics*, **2**, 163–172

Bridges, P. K. and Bartlett, J. R. (1977). Review article: psychosurgery: yesterday and today. *Br. J. Psychiat.*, **131**, 249–250

Churchill, L. R. (1977). Tacit components of medical ethics: making decisions in the clinic. *J. med. Ethics*, **3**, 129–132

Clare, A.W. (1976). *Psychiatry in Dissent*. Tavistock, London

Gardiner, Lord (1972). Minority report, Parker Committee, Report of the Committee of Privy Counsellors Appointed to Consider Authorised Procedures for the Interrogation of Persons Suspected of Terrorism. *Cmnd.* 4901, H.M.S.O., London

Garnham, J. C. (1975). Some observations on informed consent in non-therapeutic research. *J. med. Ethics*, **1**, 138–145

Gostin, L. (1975). The Mental Health Act from 1959 to 1975. Observations, Analysis and Proposals for Reform. Vol. 1. A MIND Special Report. MIND (National Association for Mental Health), London

Hitchcock, E. and Cairns, V. (1973). Amygdalotomy. *Postgrad. med. J.*, **49**, 894–904

Hunter Brown, M. and Lighthill, J. A. (1968). Selective anterior cingulotomy: a psychosurgical evaluation. *J. Neurosurg.*, **29**, 513–519

Kiloh, L. G. (1977). Commentary on the Report of Inquiry into Psychosurgery. *Med. J. Aust.*, **2**, 296–301

Kiloh, L. G., Gye, R. S., Rushworth, R. G., Bell, D. S. and White, R. T. (1974). Stereotactic amygdalotomy for aggressive behaviour. *J. Neurol. Neurosurg. Psychiat.*, **37**, 437–44

Narabayashi, H., Nagao, T., Saito, Y., Yoshida, M. and Nagahata, M. (1963). Stereotaxic amygdalotomy for behaviour disorders. *Archs Neurol.*, **9**, 11–26

New South Wales Committee of Inquiry into Psychosurgery (1977). Reported in Kiloh, L. G. (1977) *Med. J. Aust.*, **2**, 296–301

Prewer, R. (1974). The contribution of prison medicine. In *Progress in Penal Reform* (Ed. L. Blom-Cooper), Clarendon Press, Oxford

Ramsey, P. (1970). *The Patient as Person*. Yale University Press, New Haven and London

Reeder, F., Orthner, H. and Muller, D. (1972). The stereotaxic treatment of pedophilic homosexuality and other sexual deviations. In *Psychosurgery* (Ed. E. R. Hitchcock, L. V. Laitinen and K. Varnet) Charles C. Thomas, Springfield, Illinois

Royal College of Psychiatrists' Memorandum on the Use of Electroconvulsive Therapy (1977a). *Br. J. Psychiat.*, **131**, 261–72

Royal College of Psychiatrists (1977b). Confidentiality: a Report to Council. *Br. J. Psychiat.* News and Notes Supplement, January 1977, 4–8

Royal College of Psychiatrists (1977c). The responsibilities of consultants in psychiatry within the National Health Service. *Br. J. Psychiat.*, News and Notes Supplement, September 1977, 4–7

Szasz, T. S. (1974). *The Second Sin*. Routledge and Kegan Paul, London

Thompson, I. E. (1976). Implications of medical ethics for ethics in general. *J. med. Ethics*, **2**, 74–82

The Trethowan Report (1977). The Role of Psychologists in the Health Services. Report of the Sub-Committee. H.M.S.O., London

U.S. National Commission for the Protection of Human Subjects of Biomedical and Behavioural Research (1977). *Report and Recommendations on Psychosurgery*. Dept. of Health, Education and Welfare. Publication No. (OS) 77–0001. Washington, D. C.

World Health Organization (1976). *Health Aspects of Human Rights*. W.H.O., Geneva

APPENDIX

WORLD PSYCHIATRIC ASSOCIATION
Proposed Declaration of Hawaii

Ever since the dawn of culture ethics has been an essential part of the healing art. Conflicting loyalties for physicians in contemporary society, the delicate nature of the therapist—patient relationship, and the possibility of abuses of psychiatric concepts, knowledge and technology in actions contrary to the laws of humanity, all make high ethical standards more necessary than ever for those practising the art and science of psychiatry.

As a practitioner of medicine and a member of society, the psychiatrist has to consider the ethical implications specific to psychiatry as well as the ethical demands on all physicians and the societal duties of every man and woman.

A keen conscience and personal judgement is essential for ethical behaviour. Nevertheless, to clarify the profession's ethical implications and to guide individual psychiatrists and help form their consciences, written rules are needed. Therefore, the General Assembly of the World Psychiatric Association has laid down the following ethical guidelines for psychiatrists all over the world.

(1) The aim of psychiatry is to promote health and personal autonomy and growth. To the best of his or her ability, consistent with accepted scientific and ethical principles, the psychiatrist shall serve the best interests of the patient and be also concerned for the common good and a just allocation of health resources.

To fulfil these aims requires continuous research and continual education of health care personnel, patients and the public.

(2) Every patient must be offered the best therapy available and be treated with the solicitude and respect due to the dignity of all human beings and to their autonomy over their own lives and health.

The psychiatrist is responsible for treatment given by the staff members and owes them qualifed supervision and education. Whenever there is a need, or whenever a reasonable request is forthcoming from the patient, the psychiatrist should seek the help or the opinion of a more experienced colleague.

(3) A therapeutic relationship between patient and psychiatrist is founded on mutual agreement. It requires trust, confidentiality, openness, co-operation and mutual responsibility. Such a relationship may not be possible to establish with some severely ill patients. In that case, as in the treatment of children contact should be established with a person close to the patient and acceptable for him or her.

If and when a relationship is established for purposes other than therapeutic, such as in forensic psychiatry, its nature must be thoroughly explained to the person concerned.

(4) The psychiatrist should inform the patient of the nature of the

condition, of the proposed diagnostic and therapeutic procedures, including possible alternatives, and of the prognosis. This information must be offered in a considerate way and the patient be given the opportunity to choose between appropriate and available methods.

(5) No procedure must be performed or treatment given against or independent of a patient's own will, unless the patient lacks capacity to express his or her own wishes or, owing to psychiatric illness, cannot see what is in his or her best interest or, for the same reason, is a severe threat to others.

In these cases compulsory treatment may or should be given, provided that it is done in the patient's best interests and over a reasonable period of time, a retroactive informed consent can be presumed and, whenever possible, consent has been obtained from someone close to the patient.

(6) As soon as the above conditions for compulsory treatment no longer apply the patient must be released, unless he or she voluntarily consents to further treatment.

Whenever there is compulsory treatment or detention there must be an independent and neutral body of appeal for regular inquiry into these cases. Every patient must be informed of its existence and be permitted to appeal to it, personally or through a representative, without interference by the hospital staff or by anyone else.

(7) The psychiatrist must never use the possibilities of the profession for maltreatment of individuals or groups, and should be concerned never to let inappropriate personal desires, feelings or prejudices interfere with the treatment.

The psychiatrist must not participate in compulsory psychiatric treatment in the absence of psychiatric illness. If the patient or some third party demands actions contrary to scientific or ethical principles the psychiatrist must refuse to co-operate. When, for any reason, either the wishes or the best interest of the patient cannot be promoted he or she must be so informed.

(8) Whatever the psychiatrist has been told by the patient, or has noted during examination or treatment, must be kept confidential unless the patient releases the psychiatrist from professional secrecy, or else vital common values or the patient's best interest makes disclosure imperative. In these cases, however, the patient must be immediately informed of the breach of secrecy.

(9) To increase and propagate psychiatric knowledge and skill requires participation of the patients. Informed consent must, however, be obtained before presenting a patient to a class and, if possible, also when a case history is published, and all reasonable measures be taken to preserve the anonymity and to safeguard the personal reputation of the subject.

In clinical research, as in therapy, every subject must be offered the best available treatment. His or her participation must be voluntary, after full information has been given of the aims, procedures, risks and inconveniences of the project, and there must always be a reasonable relationship between calculated risks or inconveniences and the benefit of the study.

For children and other patients who cannot themselves give informed consent this should be obtained from someone close to them.

(10) Every patient or research subject is free to withdraw for any reason at any time from any voluntary treatment and from any teaching or research programme in which he or she participates. This withdrawal, as well as any refusal to enter a programme, must never influence the psychiatrist's efforts to help the patient or subject.

The psychiatrist should stop all therapeutic, teaching or research programmes that may evolve contrary to the principles of this Declaration.

8 Psychiatric 'Experiments'— Moral and Ethical Issues

Steven Hirsch

Recently, one of Britain's most well-known senior psychiatrists, Dr William Sargant (1975), challenged the value of clinical trials in medicine and psychiatry asserting that they were being carried out on . . .

> large groups of . . . mentally tortured patients, so as to convince not those at the bedside who can soon see for themselves whether this drug is working, but laboratory statisticians and armchair writers who have generally been the reactionary critics in the advancing treatment scene—especially in psychiatry.

Sargant demanded that such 'controlled' testing of drugs be brought to full public notice and claimed that clinical trials have 'taught us practically nothing'. Finally, he questioned the practice of comparing the effects of untested drugs with inert 'placebo' substances. His article raises ethical issues which are basic to clinical research, issues which concern the public, research workers and clinicians alike, and are increasingly in the forefront of people's minds when research is to be carried out.

Let me emphasise how emotive this issue can be by citing what is perhaps a special case in the extreme, but one which did occur and would in the end have to be accommodated or ruled out as being ethically acceptable.

A new treatment was introduced on the market which markedly reduced the frequency patients had to have medication administered. It rapidly gained in popularity, to an extent which would be unlikely without a large sales campaign. Associated with the treatment was a new approach to looking after patients involving community nurses and greater support and observation of the patients.There were claims, some documented, of a reduction in the relapse rate for the period following institution of the treatment compared to an equal time at risk before. The M.R.C. supported the decision to conduct a controlled clinical trial in which most of the hundred patients receiving the treatment at one centre were randomly allocated without their knowledge either to continue on the treatment or have it withdrawn by substituting a placebo. Of those who received the placebo, 66 per cent relapsed compared to only 3 per cent in the treated group and the relapsed patients were hospitalised on average 2–5 weeks, some longer.

Let us consider two questions, the first posed by Sargant (1976)—How would you feel if the psychiatrist you trusted most to treat your wife or daughter, without warning took her off the treatment she needed and let her relapse, having not had any explanation of what was happening?

Psychiatrists are trained to answer one question by asking another. Consider the next question:

How would you feel if the psychiatrist you trusted most to treat your wife or daughter, without warning or explanation of what he was doing, administered a drug that had been reported as being associated with an unduly high risk of depression and suicide and a high risk of neurological side-effects and possible brain damage; a drug which reduced facial and body movement and expression in a way which made your wife or daughter less attractive and socially acceptable?

Both questions have been asked concerning the trial about which Sargant wrote with such indignation. I would like to try to examine these issues:

Is it unethical to do clinical trials? or
Is it unethical not to do clinical trials?

Is it unethical not to tell the patient? or
Is it unethical to tell the patient?

Is the doctrine of 'informed consent' used to protect the patient or to protect the doctor?

Let us consider these issues in a systematic way.

Are Clinical Experiments on Patients ever Justifiable?

This question must be looked at in the general context of a doctor's work. Every time a doctor writes a prescription he is in effect conducting an experiment, because there is no known effective treatment in medicine that does not carry some risk. Even aspirin used indiscriminately can cause stomach haemorrhage, kidney damage or death. The problem for patients and physicians alike is to have available as much objective knowledge as possible about the benefits of any treatment and the risk of side-effects. Armed with firmly based facts, the doctor is then in a position to make a reasoned judgement, balancing the benefits against the risk and taking into account the special situation which each individual presents.

Can we regard the individual and collective impressions of physicians about the efficacy of any treatment as an adequate basis for making these judgements as Sargant suggests we should? If we define ethics as the rules and standards which govern practice within a body or association, it is generally true that it is both ethical and legal to apply treatments which are currently in use and considered acceptable practice. But equally it could be asked whether doctors should be allowed to rely on the gradual accumulation of general experience to determine the benefit and risks of any treatment. The controlled clinical trial offers a more rapid means of assessment, during which cautious observation is maximised and the risk of untoward effects remaining undetected is minimised. If we reserve the term 'ethics' to refer to accepted rules and practice—we could ask whether we have a higher moral obligation to carry out clinical trials in order to be able to most rapidly and precisely determine a drug's advantages and disadvantages; otherwise we would unnecessarily be putting our patients at risk. Today, the need for speedy and accurate evaluation is greater than ever because of the rapidity with which drugs are introduced to all fields of medicine.

While we might rely on clinical experience in some cases, such as the case of penicillin for pneumonia or ECT for severe depression, most treatments in psychiatry do not dramatically alter the expected course of the illness so rapidly and in such a high percentage of cases that their indisputable beneficial effect is immediately evident. To extend the example of penicillin, its value for acute pneumococcal pneumonia in the early days is not replicated by its value in acute-upon-chronic bronchitis, and the value of antibiotics as maintenance treatment for bronchitis to prevent relapse is even more difficult to judge.

The need for clinical trials is all the greater in psychiatry given the breadth and elasticity of our diagnostic categories and the wide variation of clinical outcome. The course of most disorders depends on a combination of genetic constitution, persistence of social stress, and the type of relief available. Current treatments are not wholly successful—some patients do not respond, and one to two-thirds have an eventual spontaneous remission if left untreated; the real benefit of treatment being to significantly shorten the period of suffering. Physicians may be convinced by their first-hand experience because of an apparent benefit which is subsequently shown to be due to the fact that they are treating the group most likely to respond spontaneously. This would explain why Sargant and other esteemed psychiatrists convinced of the effectiveness of insulin coma treatment for schizophrenia in the early 1940s and 1950s were later proved wrong when, against great opposition this treatment was subjected to a controlled trial which showed that it was no better than a simple anaesthetic followed by benzedrine. (The evidence that insulin treatment is ineffective is not watertight but the example serves the purpose of this argument. Patients recommended as showing a good response—good premorbid personality, sudden onset, etc.—were those most likely to remit spontaneously. The trial referred to showed that it was not a specific treatment for paranoid schizophrenics but its popularity waned for other reasons as well, such as the advent of safer but effective phenothiazines.) Since nearly 1 per cent of patients subjected to insulin coma treatment died, it would seem hard to argue that such 'experiments' are not in everyone's interest.

My argument has been that we have the highest moral obligation to carry out clinical trials rather than rely on accumulated clinical experience. Unfortunately, most trials of new treatment are based on open design in which the observer is aware of what treatment is being administered and there is no comparison group. This is useful in the early days of a new treatment when dosage schedules are being determined and toxicity studies are being carried out. However, in most circumstances open trials could be regarded as unethical—they expose patients to a relatively untested substance without being able to demonstrate whether or not the treatment is more worthwhile than known safe established substances or no treatment at all. For this you would need a 'controlled trial'.

What do We Mean by a 'Controlled Trial'? Is It a Form of Experiment?

Controlled trials are intended to eliminate unspecific influences. 'Experiment' is an emotive word if used to refer to research involving people. It conveys the idea of trying something out to see what will happen. If we were giving patients a completely untested treatment for the first time it would be an experiment, but the word is misleading if we are referring to a treatment which has already been in use and our concern is whether it really has the effect that is claimed. The controlled trial involves a comparison of the new treatment to an established treatment with known benefits or to some inactive substance. Most trials are carried out in order to establish whether the drug has the same, greater, or less effect than a known preparation.

The controlled trial is intended to eliminate the effect of unspecific influences by including controls. Controls are used to eliminate the influence of known objective influences by having them present to a nearly equal degree in all groups involved in the comparison. The effect of unknown objective influences is meant to be eliminated by randomisation of patients to different treatments involved in the comparison, thereby equally distributing unknown influences by chance. Subjective influences are meant to be eliminated by the double-blind technique so that neither the experimenter nor the patient can be affected by the knowledge that he is being treated by the experimental, inactive, or known established substance (I will return to this point below). If neither the experimenter nor the patient knows which preparation is which, and the patients are randomly allocated to either treatment, the effect of other factors such as age, weight, severity of symptoms, length of previous illness and psychological factors influencing recovery can be equalised between the two groups and the more effective treatment can be reliably identified. This unbiased comparison of the treatments provides the doctor with the facts necessary to make an informed decision regarding future medication. This is the best protection we, the public, can have against the zealous enthusiasm of those who advocate and publicise unproven treatments and expose us to the kind of dangerous results which arose from the unbridled use of insulin coma and leucotomy in the 1950s. Because the quality of the evidence is so much better from controlled trials, they greatly shorten the period during which patients are exposed to unproven treatments. In fact, this form of research design was so powerful a method of more precisely and quickly determining a treatment's comparative beneficial and detrimental effects that the discovery of the controlled double-blind technique was kept a military secret during the Second World War.

Placebo Treatment

In the course of testing the effects of unproven treatments, is it ever justifiable to use inert 'placebo' treatment when the patient thinks he or she is receiving active medication?

Because a significant proportion of patients recover spontaneously, it is necessary to compare the recovery rate following a new treatment with the spontaneous recovery rate which occurs on placebo if one is to show that the treatment is better than 'letting nature take its course'. There is also a placebo effect in all medication which needs to be controlled for. (If it is necessary to measure the extent of the placebo effect, a group receiving no treatment, for example being kept on the waiting list, must be included. The placebo group actually measures the combined influence of spontaneous remission plus non-specific placebo effect.) Patients who think they are getting treated often improve more than those not treated at all. If there is no established treatment which has previously been shown to be better than placebo, then any new medication must be compared against placebo to show that the benefit is not due to spontaneous recovery or psychological factors. If a new treatment is only compared with an established one, both may result in remarkably high rates of recovery simply because the patients under study would have responded spontaneously anyway. Thus the placebo also provides a measure of the degree of spontaneous recovery. Let us illustrate the point with a simple example. Suppose a new antidepressant were introduced on 50 medical students who had failed their examinations—and this is the only criteria of giving them the medication—if the treatment was compared to valium on the one hand and imipramine on the other, anxiety and depressive symptoms would be expected to resolve equally quickly in all groups, suggesting that the new antidepressant was as good as valium or imipramine. If a placebo had been used in the trial the fact that the symptoms remitted spontaneously and in equal rapidity and degree with all treatments would not have led to the error of overestimating the efficacy of the active drugs because of an under-estimation of the spontaneous tendency to remit. A possible false conclusion that the new treatment was a good tranquilliser or antidepressant would have been avoided.

If we agree that it is unethical not to do clinical trials, then the most difficult issue still remains.

Should the Patient always be Informed that He or She is a Subject in a Drug Trial?

A general rule which is also included in the code of ethics of the Medical Research Council is that a patient's consent should be obtained before being included in a research project of this kind. However, the Council recognises that exceptions occasionally arise when the process of obtaining the patient's consent would seriously interfere with the general clinical management of the patient. An example of this is provided by the trial criticised by Sargant. While there was some evidence to suggest that monthly injections of fluphenazine reduced the relapse rate of patients with chronic schizophrenia, an equally plausible possibility was that the improved prognosis was due to the increased contact with supporting services which the treatment entailed in the setting up of Modecate clinics. If the patients were given to think that there was some doubt about the efficacy of their injections they might withdraw from treatment altogether. To awaken doubts within the patient could itself cause relapse whether active treatment continued or not. It could undermine one of the critical clinical variables against which the pharmacological efficacy of the treatment was being tested, which was the patient's confidence in the clinic. This was not only essential to the trial but also to the future clinical management of the patient who suffered from chronic schizophrenia. As it turned out, though many relapsed the resurgence of their symptoms was quickly spotted and their confidence in the clinic and willingness to attend was generally unaffected.

The question whether or not we should obtain a patient's consent to be included in a drug trial is part of a wider ranging issue involving a clinician's general obligation to inform patients of the possible, or even rare, risk related to any medical treatment. This arises from what has come to be called the patient's right to 'informed consent'—that it is unethical to perform a medical procedure or administer a medical treatment without fully informing the patient of all risks or harm which could ensue. This can be seen as part of society's growing demand for self-determination of the individual and paradoxically may have been abetted in medicine as a result of the explosive increase in experimental investigations on human subjects (Helmchen and Muller, 1975).

Professor John Wing has responded (1975) by pointing out that the clinical trial should be understood in the setting of a doctor's over-all clinical activity, of which the decision to conduct a trial or to enter a patient into a trial and *pari passu* the decision to tell the patient about the trial is a special case. In medicine it is virtually impossible 'for the clinician to tell the patient everything that is in his mind. He must select. Further, the patient can only rarely be as well informed as the clinician. Even when in exceptional cases the patient himself is a doctor, and has taken a second opinion, looked up textbooks, consulted original papers and has obtained the best statistics as to the cure rates and side-effects and so on, he will usually still need advice as to the best course of action'.

Patients want advice; providing uninvited information by the doctor could be interpreted as the doctor's lack of willingness to take responsibility, thereby undermining the doctor–patient relationship which is an essential element in medical treatment. However, critics favouring the doctrine of informed consent may argue that such a view smacks of elitism and professionalism casting aspersion on patients as being unable to cope with the truth or decide for themselves. Having heard the facts it should be up to the patient if s(he) wants to say—'you decide doctor'.

I would offer this analysis of the problem: In Britain and most other cultures the treatment of the individual by the doctor has been based on an implicit willingness by the patient to be guided by the doctor's judgement, as well as an expectation that the doctor will act with the patient's best interest uppermost in his mind. This amounts to an implicit contract by which the patient seeks advice and invests his rights and responsibilities in the doctor—'I'm in your hands doctor'. What could be more trusting than allowing another human being to open your chest to replace a heart valve? The responsibility whether to tell and what to tell is implicitly assigned by the patient to the doctor, according to and determined by current morals and standards. Common practice does not demand that a severely depressed patient be told that there is only a 60 per cent chance the medication he will receive for the next month will work, or that the severe schizophrenic be told that the phenothiazines may result in irreversible damage to his brain. Although in the United States the doctrine of informed consent is gaining ascendancy, it is not at all clear that this is because of basic medico-ethical reasons. Rather, it is likely that the reason is medico-legal to protect the doctor against legal suit—to divert responsibility for medical decisions to the patient. On this basis one could conclude that rigid observance of the doctrine of informed consent is unethical and medically irresponsible. However, if public opinion in the United Kingdom moves in the direction it has in the United States, then the handover of responsibility by the patient to the doctor currently implied in the contract between the doctor and patient will also be revised.

Considering drug trials, one must assume that if a drug is subject to a controlled trial it is because there is a real doubt about its value. It could be said that the question whether to tell the patient that he or she may be receiving alternatively a drug or placebo is the same question as whether to tell the patient that there are doubts about the effectiveness of the treatment, and that it may have severe (however rare) side-effects. Many will still feel that in the end the physician must be guided by the overriding principle of doing what is best for the patient. If the comparative benefits and disadvantages of the treatment are still uncertain, then this could include putting the patient in a clinical trial.

Withdrawal of Medication

What about the special situation of withdrawing a patient from a medication he or she has been taking for some time, yet not telling him or her?

This arises when a treatment which carries a serious risk of side-effects becomes established before it has been proven to be effective and is a special case. It has occurred with drugs used for long-term maintenance treatment. In several cases the strategy used to test their effectiveness has been to randomly substitute an inert drug for the medication under test, sometimes without telling the patient. However, there is nothing immoral about depriving the patient of a treatment which we do not know is effective and substituting an inert placebo which, at its worst, has no side-effects. In the case of the M.R.C. trial already mentioned, there had been serious reports of depression and suicide following the use of long-acting fluphenazine, and it was known to have a high incidence of neurological side-effects though these are probably controllable. The trial showed that the benefits outweighed the risk of side-effects and suggested that depression was not a problem. By way of contrast, in the insulin coma trial, patients who received placebo were saved the risk of convulsion and death to which the active treatment group were exposed and it turned out that the treatment though dangerous was ineffective, thereby saving both patients in the trial and thousands of others from these risks ever since.

The ethical problems surrounding the extent of our obligation to inform patients are complex and difficult. Sometimes doctors may feel obliged to carry out a study and not tell the patient on the grounds that this is in the best interest of the public as a whole. This practice will understandably raise the anxieties of some doctors and members of the public, especially when the treatment is widely in use. This and many of the other more difficult ethical problems I have discussed would be avoided if the pharmaceutical industry were able to ensure that drugs are proven to be effective by systematically controllable trials on volunteers, prior to their general release for use by the public.

For completeness a final point should be clarified. In the report on 'Responsibility in Investigations on Human Subjects' (Medical Research Council, 1962–63) the M.R.C. makes a distinction between treatments which are of potential benefit for the patient and are undertaken as part of their cure, and procedures undertaken on patients or healthy subjects for the purpose of contributing to basic medical knowledge, but not of themselves designed to benefit the particular individual on whom they are performed. I have been discussing only the former which falls within the ambit of medical care and the rules which govern professional conduct in medicine. The latter constitute investigations upon volunteers and should always be carried out with their full knowledge and consent. When blind trials are carried out, doctors should always be in the position to withdraw the patient from the blind comparison and treat openly whensoever he thinks this is in the patient's best interest. No child under 12 or person of incompetent capacity shall be regarded as having the capacity to consent to any procedure which could bring him harm or injury.

To précis the Medical Research Council, at the end of the day the trust of patients in their doctors is such that most will consent to any proposal that is made. 'It must therefore be frankly recognised that for practical purposes an inescapable moral responsibility rests with the doctor concerning what investigations or treatments are or are not proposed to a particular patient or volunteer.'

References

Helmchen, H. and Muller, B. (1975). Oerlinghausen. *J. med. Ethics*, **1**, 168–173
Medical Research Council (1962–63). Cmnd 2382, pp. 21–25, H.M.S.O., London
Sargant, W. (1975). *The Times*, 29th August
Sargant, W. (1976). *World Medicine*, 14th January
Wing, J. (1975). *J. med. Ethics*, **1**, 174–75

SECTION 2
ISSUES OF
CONTEMPORARY
CONCERN

9 Overprescribing of Psychotropic Drugs

J. Guy Edwards

During recent years we have seen startling increases in the manufacture, distribution, prescription and cost of psychotropic drugs. Many figures have been quoted from Department of Health and Social Security and other sources (for example Trethowan, 1975) to illustrate these increases. The figures quoted are often said to be out of proportion to the prevalence of the psychiatric disorders for which they are prescribed. This, however, cannot be accepted as a statement of fact, because the prevalence of mental illness in general, let alone that of specific psychiatric disorders that call for drug treatment, is not known. The figures are, none the less, suggestive.

Even more suggestive are those data on the use of psychotropic drugs obtained from community surveys (Jeffreys *et al.*, 1960; Parry, 1968; Manheimer *et al.*, 1968; Linn, 1971; Mellinger *et al.*, 1971). To cite but one example, we found that almost 18 per cent of a random community sample in the Washington Heights area of New York City indicated that they often took sleeping pills or other drugs to calm their nerves. A detailed breakdown of statistics concerning drug use in a community sample, such as that made by Parry *et al.* (1973), may suggest that over-all drug use, being sporadic and irregular, is conservative. Alternatively, extrapolations made from other data, such as those of Dunlop (1971) who roughly computed that the number of prescriptions for hypnotics in Britain represented enough drugs, if taken, to make every tenth sleep in the U.K. hypnotic-induced, make us suspect that there is a problem of overprescribing. Whatever the case, we should assess the data in relation to those other problems concerning drug use that are discussed below. If then we accept that there is a problem of overprescribing, we should assess the extent to which we, as psychiatrists, contribute to it and consider ways in which we may be able to minimise the problem.

Causes for Concern

The price that has to be paid for advances in psychopharmacology has been a wide range of unwanted effects. We should be concerned, not only about the well-known effects, however frequently or infrequently they may occur, but also about the risk of indirectly occurring effects and the possibility of reactions yet to be discovered. There is evidence to suggest, for instance, that benzodiazepines can precipitate hostility in situations where people are grouped together and a frustrating stimulus is introduced (Salzmann *et al.*, 1974). It is possible, therefore, that the excessive use of these drugs contributes to the apparent increase in hostility in society. While such an idea must remain speculative, it serves to remind us of the possible broader sociological implications of our prescribing. Likewise, we should be concerned about the potential effects of drugs on driving and their contribution to road traffic accidents.

There is also evidence to suggest a relationship between the use of psychotropic drugs in parents and the abuse of psychodysleptic agents in their children (Smart and Fejer, 1972). Although a causal connection has not been definitely established, it suggests the possibility that children model their drug-taking behaviour on that of their parents. If this is the case, by unnecessary prescribing we may indirectly contribute to the drug abuse problem which we so readily condemn. Then there is the relationship between overprescribing and self-poisoning. It is well known that many patients do not take their treatment as prescribed. Drugs that are not taken are often hoarded. Hoarded drugs become a ready source of accidental self-poisoning for children or deliberate self-poisoning for potentially suicidal people.

Another potential implication of overprescribing was stressed by Trethowan (1975);

> . . . anxiety, like pain, is biologically purposive in that it draws attention to a threat. When this threat is not a real but a neurotic one it points to a conflict that needs to be resolved. If the sufferer is given too ready a means to suppress his anxiety his motivation to try and resolve the conflict that underlies it may also be suppressed. In short, to overcome anxiety a patient must be allowed to experience it, albeit in tolerable doses. Merely to suppress anxiety is to run the risk of suppressing the will needed to try and overcome it.

Finally, there is a question of cost. Although the cost of prescribing per head of population in Britain is lower than elsewhere in the European Economic Community, the expenditure on drugs has risen at an alarming rate during the past decade. The cost of drugs prescribed by family doctors, for example, has increased from £140 million in 1968 to almost £415 million in 1977 (*Lancet*, 1977).

Factors Contributing to Overprescribing

The prescribing of drugs is a much more complex social process than we might readily imagine and many factors are involved. These include:

Time and Training

There are too few doctors and too many patients. Under the circumstances, we often have inadequate time to provide alternative forms of treatment, even when they are more appropriate than pharmacotherapy. Added to this is the fact that doctors, particularly general practitioners, have often had inadequate training to deal with the numerous personality and social problems that pour into their surgeries. Thus, in our overcrowded clinics '. . . we have all, I guess, overprescribed in order to get luncheon or supper—and once started the habit is apt to grow' (Dunlop, 1973).

Demand for Drugs

Man has sought drugs from time immemorial, not only to seek relief from mental and physical anguish, but also in an attempt to transcend the emotional and intellectual boundaries of normality and to seek entry into the realms of euphoria, ecstasy, fantasy and the unknown. Drugs are also seen by many as the ready-made panacea for minor mood changes and somatic sensations that people conceive as being incompatible with a normal healthy existence. Just as people in other cultures expect their culturally-familiar treatments, our patients expect drugs. We often do not have the time or skill to resist the demands made upon us.

Fashions in Prescribing

We are often the victims of prescribing fashions. In many instances these have been fostered by the pharmaceutical industry which has a vested interest in our prescribing habits. The fact that its total promotional budget is about £30–40 million (Stimson, 1976a), reflects this interest.

Difficulties in Diagnosing

When difficulties in diagnosing occur, as they often do in psychiatry, we tend to administer symptomatic, rather than diagnosis-orientated, treatment. Symptoms in psychiatry can be identical to those that occur in normal people and those with problems that do not call for drug treatment. Prescribing in the face of these difficulties often results in a certain amount of unnecessary drug treatment.

Preventive Psychiatry

The early or premonitory symptoms of endogenous illnesses that call for drug treatment are often identical to those that occur in normal and neurotic states for which drugs should be avoided. If we attempt early treatment of endogenous illness in the hope of preventing its complications, we will inevitably prescribe drugs for a number of patients who should not receive them.

Faulty Prescribing Habits

We may contribute to the problem of overprescribing by:

(1) Attempting to provide chemical solutions to non-medical conditions.

(2) Introducing drug treatment prematurely.

(3) Succumbing to those influences that attempt to determine our drugs of choice.

(4) Failing to use optimum dosages.

(5) Administering drugs in divided doses at unnecessarily frequent intervals of time.

(6) Prescribing unnecessary drug combinations.

(7) Changing treatment more often than necessary.

(8) Giving drug treatment for excessive periods of time.

Not only do we overprescribe ourselves through these faulty habits, but, in adhering to them, we often set a bad example to our general practitioner colleagues who are influenced by our prescribing policies, and thereby contribute, through them, to the even larger problem of overprescribing in general practice.

By focusing our attention on our prescribing habits, we can make significant contributions towards easing the problem of overprescribing.

Some Practical Solutions

To Prescribe or Not to Prescribe

After assessing our patients we have to decide, among other things, whether or not to prescribe drugs. In practice, the endpoint of the doctor–patient encounter is the writing of a prescription in about two-thirds of cases (National Disease and Therapeutic Index, 1968), and we are all familiar with the patient who complains that the doctor starts writing the prescription before he has had chance to say what his problems are. Many of these prescriptions will have been given for sound rational reasons, but we know also that many others are issued, not for scientific pharmacological reasons, but because of the pressures that are put upon us. Our first aim, therefore, should be to become more aware of these pressures and to resist them wherever possible.

We should not prescribe drugs unless there is evidence to suggest that the benefits are likely to outweigh the risks. In prescribing psychotropic drugs for the many patients with normal emotional reactions that pour into our clinics there is no such evidence. We should particularly resist prescribing when other forms of treatment, for instance marriage guidance counselling, are more appropriate. To translate every problem into a medical or psychiatric condition and to create diagnoses out of ordinary life-situations is to do the patient an injustice. In addition to the risks of drug treatment, including dependency, providing drugs may mask the real problem and thereby remove the stimulus to seek constructive help.

We should also resist the demands put upon us by patients whose sole expectation is the inappropriate provision of a prescription. While being aware of the ways in which we may be manipulated by drug abusers (Edwards, 1974), we should not over-estimate patients' demands in general and feel over-confident in thinking that we know what our patients really want (Stimson, 1976*b*). If we accept that many patients will be satisfied with the opportunity of airing their problems, with explanations of the cause, with reassurance and/or advice, we can avoid writing many unnecessary prescriptions.

Finally, we should remember that the giving of drugs, unless clearly based on sound criteria, often means that the patient is '. . . getting less value from the doctor's input because the memory and judgement of the doctor are to some extent devoted to sorting out the properties of the profession's cluttered armamentarium' (Muller, 1972).

Starting Treatment

If we have determined that drug treatment is indicated, we next have to decide when to start treatment. Most of us agree that, if drug treatment is to have a rational basis, the patient should be thoroughly assessed. We also agree that such an assessment often calls for more than a single interview. Yet we initiate treatment, often with drugs that take several weeks to produce their desired effects, after short assessments in busy clinics and after even shorter assessments during busy nights on call. Our tendency to do this is reinforced by the dramatic improvements that follow. These include improvements that follow a day or two's treatment with a drug that takes a week or two to produce its main pharmacological effect.

We overlook the fact that merely seeing a doctor, the taking of a history, examination of the mental state or admission to hospital are often therapeutic in themselves. Drug treatment then usurps the credit that should rightly be given to the suggestion, reassurance, faith, optimism and other non-specific effects that are derived from these events. We should remember also that spontaneous recoveries, even in severe and serious illnesses, are by no means uncommon. Thus, unless there are strong indications for giving immediate symptomatic relief, delaying treatment allows for a more accurate assessment and a more rational basis for treatment. It may also spare the patient unnecessary, and sometimes even dangerous, treatment.

Placebos

After the preliminary assessment of a patient, we also have to decide if an active or inert substance is called for. Attitudes towards placebos differ widely. Some doctors feel that it is unethical to deceive a patient by giving an inert substance, while others, such as Findley (1953), believing that the placebo '. . . has been . . . and will continue to be the most important therapeutic weapon which the physician has', stated: 'It should be accorded more respect than it gets. For the vast majority of his patients it and himself are all that even the modern physician has to offer'. Doctors who share these sentiments sometimes prescribe placebos deliberately, but more often the sceptical physician either 'plays it safe' and, not having the confidence to prescribe a placebo, gives an active drug in the belief that its main action is a placebo, rather than a pharmacological, effect. There are, of course, no absolute rules that can be laid down concerning the prescribing of placebos. Each doctor has to be guided by his knowledge and personal ethics. None the less, it should be incumbent upon us to familiarise ourselves with the placebo effect. This subject has been reviewed by Honigfeld (1964), Shapiro (1968) and others.

I do not wish to advocate widespread use of placebos, but there will be occasions when we are faced with a situation in which we feel obliged to give a distressed patient a prescription of some kind or another. Under these circumstances we may find comfort in the knowledge that, when there are no definite indications for pharmacotherapy, it is safer to prescribe inert substances than potentially hazardous ones, however undesirable the prescribing of either may be. A satisfactory placebo response in a transitional state may well prevent a patient from embarking upon a course of treatment with a habit-forming drug and thereby prevent his swelling the ranks of the many drug-dependent people in our midst.

Those opposed to the use of placebos should be reminded that most of the remedies given through the ages were, until relatively recent years, pharmacotherapeutically inactive. Galen's Pharmacopoea contained 820 substances— all pharmacologically inert in the conditions for which they were given (Shapiro, 1968). From the time of Hippocrates to the end of the eighteenth century only five specific remedies were introduced (George, 1974). They should also be reminded that many physicians, perhaps themselves included, already practice placebo therapy, by prescribing drugs of unproven pharmacological value or active drugs in conditions unresponsive to their pharmacological actions. Alternatively, effective drugs may be given in ineffective dosages. Tricyclic antidepressants, for instance, are given in doses as small as 10 mg two or three times a day.

Choice of Drugs

In practice deliberate placebo treatment is not as frequently used as active chemotherapy, and we have to decide which pharmacological agent to use. A considerable body of knowledge has accumulated on the factors that determine our choice of drugs (Coleman *et al.*, 1966; Sainsbury Committee, 1967; Worthen, 1973; Miller, 1974; and Hemminki, 1975). The process of adoption of a new drug is complex. Different types and categories of doctors rely on different sources of advice for different illnesses. Although these influences, both in number and type, remain constant, the importance of individual influences changes with time (Worthen, 1973). Commercial sources inform the physician of the existence of a product, while professional influences act as a 'legitimising channel', bestowing approval on its use (Sainsbury Committee, 1967; Worthen, 1973; Eaton and Parish, 1976).

The diffusion process by which a new drug is introduced into a community has been studied by Menzel and Katz (1955–56) and Coleman *et al.* (1957, 1959). There appear to be physician leaders whose recommendations influence the diffusion rate. A social intermediary, such as a drug firm representative or colleague, also influences the diffusion process, and does so to a greater extent than impersonal media, such as journals or advertisements. The more personal and professional ties a doctor has within a medical community, the more likely he is to adopt the drug. The active role of the patient in persuading the doctor to use a particular drug has been stressed by Webb and Stimson (1976). Marked regional differences in prescribing have been reported by Martin (1957), Lee (1964) and Lee *et al.* (1965). The latter demonstrated striking differences between doctors in the prescribing of amphetamines and antidepressants.

It is unfortunate that we are caught up in a process that is influenced by biased opinion rather than one based entirely on scientific criteria. Despite attempts to counterbalance some of this opinion by the Department of Health and Social Security, such as by issuing the British National Formulary and Prescribers' Journal, we invariably succumb to the pervasive influence of new fashions in prescribing, a process that is fostered by our frustration with the older remedies. Doctors, like other professional groups, have always been the victims of fashion. Sir William Gull, a nineteenth-century physician, concerned over the many treatments said to be useful for rheumatic fever, published a tongue-in-cheek paper extolling the virtues of mint as a cure. He selected mint at random, but was surprised to see that mint water became fashionable—and apparently effective (Coleman, 1975). In psychiatry too we have seen fashions come and go. To a large extent this is due to treatment having a shaky scientific basis. Greenblatt and Shader (1971), for example, pointed out that the initial enthusiasm for meprobamate, with patients in the United States queuing for hours to get their rations, was unjustifiably based on casual observations, isolated case reports, trials on a handful of patients and uncontrolled studies. Eighty to ninety per cent of the reports were of research findings based on inadequate methods.

Time and time again we see the same repetitive sequence: frustration over the relative lack of effectiveness of current treatment ⟶ the introduction of a new drug ⟶ claims of greater effectiveness and/or fewer unwanted effects ⟶ a wave of enthusiasm and a new fashion ⟶ attrition of the enthusiasm or the discovery of a serious unwanted effect ⟶ frustration with current treatment.

The enormous choice of drugs available is an index of the relative lack of success of any one of them and the wide range of preferences held says more about the physician than about the drug. The histories of patients who have been given drug after drug over periods of many years, with little or no change in their clinical state, except that expected from the fluctuations that normally occur in the conditions being treated, testify to this. It is not in the patient's best interest for every available drug to be given, when he fails to respond to the doctor's drug of choice. Instead of trying endlessly to find the right drug, if appropriate drugs have been administered skilfully without a satisfactory response, a more intensive assessment of the patient will often reveal that the problem is, for example, a personality or social problem rather than one that would be expected to respond to pharmacotherapy.

We should not allow ourselves to be influenced by those who have an invested interest in a particular drug, and we should resist the persuasive try-it-for-yourself approach. Paradoxical as it may sound, the main danger of 'trying it for yourself' is that good results will probably follow. When dealing with conditions that run a fluctuating course, or that are influenced by many non-specific factors including changes of drugs and the enthusiasm of the physician, the laws of chance will guarantee that good results will occur in a large number of cases. The danger is that they are then attributed to the drug as a *post hoc* error of thinking, and a stimulus is thereby given to the spread of a new fashion.

There appears to be a relationship between the number of different preparations that a doctor uses and the number of prescriptions that he writes (Wilson *et al.*, 1964). If we are concerned about overprescribing, one way of facing the problem would be to adopt a conservative approach to treatment. It is far better—and far more difficult—to learn how to use a few drugs skilfully and to familiarise ourselves with their pharmacological actions, wanted and unwanted effects, and interactions with other drugs than to use every new drug that appears on the market. In deciding which drugs to use, a sound policy is to use those established drugs that have been in use for the longest periods of time, as any longer-term unwanted effects are more likely to be known. We should adhere to this principle until at least two or three meticulously conducted trials, fulfilling those criteria which have now become well established in psychopharmacological research, have shown *unequivocal* advantages of the new drug over the old unless serious adverse reactions to the old drug are reported in the meantime. We should regard new drugs as experimental agents for a number of years after they have been marketed.

To some these recommendations may sound restrictive. They may even be seen as implying that we are unable to tell a good drug when we see one. I have no doubt that we are capable of recognising changes in a patient's mental state, but, in so far as it requires a large sample of patients to demonstrate advantages over placebo or differences between drugs, it follows that none of us has the mental apparatus to establish a causal relationship between these changes and the administration of a drug in individual patients, or to recognise marginal differences between drugs.

Clinical trials

As our choice of drugs ought to be dependent upon the result of clinical drug trials, a word about trials is appropriate.

New drugs are often presented as major advances, yet a critical appraisal of the research undertaken does not usually justify such claims. Even when the claims are based upon the results of a meticulously executed trial, it should be appreciated that statistically significant differences between the experimental and control groups can occur by chance. Some of these are recognised as chance findings, but others excite interest and their widespread and skilful presentation contributes to the spread of new fashions. We should, therefore, review the results of several trials before deciding upon whether or not alleged advantages are real or chance findings. In so doing, we have to take many factors into consideration, because a clinical trial is a far more complicated procedure than is often realised.

We should consider particularly the criteria for including patients in the trial. Because of the difficulties in defining psychiatric conditions, these should be fully described and we should not interpret the results of the trial until we know what they are. An example will illustrate the importance of this. In a published study of an antidepressant drug trial, one investigator's criteria for inclusion were 'depressive states . . . both psychotic and neurotic, together with some related disorders, including: subjective post-traumatic syndromes; depressive headaches; some cases of phobic, obsessional and hysterical neuroses, with or without associated depression; two cases of emotional anorexia; (and) one psychosomatic condition'. This was not a trial in 'depressive illness', but in a medley of conditions. It is also worrying when one hears of a general practitioner participant in a multi-centre trial say, when asked what were his criteria for inclusion: 'I ask them if they're depressed and, if they say "yes", they're in'.

Problems in the interpretation of the results of a trial also arise because of the previous medication given to the patient. If the patient has failed to respond to a particular drug in the past and that drug is used as a control, a bias against it is introduced. Although the careful investigator takes account of this, patients often do not know what prior medication they have received and medical record keeping is not all that it should be.

Then there are the problems of matching patients. It may not be so difficult to match for sex and age, but matching for all those variables that can affect the outcome of treatment—biological, psychological and social, including life-events and adherence to treatment—provides formidable obstacles. Yet, unless there is satisfactory matching, we simply cannot draw clinically relevant conclusions from the results of the research.

Although the importance of rating scales should not be underestimated, we should remember that a scale is only as good as the person who uses it. We should also be aware that statistically significant differences between scores on rating scales are often erroneously mistaken for clinically significant results. A statistically significant change in the rating of, for example, depression of mood may be clinically insignificant in relation to the over-all disability caused by the depressive illness. Residual symptoms, producing a low score on a rating scale, may be the major problem in preventing a patient from returning to useful employment, with all that this implies regarding his sense of responsibility and usefulness in fulfilling his normal social role. The persistence of such symptoms can determine over-all treatment success or failure. Conversely, as Lader (1976) pointed out, drug X may not be statistically different from drug Y because it makes three-quarters of the patients worse but cures the rest. This is of great clinical significance.

We should, therefore, be sceptical about claims that are based on a small number of trials. Scepticism should be inculcated from our early formative professional years, and continually reinforced. The value of undergraduate education in this respect has been demonstrated by Garb (1958) and Daniel and Leedham (1966).

Dosage, Route and Frequency of Administration

After choosing a drug, we next have to decide upon its mode of administration. The dose of drugs prescribed should be the lowest that will produce the desired response, unless unwanted effects occur before this is reached. If they do, we have to steer a course between wanted and unwanted effects. There are so many variables that determine the response to drugs that no simple guidelines provide the answer to all clinical problems, and the dose has to be tailored to the individual patient's needs. When we have an illness, such as schizophrenia, that is adequately controlled by a drug, we do not always realise that the same degree of control could be obtained with a smaller dosage. In fact, it is worth attempting to reduce the dose in practically every patient requiring long-term treatment, unless an attempt to reduce it has already been made without success. Alternatively, we could discontinue the drug for short periods of time, such as on weekends.

It is not only the prescribing of too large a dose that contributes to overprescribing. Overprescribing may also be caused by giving too small a dose because, through not obtaining the desired response, the drug may be continued for an unnecessary length of time. The problems of giving too much or too little or too often arise from our having a fixation on familiar-sounding doses and, being the victims of habit, a reluctance to exceed these.

Although most psychotropic drugs are given orally, during recent years there has been a greatly increased use of the intramuscular route for the administration of long-acting depot neuroleptics, given largely in the hope of decreasing the chances of relapse due to non-adherence to treatment. After deciding to use this route, doctors sometimes give oral medication in addition to the depot neuroleptic when progress is not to their satisfaction. Arguments that we sometimes hear to justify this are that the intramuscular medication makes the patient sufficiently co-operative to take his oral drugs or that a larger dose of the intramuscular preparation would be dangerous. A more likely explanation is that we are again demonstrating how we are the victims of habit, in this case by being reluctant to increase the dose of the depot preparation, but being prepared to add oral drugs instead, which often amounts to the same thing. The oral drugs added to the intramuscular regime of a patient unlikely to adhere to treatment will probably not be taken as prescribed. As in the case of giving too small a dose, through not obtaining the desired response, the drug may then be continued for an excessive period of time, thereby contributing to the problem of overprescribing.

Yet another of our habits is to prescribe drugs ritualistically in a stereotyped three- or four-times-a-day way, often with little regard to the pharmacological properties of the drug and empirical observations made upon its use. While acutely disturbed patients may need monitoring of therapeutic and unwanted effects after such frequently prescribed dosages, there is no rationale for maintaining all patients needing long-term treatment on such frequent dosages, especially in the case of those drugs with a relatively long half-life. Studies demonstrating the effectiveness of once-daily medication have best been demonstrated in the management of schizophrenia; they have been reviewed by Lee *et al.* (1974). The advantages of once-daily medication are better adherence to treatment; less embarrassment for the patient in not having to take medication during the daytime; the possible association in the patient's mind of less sickness; help with sleep difficulty and the decreased need for hypnotics if the single dose is given at night; less trouble with the more immediately occurring side-effects, which may occur during sleep if the drug is given at night; and economy of nurses' time. Once-daily medication may have particular advantages for the elderly, especially if there is a memory deficit and anxiety caused by having to remember a complicated regime. However, with elderly patients we should be particularly alert when giving large once-daily dosages because of the increased propensity of unwanted effects.

Notwithstanding the advantages of giving medication once daily, we still prescribe drugs in divided doses at unnecessarily frequent intervals, and thereby contribute to the problem of non-adherence to treatment. This, in turn, may mean that the desired effect of the drug is not obtained and the drug is given for an excessive period of time.

Drug Combinations

During the course of treatment we may consider whether we should treat our patients with a single drug or combinations of drugs. Polypharmacy has been a fashionable habit of doctors for centuries, although, up until the introduction of large numbers of potentially dangerous drugs into clinical practice, it often amounted to little more than poly-placebo therapy. This addiction to blunderbuss therapy was stressed by Dunlop (1971) when he referred to the Frenchman's idea of Scotch whisky toddy: 'You put in whisky to make it strong and water to make it weak and lemon to make it sour and sugar to make it sweet and then you say *à vous* and drink it off yourself'. Elsewhere referring to the *furor therapeutikus* of those who prescribe compound haematinics, he wrote: 'Doctors who prescribe these haematinics resemble bad sportsmen who shut their eyes and brown the covey with a discharge of shot in the hope that something will fall down, sending away a lot of the birds with dangling legs' (Dunlop, 1972).

D'Arcy (1976) has cited from the literature examples of patients being prescribed large numbers of drugs on single prescriptions. The record seems to have been held by Hammond (1974) who dispensed one EC10 form on which 12 items were prescribed for a single patient. What is also worrying is that, in a study of physicians in the Montreal area, including hospital residents, general practitioners and specialists, the majority did not know the number or names of the ingredients in the drug combinations that they were accustomed to prescribe. The greater the number of ingredients, the less likely they were to know the constituents (Biron, 1973). The dangers of prescribing drugs to the elderly are well known, yet those of us who boast better memories than our demented and psychotic elderly patients could not possibly hope to remember the combinations that are often prescribed. The complicated instructions issued are often of little help.

The same criticisms that have been directed towards polypharmacy in general medicine apply to psychiatry. While there is no agreement on whether drug treatment should be determined by the diagnosis or the symptoms, most doctors, at least sometime during their careers, prescribe specific drugs for specific symptoms. Thus, they prescribe, for example, a neuroleptic for the formal thought disorder and an antidepressant for the associated depressive symptoms in a schizophrenic patient. Doctors also prescribe two or more drugs in the hope of obtaining an additive or synergistic effect or of obtaining more manoeuvrability in steering a course between therapeutic and adverse effects. It is difficult enough to draw conclusions from the administration of one drug and its clinical response, let alone combinations of drugs, and here too we are at risk of erroneously confusing *post hoc* and *propter hoc* events. An apparent response to the addition of a second drug may be due to the continued or accumulative effect of the first drug prescribed, rather than due to the giving of the second drug. Even if the effect is additive, the same result might have been obtained by increasing the dose of the first drug. Add to this the non-specific psychological effect of change—in this case the addition of a drug—and the logical confusion is not difficult to understand.

It cannot be stated categorically that drug combinations are always contraindicated in psychiatry, but the addition of a second or third drug to our drug of choice may be an example of our treating our own anxieties over what we regard as a delay in obtaining the expected therapeutic response. Not only do these additional drugs contribute to the problem of overprescribing, but they add to the risk of unwanted interactions with other drugs in ways which have been reviewed elsewhere (Edwards, 1977). If we wish to avoid unnecessary prescribing, drug combinations are best avoided.

Adherence to Treatment

Throughout the period of treatment, we should remain constantly aware that many patients do not take their drugs as prescribed. It has already been stated that, if a patient does not respond satisfactorily to drugs, they may be prescribed for longer than would otherwise be necessary. One of the causes of an unsatisfactory response is non-adherence to treatment. The subject has been reviewed by Blackwell (1973, 1976), Sackett and Haynes (1976) and others. Non-adherence occurs to a greater extent than we often realise. Hare and Willcox (1967) showed that it occurs in as many as 48 per cent of out-patients. Experienced psychiatrists may make errors in 20 per cent of their predictions of which patients are taking their medication (McClellan and Cowan, 1970).

We can obtain better co-operation from patients if we have a caring attitude (Reynolds *et al.*, 1965; Irwin *et al.*, 1971), if we meet patients' expectations and desire for information (Francis *et al.*, 1969) and by providing a more personalised service (Finnerty *et al.*, 1973). There is ample evidence to show that adherence is adversely effected by complicated drug regimes, such as drugs being given in several divided doses a day or in non-fixed combinations with other drugs (Mallahy, 1966; Gatley, 1968; Porter, 1969). We should recognise the importance of giving clear written and oral instructions, repeating them and asking the patient to restate them (*British Medical Journal*, 1977).

Changing Treatment

During treatment we also have to decide if and when treatment should be changed. In everyday practice we frequently see patients whose drug treatment has been changed at very frequent intervals, sometimes after only a few days. Drugs given for so short a period of time that they have not been given a chance to produce their expected therapeutic effects, as in the case of drugs being given in inadequate doses, contribute to the problem of overprescribing. Changes are often made because the patient is unable to tolerate a particular drug, but they can also be seen as another example of doctors treating themselves because of their frustration at not seeing a satisfactory response as quickly as they would have liked.

Patients sometimes appear to respond selectively to one drug or category of drugs but not to others, but this does not occur with sufficient frequency to explain the large number of changes in drug treatment that are often made. Furthermore, patients not responding to one drug may appear to respond to a second drug which is almost pharmacologically identical or whose action may be mediated through identical metabolites. This apparent response is not necessarily due to the introduction of the second drug. As in the case of adding drugs, it could have been brought about by the accumulative effect of drugs with similar central actions, the psychological effect of change or even the passage of time. Evidence that change can be important was provided by one study that demonstrated three dissimilar placebos, each given for two weeks, having a better effect than one placebo given for six weeks (Rickels *et al.*, 1964).

We should therefore not change a drug until it has been given in an adequate dose for a sufficient length of time to have produced its desired effect. Until then we cannot say that a patient is unresponsive to it. We should also ensure that, in changing drugs, we are not treating our own anxieties.

Discontinuing Treatment

Finally, we have to decide when to discontinue drug treatment or whether it should be continued indefinitely.

Unless we do this, there is a serious risk that, once a drug has been introduced, repeat prescriptions may be given with no end in sight. Coleman (1975) has seen patients who have received repeat prescriptions for period of up to 12 years without a full consultation with their doctors. Some patients may need 'maintenance treatment' indefinitely, but others, who have reached a satisfactory level of improvement and have maintained it for an appreciable length of time, can cope just as well without drugs. Here, as elsewhere, there are no hard-and-fast rules, and we have to be guided by the predicted natural history of the condition being treated. In the case of a first bout of depression precipitated by stress in a previously well-adjusted, healthy, young individual, antidepressant treatment may be discontinued almost as soon as the depression has resolved. At the other extreme, a chronic relapsing schizophrenic patient may require neuroleptics indefinitely. Between these two extremes are all types of patients and illnesses that require treatment for varying lengths of time.

Most research into discontinuing treatment has been carried out in schizophrenic patients. Some investigators believe that neuroleptics should be continued indefinitely because of the serious risk of relapse, whereas others have been more cautious and have stressed the long-term risks and contribution of continued drug use to the problems of overprescribing. While there are these risks, we should at least consider the possibility of shortening the duration of treatment. If we do this, it is not only important to know the probability of a relapse, but also the psychiatric and social consequences, and the chances of regaining rapid therapeutic control. We would be more hesitant to risk a relapse if it might lead to dangerous behaviour or disastrous social consequences than, say, a worsening of apathy and withdrawal in a longstay patient, especially if the re-introduction of the drug leads to a rapid remission.

Gardos and Cole (1976) have reviewed the published work on the effects of withdrawal of neuroleptics on the relapse rates of schizophrenic patients. They estimated that the proportion of schizophrenics in the community that do not need to continue treatment with antipsychotic drugs, either because they progress satisfactorily without them or because they do not progress so well on drugs for such reasons as not being given optimum dosages, non-adherence to treatment and unwanted effects, may be as high as 50 per cent. They also inferred tentatively that relapse following discontinuation of drugs can be reversed in most instances by the prompt resumption of treatment.

It can be argued, therefore, that we should give many, if not most, schizophrenic patients who are maintained on antipsychotic medication the benefit of a trial without drugs. Within the broader context of the problem of overprescribing, discontinuing antidepressants and anxiolytic drugs in the numerous people receiving them for prolonged periods of time for the treatment of non-medical problems, is likely to be more rewarding. While in depressive illnesses tricyclic antidepressants may confer benefits for 6–8 months (Mindham *et al.*, 1973; Paykel *et al.*, 1975) or even for 2 years (Prien *et al.*, 1973), there are no scientific grounds for prescribing them indefinitely.

Conclusions

(1) There is considerable circumstantial evidence that psychotropic drugs, like other drugs, are overprescribed. Their unwanted effects contribute to a serious public health hazard. In addition to this, overprescribing throws heavy demands upon an already restricted national budget. We can contribute significantly towards the reduction of these problems by becoming more aware of the broader social implications of our prescribing and by adopting more thoughtful prescribing policies. These should be applied at each point in the doctor–patient encounter.

(2) The effect of a drug upon an individual is a complex interaction that depends on the drug, the patient's pathophysiological state, psychological and social factors. There are so many variables involved that we should not prescribe drugs until we are familiar with their major pharmacological actions, unwanted effects and interactions with other drugs, the patient's medical and psychiatric history, and those other factors that will influence the outcome of treatment. Before prescribing we should be convinced that the chances of benefit outweigh the risks—including the indirect and longer-term consequences.

(3) We should not 'psychiatrise' all the problems that come our way in order that they may fit the potent treatments that are available. We should learn more about normality, have the courage to diagnose it, and resist offering chemical 'solutions' to non-medical problems. We should not assume that every interview must end with a prescription. Giving drugs to people with personality and social problems may, in the longer term, add to their difficulties.

(4) We should be aware of, and able to resist, the influences of those who have a vested interest in our prescribing policies and those who have not demonstrated their relative freedom from bias.

(5) Unless there are definite indications for immediate symptomatic relief, a

planned withholding of drugs will often be rewarded by a significant favourable response to the initial interview, or even a spontaneous recovery. The patient may thereby be spared an unnecessary course of treatment with a potentially hazardous compound.

(6) Rather than prescribe drug after drug in the constant search for the 'right' one or be the victims of fashion trying every drug that appears on the market, we should learn the more difficult task of using a few drugs skilfully.

(7) When we are faced with a situation in which we see no alternative to prescribing 'something'—a situation that does arise in a busy medical practice—we should consider prescribing, in the short term, a placebo rather than a potentially dangerous substance, however undesirable the prescribing of either may be.

(8) We should familiarise ourselves with the numerous factors that can influence the results of clinical drug trials. By so doing, we will be in a stronger position to assess their results more critically, and less influenced by the results of any one or two trials. We should not use new drugs, which may have unwanted effects lying in store for our patients and which are usually more expensive than established remedies, until at least two or three trials, fulfilling the well-established criteria called for by sophisticated research methodology, have shown *unequivocal* advantages of the new drug over the old.

(9) In administering a drug, we should tailor the dose to the patient's clinical needs. Giving too large a dose increases the risk of toxicity. Giving too little can result in the drug being given for an excessive length of time, because it has not been given in a dose large enough to produce its desired effect. We should not prescribe drugs in divided daily dosages in those instances where once-daily medication offers advantages.

(10) We should also avoid drug combinations wherever possible. By doing this and following the other recommendations outlined above, we will help to decrease the chances of non-adherence to treatment.

(11) We cannot say that a patient is unresponsive to a drug until it has been given in an adequate dose for a sufficient length of time to have produced its desired effect. While a change in treatment may then be indicated, changing from drug to drug—especially from one to another that is pharmacologically identical—is not in the patient's best interests. A more detailed assessment will often be more rewarding.

(12) It is only in a very small minority of patients that drug treatment will need to be continued indefinitely. In the vast majority, we should have a target for discontinuing treatment constantly in mind. Some of those patients whose treatment cannot be withdrawn when that target is reached may have a problem of dependency, with withdrawal symptoms masquerading as a relapse of the symptoms for which the drug was originally given.

References

Biron, P. (1973). A hopefully biased pilot survey of physicians' knowledge of the content of drug combinations. *Can. med. Ass. J.*, **109**, 35–39

Blackwell, B. (1973). Rational drug use in psychiatry. In *Rational Psychopharmacotherapy and the Right to Treatment* (Ed. F. J. Ayd), Ayd Medical Communication, Baltimore

Blackwell, B. (1976). Treatment adherence. *Br. J. Psychiat.*, **129**, 513–531

British Medical Journal Leading Article (1977). Keep on taking the tablets. *Br. med. J.*, **1**, 793

Coleman, J., Katz, E. and Menzel, H. (1957). The diffusion of an innovation among physicians. *Sociometry*, **20**, 253–270

Coleman, J., Katz, E. and Menzel, H. (1966). *Medical Innovation—a Diffusion Study*. Bobbs-Merril Company, Indianapolis

Coleman, J., Menzel, H. and Katz, E. (1959). Social processes in physicians' adoption of a new drug. *J. chronic Dis.*, **9**, 1–19

Coleman, V. (1975). *The Medicine Men: Drug Makers, Doctors and Patients*. Temple Smith, London

Daniel, E. E. and Leedham, L. (1966). Effect on student attitudes of a programme of critical evaluation of claims for drugs. *J. med. Educ.*, **41**, 49–60

D'Arcy, P. F. (1976). Iatrogenic disease: a hazard of multiple drug therapy. *R. Soc. Hlth J.*, **96**, 277–283

Dunlop, Sir Derrick M. (1971). The use and abuse of psychotropic drugs. *Scot. med. J.*, **16**, 345–349

Dunlop, Sir Derrick M. (1972). Drug interactions. *Community Health*, **4**, 8–13

Dunlop, Sir Derrick M. (1973). Medicines, governments, doctors and pharmacists. Lister Memorial Lecture. *Chemistry and Industry*, Feb. 3, 127–131

Eaton, G. and Parish, P. (1976). General practitioners' views of information about drugs. *J. R. Coll. gen. Pract.*, **26**, Supplement No. 1, 64–68

Edwards, J. G. (1974). Doctors, drugs and drug abuse. *Practitioner*, **212**, 815–822

Edwards, J. G. (1977). Unwanted effects of psychotropic drugs. I—Some general considerations. *Practitioner*, **218**, 556–562

Findley, T. (1953). The placebo and the physician. *Med. Clinics N. Am.*, **37**, 1821–1826

Finnerty, F. A., Mattie, E. C. and Finnerty, F. A. (1973). Hypertension in the inner city. I. Analysis of clinic dropouts. *Circulation*, **47**, 76–78

Francis, V., Kotsch, B. M. and Morris, M. J. (1969). Gaps in doctor – patient communications. Patients' response to medical advice. *New Engl. J. Med.*, **280**, 535–540

Garb, S. (1958). The reaction of medical students to drug advertising. *New Engl. J. Med.*, **259**, 121–123

Gardos, G. and Cole, J. O. (1976). Maintenance antipsychotic therapy: is the cure worse than the disease? *Am. J. Psychiat.*, **133**, 32–36

Gatley, M. S. (1968). To be taken as directed. *J. R. Coll. gen. Pract.*, **16**, 39–44

George, C. F. (1974). The investigation of new drugs in man. *Br. J. Hosp. Med.*, **11**, 780–787

Greenblatt, D. J. and Shader, R. I. (1971). Meprobamate: a study of irrational drug use. *Am. J. Psychiat.*, **127**, 1297–1303

Hammond, C. V. (1974). Polypharmacy. Personal communication with and quoted by D'Arcy, P. F.

Hare, E. H. and Willcox, B. R. C. (1967). Do psychiatric in-patients take their pills? *Br. J. Psychiat.*, **113**, 1435–1439

Hemminki, E. (1975). Review of literature on the factors affecting drug prescribing. *Soc. Sci. Med.*, **9**, 111–116

Honigfeld, G. (1964). Non-specific factors in treatment. I. Review of placebo reactions and placebo reactors. *Dis. Nerv. Syst.*, **25**, 145–156

Irwin, D. S., Weitzel, W. D. and Morgan, D. W. (1971). Phenothiazine intake and staff attitudes. *Am. J. Psychiat.*, **127**, 1631–1635

Jeffreys, M., Brotherston, J. H. F. and Cartwright, A. (1960). Consumption of medicines on a working-class housing estate. *Br. J. prevent. soc Med.*, **14**, 64–76

Lader, M. H. (1976) Basic trial design. *Br. J. clin. Pharmac.*, **3**, Supplement (2), 375–379

Lancet. Commentary from Westminster (1977). Curbing expenditure on drugs. *Lancet*, **i**, 962–963

Lee, J. A. H. (1964). Prescribing and other aspects of general practice in three towns. *Proc. R. Soc. Med.*, **57**, 1041–1043

Lee, J. A. H., Draper, P. A. and Weatherall, M. (1965). Primary medical care: prescribing in three English towns. *Milbank Memorial Fund Q.*, **43**, 285–290

Lee, J. H., Branchey, M., Haher, E. J., Varga, E. and Simpson, G. M. (1974). Once versus thrice daily thiothixine in the treatment of schizophrenic in-patients. *Br. J. Psychiat.*, **125**, 73–78

Linn, L. S. (1971). Physician characteristics and attitudes towards legitimate use of psychotherapeutic drugs. *J. Hlth soc Behav.*, **12**, 132–140

Mallahy, B. (1966). The effect of instruction and labeling on the number of medication errors made by patients at home. *Am. J. Hosp. Pharmac.*, **23**, 283–292

Manheimer, D. I., Mellinger, G. D. and Balter, M. B. (1968). Psychotherapeutic drugs: use among adults in California. *Cali. Med.*, **109**, 445–451

Martin, J. P. (1957). *Social Aspects of Prescribing.* Heinemann, London

McClellan, T. A. and Cowan, G. (1970). Use of antipsychotic and antidepressant drugs by chronically ill patients. *Am. J. Psychiat.*, **126**, 1771–1773

Mellinger, G. D., Balter, M. B. and Manheimer, D. I. (1971). Patterns of psychotherapeutic drug use among adults in San Francisco. *Archs gen. Psychiat.*, **25**, 385–394

Menzel, H. and Katz, E. (1955–56). Social relations innovation in the medical profession: the epidemiology of a new drug. *Public Opinion Q.*, **19**, 337–352

Miller, R. R. (1974). Prescribing habits of physicians: a review of studies on prescribing of drugs. *Drug Intelligence clin. Pharm.*, **8**, 81–91

Mindham, R. H. S., Howland, C. and Shepherd, M. (1973). An evaluation of continuation therapy with tricyclic antidepressants in depressive illness. *Psychol. Med.*, **3**, 5–17

Muller, C. (1972). The over-medicated society: forces in the marketplace for medical care. *Science*, **176**, 488–492

National Disease and Therapeutic Index, Reference, File, Diagnosis. July 1967–June 1968. Lea Associates Inc., Amber, Pennsylvania

Parry, H. J. (1968). Use of psychotropic drugs by U. S. adults. *Public Hlth Rep.*, **83**, 799–810

Parry, H. J., Balter, M. B., Mellinger, G. D., Cisin, I. H. and Manheimer, D. I. (1973). National patterns of psychotherapeutic drug use. *Archs gen. Psychiat.*, **28**, 769–783

Paykel, E. S., Dimascio, A., Haskell, D. and Prusoff, B. A. (1975). The effects of maintenance amitriptyline and psychotherapy on symptoms of depression. *Psychol. Med.*, **5**, 67–77

Porter, A. M. H. (1969). Drug defaulting in a general practice. *Br. med. J.*, **1**, 218–222

Prien, R. F., Klett, J. and Caffey, E. M. (1973). Lithium carbonate and imipramine in prevention of affective episodes: a comparison in recurrent affective illness. *Archs gen. Psychiat.*, **29**, 420–425

Reynolds, E., Joyce, C. R. B., Swift, J. L., Tooley, P. H. and Weatherall, M. (1965). Psychological and clinical investigation of the treatment of anxious out-patients with three barbiturates and placebo. *Br. J. Psychiat.*, **111**, 84–95

Rickels, K., Baumm, C. and Fales, K. (1964). In *Neuro-psychopharmacology*, Vol. 3

(Ed. P. B. Bradley, F. Flugel and P. Hoch), Elsevier, Amsterdam

Sackett, D. L. and Haynes, R. B. (1976). An annotated bibliography on the compliance of patients with therapeutic regimens. In *Compliance with Therapeutic Regimens,* Johns Hopkins University Press, Baltimore

Sainsbury, Lord (Chairman) (1967). *Report of the Committee of Enquiry into the Relationship of the Pharmaceutical Industry with the National Health Service.* (1965–1967), H.M.S.O., London

Salzman, C., Kochansky, G. E., Schader, R. I., Porrino, L. J., Harmatz, J. S. and Sweet, C. P. (1974). Chlordiazepoxide-induced hostility in a small group setting. *Archs gen. Psychiat.*, **31**, 401–404

Shapiro, A. K. (1968). The placebo response. In *Modern Perspectives in World Psychiatry* (Ed. J. G. Howells) Oliver and Boyd, Edinburgh

Smart, R. G. and Fejer, D. (1972). Drug use among adolescents and their parents: closing the generation gap in mood modification. *J. abnorm. Psychol.*, **79**, 153–160

Stimson, G. V. (1976a). The extent of advertising of pharmaceutical products. *J. R. Coll. gen. Practit.*, **26**, Supplement No. 1, 69–76

Stimson, G. V. (1976b) Doctor – patient interaction and some problems for prescribing. *J. R. Coll. gen. Practit.*, **26**, Supplement No. 1, 88–96

Trethowan, W. H. (1975). Pills for personal problems. *Br. med. J.*, **4**, 749–751

Webb, B. and Stimson, G. V. (1976). People's accounts of medical encounters. In *Sociology of Everyday Medical Life* (Ed. M. Wadsworth and D. Robinson), Martin Robertson, London

Wilson, C. W. M., Banks, J., Mapes, R. and Courte, S. M. T. (1964). The assessment of prescribing: a study in operational research. In *Problems and Progress in Medical Care* (Ed. G. McLachlan), Oxford University Press, London

Worthen, D. B. (1973). Prescribing influences: an overview. *Br. J. med. Educ.*, **7**, 109–117

10 The Self-poisoning Patient: Treatment and Prevention

H. Gethin Morgan

The main purpose of this chapter is to discuss the causes and management of deliberate self-harm (DSH) which has increased progressively since the early 1960s until it now constitutes 20 per cent of all emergency medical admissions to hospital (Smith, 1972). The clinical and demographic characteristics of the problem have been well documented elsewhere (Aitken *et al.*, 1969; Morgan *et al.*, 1975b) but the main features will first be summarised before proceeding to a fuller discussion of causes and management.

Clinical and Socio-economic Characteristics

The greatest incidence of DSH occurs in late teenagers and young adults, and apart from in the elderly, females outnumber males at all ages (figure 10.1).

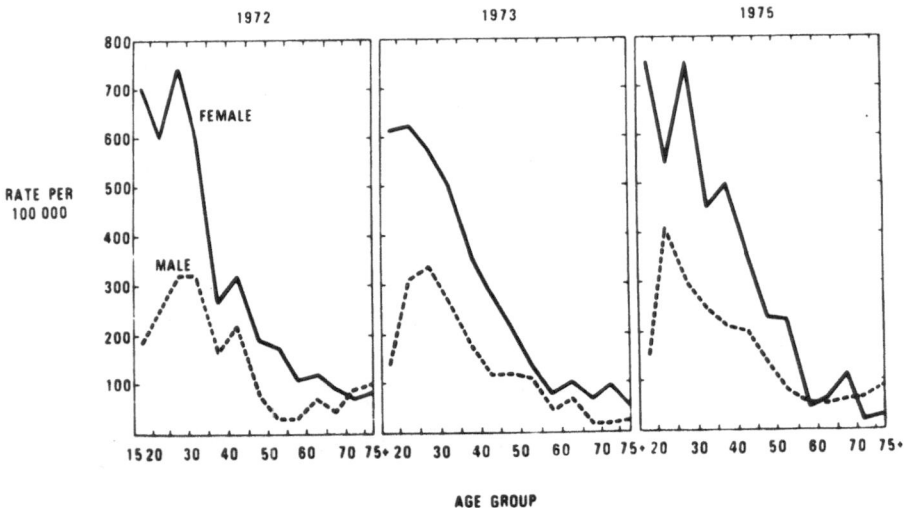

Figure 10.1   Deliberate self-harm rates: Bristol County Borough (persons referred to hospital casualty)

The majority (93 per cent) of these patients seen in hospital have taken some form of drug overdose, the small remainder having resorted to laceration, and in a very small proportion, poisoning with coal gas or non-ingestants (table 10.1).

Table 10.1
Deliberate self-harm: breakdown of methods used

Method	Number of Patients	%
Self poisoning		
Drug overdose	1 440	91.8
Non-ingestant	7	0.5
Gas	8	0.5
Laceration	76	4.8
Other (immersion, hanging, jumping)	16	1.1
Drug overdose and any other	22	1.3
Total	1 569	100

(Persons Attending Accident and Emergency Departments, Bristol County Borough, 1972 and 1973)

Most of the drugs originate from medical prescription, 50 per cent being psychotropic drugs (tranquillisers, antidepressants or sedatives) prescribed for the self. Only a small proportion of patients are found to be suffering from psychotic mental illness, the majority showing the picture of an acute reaction in the face of an intolerable situation, frequently in the nature of an interpersonal conflict. At the time, emotional upset is often severe, and measures of anxiety and depression are similar to those found amongst psychiatric in-patients (Morgan et al., 1975b). The problem is particularly common in city areas of underprivilege and over-crowding (Morgan et al., (1975a). Many patients express a marked feeling of personal isolation, without

Table 10.2
Attitudes to self-harm at time of act (% interviewed patients)

Attitude	Male	Female
Wanted to die	46.3	34.4
Expected to die	28.9	25.5
Preparations made for death, e.g. making a will	5.8	3.6
Active precautions taken against discovery	7.4	1.6
Regrets not killing self (at time of interview)	17.4	10.5
Left suicide note	21.5	16.2
Planned act more than 6 hours before	11.6	10.9

close friends with whom they can share personal problems. Only a minority (46 per cent males, 34 per cent females) admit to conscious suicidal ideas either at the time or subsequent to the act of self-harm, and it is inappropriate to refer to this complex problem as 'attempted suicide' (table 10.2). The term 'deliberate self-harm' is suggested because of its descriptive general meaning, free from implied motivation. Abuse of alcohol is closely related to the problem, both through the disinhibiting effect of recent drinking, as well as the problems inherent in chronic alcohol addiction (table 10.3).

Table 10.3
Pattern of alcohol intake in previous three months (% interviewed patients)

Alcohol intake	Whole series	Male	Female
Always abstinent	9.8	9.1	10.1
Uncomplicated social drinking	66.6	47.9	74.9
Increased social drinking	10.1	16.5	6.9
Problem drinking	12.5	24.0	6.9
Uncertain	1.6	2.5	1.2
Alcohol intake within 6 hours preceding self-harm			
Usual amount	19.3	28.1	15.0
More than usual amount	15.5	24.6	10.0

Causes

Any consideration of causation must take into account the complexity of motivating factors as well as the remarkable increase in this form of behaviour during the past 15 years. Table 10.4 illustrates the various groups of factors involved, arranged according to whether they are immediate (motivating) or in the more distant past (antecedent) and whether they are personal, interpersonal or social in nature.

A major problem revolves around assessment of the degree of conscious intent inherent in an act of self-harm, which so easily arouses the suspicion that it is perverse and deliberate in the sense that it could have been avoided with a little more personal control. In fact, it is usually an example of acute impulsive albeit reckless behaviour under stress, and in our search for causes it is relevant that we should look at those changes in society during the past two decades which have greatly increased the likelihood that vulnerable individuals will harm themselves deliberately. The situation was summarised succinctly by the *Lancet* (1974): 'Some pervasive influence is affecting increasing numbers of people. That influence may be the knowledge that the wish to die, made obvious, can be a very powerful way of releasing intolerable stresses or generating concern'.

Table   10.4
Causes of deliberate self-harm

	Antecedent	Motivating
Personal	Psychological: Reactive Depression Personality Disorder Alcoholism	True suicide intent Search for sympto-matic relief
Interpersonal	Conflict with other key individual Marital failure Lack of close relationships Delinquency Antisocial behaviour Separation from parent in childhood	To influence attitudes and behaviour of others To communicate de-gree of personal dis-tress or anger
Social	Environmental (accommodation, econ-omic, employment) Lack of support (family community) Problems of youth Society's attitude to self-harm Prescription of psychotrophic drugs	To influence social agencies To avoid adverse re-percussions of own behaviour

Presumably there have indeed been major changes in the way we perceive such behaviour and react to it, if only because since the Suicide Act of 1961 all legal sanctions against deliberately harming the self have been removed. Loosening of social ties, decrease in social regulation and in shared values are difficult to measure, but they may indeed be relevant to the self-harm problem. Bagley has demonstrated that in the United States there is an inverse relationship between the incidence of DSH and the general pattern of social regulation and control in a number of component States. Bagley ascribes the upsurge of DSH, as well as other behavioural problems, to the 'relaxation of authoritarian moral standards, a loosening of the ties . . . which constrain the actions of individuals' (Bagley, 1974). This same point is illustrated by two findings in our Bristol studies, namely the relevance of population mobility as measured by frequent changes of address, and the general lack of close personal support expressed by these patients.

It has long been recognised that self-harm has its greatest incidence in teenage girls and young women in their early twenties. This has never fully been explained, though presumably it is related in some degree to the fact that the problems facing youth in to-day's society are felt most keenly by the female. In Bristol there have been recent significant increases in incidence in young men and the most likely social stresses involved appear to be increased abuse of alcohol and a high rate of unemployment (Morgan and Turner, unpublished).

The part played by medical prescription of psychotropic drugs also warrants close scrutiny. There has been a remarkable increase in the quantity of drugs prescribed in this way during the same period that DSH has increased progressively to reach its present epidemic-like proportions. Further, the type of drug used in DSH reflects the pattern of their availability through medical prescription (figure 10.2).

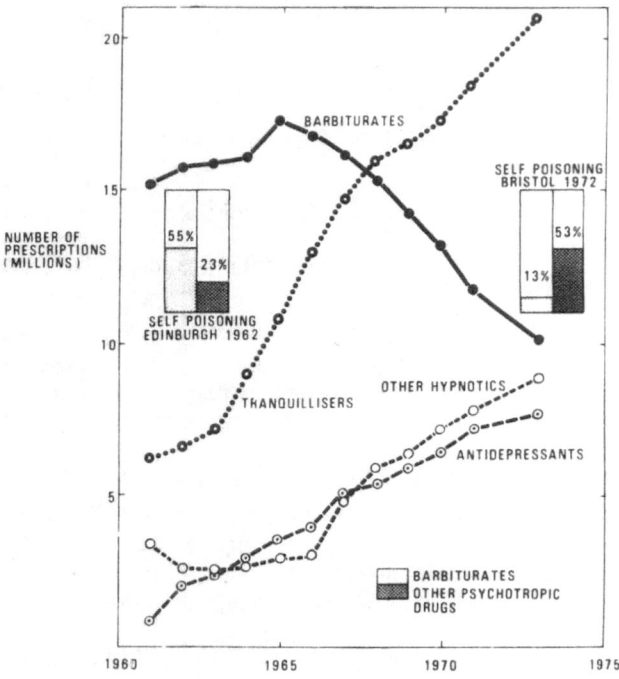

Figure 10.2   Trends in national prescriptions of psychotropic drugs and methods of non-fatal self-poisoning 1961–73 (sources: Annual Report D.H.S.S., Kessel (1965), Morgan *et al.* (1975))

Undoubtedly, these drugs when used correctly are a major therapeutic advance. When utilised inappropriately, however, especially as a panacea without adequate concomitant personal support for unhappy people with severe life difficulties, they constitute an ineffective solution. The scene is then set for deliberate overdose when crises continue, the drug ammunition being immediately available to be taken in a state of despair or anger, which is at least partly directed at the failure of others to help and at their pretence that a tablet could ever in itself resolve the complex problems involved. It is indeed a sad state of affairs that pharmaceutical companies have not fostered research on the way prescription of these drugs is complicated by deliberate overdose. We will return to this later in discussing primary prevention.

Management

A drug overdose usually means that the person concerned is transferred immediately to the nearest hospital accident department. Presumably this reflects concern about the unpredictability of physical complications. In fact, the overdose problem now places enormous demands on hospital resources, though major physical complications occur infrequently. In Bristol 81 per cent of such patients who are seen in accident departments are admitted as in-patients to medical wards. Self-inflicted lacerations in young women are more likely to be sent home directly after initial assessment, again presumably because it is easier to be reassured about immediate risks when there is no added uncertainty regarding late complications from drug overdose.

Apart from those services which have special units devoted to the management of DSH, throughout most of this country the overdose patient is admitted to general medical wards. Provided the psychiatrist is prepared to supply an efficient and rapid assessment, most physicians are prepared to tolerate this situation. The DSH patient sometimes gets a mixed reception, occasionally being seen as a nuisance which interferes with more important medical problems. Whilst most staff seem to favour a special overdosage unit in principle, few seem keen to work there (Griffin, 1973). There is clearly a danger that such a unit could become yet another low-status psychiatric facility, this time within the general hospital itself, doing little to resolve staff prejudice against such patients. A special unit undoubtedly facilitates assessment and management of the overdose, but on the other hand dispersal of the problem throughout the hospital ensures that it is not separated out of sight out of mind for those who are prejudiced against such behaviour. It is probably better for such individuals to work through their own difficulties, both by seeing the overdose problem managed and by having regular contact and support from the psychiatric staff concerned.

Physical Treatments

These cannot be reviewed in detail here. Although only a minority suffer major physical complications, the large number of DSH patients means that complications are not uncommon, including organic brain syndromes due to cerebral anoxia related to hypoventilation or cardiac arrest, chest infections complicating aspiration of stomach contents and various physical injuries following lacerations or falling.

Psychosocial Assessment and Management: (a) Immediate

Most patients are ready to discuss their problems by the next day. It is important to remember, however, that there may be immediate social problems at the time of the overdose, especially when the patient is a single parent with dependent children whose needs have to be safeguarded, if necessary by involving the help of relatives or the local authority's social services department.

The first aim of psychosocial assessment is to estimate the immediate risks involved so that one of the several management options may be chosen, ranging from the return of clinical care to the general practitioner, out-patient psychiatric appointment or psychiatric day care to informal or compulsory admission to a psychiatric in-patient unit. Assessment is best carried out by a psychiatrist and social worker pair. There is generally some haste involved, as the physician usually requires the patient to be discharged quickly, and in the circumstances it may not be easy to obtain a full history, particularly when relatives are not present. The social worker can be invaluable, not only in clinical assessment but also in immediate liaison with other agencies which may have been involved previously, as well as contacting relatives by telephone, if necessary. This is a good example of how close on-the-spot collaboration between the psychiatrist and social worker does much to improve clinical management.

Suicide Prevention
Although only a minority of patients will be found to have entertained serious ideas of self-destruction, a certain number are indeed failed suicides, in danger of attempting to take their lives unless adequate supervision and treatment is initiated. Assessment demands skills in the detection of suicide risk.

Whatever may be the underlying mental illness or social crisis, the suicidal has reached a state of despair from which his view of life in general and his own situation in particular is usually grossly distorted. The most common emotional concomitants are depression, anger, and frustration, often with a sense of repeated failure following which it seems pointless to persist. When faced with a patient in this frame of mind, it is important to remember that unless one's approach is correct, important clues may be missed, particularly when the patient sees the interview as an irrelevant and pointless intrusion into his private feelings of hopelessness. It is important to say little, but as soon as possible to state that one recognises the patient's state of despair. The interview may have to move slowly as the the patient comes out of his shell and feels that he is talking to someone who can perhaps understand his despair, and who by avoiding facile reassurance makes him feel he will be taken seriously. He may not have been able to discuss his feelings with relatives for fear of losing face. Discussion of suicidal ideas must be embarked upon carefully: for example, after commenting on the state of despair and sympathising with the patient, noting feelings of hopelessness about the future, the conversation moves to the present, and the patient is asked whether he has ever felt unable to go on with life. Following this it should then be possible to discuss freely any ideas of self-destruction which the patient may have entertained. At this point, the suicidal patient may show an emotional catharsis with a feeling of relief on being able to share such painful feelings.

The more the clinical and socio-economic characteristics of the patient conform to the suicide stereotype, the more one should suspect suicide risk, even when it is denied. The most important personal factors are increasing age, male sex, widowed, divorced or separated, unemployed, incapacitating physical disability, especially terminal illness in the elderly, life events of a loss nature, depression and/or alcoholism, self-blame and persistent insomnia, especially with a previous psychiatric history involving suicide attempts. Precipitating social crises are of course also relevant: when these have temporarily subsided, then the immediate risk is less than when the episode of self-harm has alienated relatives even further, tending as they do to equate self-harm with blackmail aimed at altering their own attitudes and behaviour. The act of self-harm may give valuable clues regarding the true suicidal intent, which is more likely when the overdose was massive, laceration was severe and extensive or was due to unusual methods such as the use of a fire-arm, precautions had been taken to avoid discovery and to ensure success, and the episode was well planned rather than impulsive.

Concomitant Mental Illness
Suicidal behaviour may complicate a wide variety of abnormal mental states, both psychotic and otherwise. The depressive or paranoid psychosis and chronic alcoholism may be missed because of denial on the patient's part. This may also make assessment particularly difficult in the elderly, who often refuse to admit that they have taken other than the usual dose of night sedative. There may be no demonstrable symptoms of mental illness, though this does not mean that the patient is free from suicide risk: given sufficient impulsivity of personality, and a return to a social situation fraught with chronic tension and interpersonal conflict, perhaps with symptomatic drinking of alcohol, then emotional tension may build up again very rapidly and lead to further suicidal behaviour.

Interpersonal and Socio-economic Factors
These need to be defined in order to tackle them in subsequent treatment and to include other key persons who may be involved in the patient's difficulties. Full discussion of these at the first interview is often itself therapeutic, being part of the sharing of the burden with others who want to help: it is indeed wrong to avoid discussion of matters merely because they cannot be changed easily. As the majority of patients will have reacted to some adverse event immediately prior to the episode of DSH, this aspect of the history is crucial.

Choice of Treatment Programme
The minority will require psychiatric hospitalisation, especially when florid illness and continuing suicidal ideas or a worsening social situation are present. Most are fit to take up out-patient appointments, or to return to the care of their general practitioners. Sometimes a decision regarding the best form of treatment is difficult because of the various ambiguities in the situation. It is then useful to ask for reassurance that a patient will come for

help if in difficulties before the next appointment and that discharge from hospital is mutually agreed to be a sensible step. One who is deeply committed to suicide may still not admit to it, but frequently a patient will discuss feelings freely, especially when a good rapport has been established by correct interview technique. Needless to say, in any doubtful situation ease of availability of help is essential and the patient should be in no doubt where to turn for assistance if in difficulty. 'Hot lines' of this nature are not often abused, particularly when the goal of the next appointment has been mutually agreed.

Whilst it is important to admit the seriously ill for in-patient psychiatric care, an immediate return home is probably the best for the majority of these patients. It can be extremely difficult to treat situational problems from a psychiatric ward, and too liberal use of hospital admission can delay rather than promote their resolution, often leading to secondary relationship problems in the ward itself. A period of care in a psychiatric day hospital may of course be a good compromise.

Psychosocial Assessment and Management: (b) Subsequent

This aims at predicting repetition of deliberate self-harm and the treatment of underlying personal, interpersonal, and socio-economic difficulties. The present discussion will not concern itself with management of the patient needing psychiatric admission for treatment of major mental illness but will concentrate on treatment of those who are referred after an episode of DSH to the out-patient clinic. In Bristol, 55 per cent are referred in this way. Of these, 71 per cent keep their appointments and only 44 per cent of those referred actually complete a course of out-patient treatment satisfactorily (Morgan *et al.*, 1976). Clearly we need to examine other ways of helping the considerable proportion who do not feel psychiatric care of this kind is relevant to their problem. Even in those who attend there is much conflicting evidence concerning not only the optimal form of treatment but even whether the psychiatric approach is helpful at all. Greer and Bagley (1971), in a study of patients attending a hospital in London, produced evidence to suggest that psychiatric intervention is beneficial. Chowdhury *et al.* (1973) on the other hand, carried out a follow-up study in Edinburgh and demonstrated that psychosocial support did not reduce the repetition rate, though it did lead to some improvement in the general social state. The Bristol follow-up study (Morgan *et al.*, 1976) showed that subsequent psychiatric treatment was positively associated with repetition of self-harm in the following year but this was probably due to the fact that patients with more severe psychiatric histories and a previous history of self-harm were preferentially selected for such treatment.

Faced with inconclusive evidence regarding the efficacy of secondary prevention, it is not surprising that there are extreme divergencies of opinion regarding the best form of treatment of DSH. It is still common for those who are less sympathetic to the problem to believe that it may be best to pay these patients as little attention as possible, or even that routine stomach wash-outs are a useful deterrent. The image of deliberate manipulative behaviour which could have been controlled by firm, uncompromising management is never far away. Even psychiatrists sometimes find it difficult to accept that these patients are relevant to their expertise, regarding them as insoluble personality disorders or social problems. It may be more accurate to see them as highly vulnerable individuals who, given a few more years of chronic frustration, will end up with more florid psychiatric syndromes.

There are clear clinical predictors of DSH repetition, which itself occurs in 32 per cent of men and 23 per cent of females within a year. The findings in Bristol are summarised in table 10.5 and they resemble those from Edinburgh studies (Buglass and Horton, 1974). A previous history of DSH is itself closely

Table 10.5
Factors significant for repetition within 12 months of initial episode

	Repeaters ($N = 56$)	Non-repeaters ($N = 159$)
Factors significant at $P < 0.001$		
(a) Preious psychatric treatment	49	62
(b) Previous act of deliberate self-harm	42	65
(c) Criminal record (conviction other than parking offences)	33	38
Factors significant at $P < 0.01$		
(d) Social class IV and V	29	49
(e) Separation from spouse/cohabitee	16	19
(f) Separation from mother before age 15	18	22
(g) Initial episode not precipitated by any upset	23	35
(h) Regret surviving	14	16
(i) Personality disorder	24	35
(j) Serious drink problems	14	15
(k) Drug dependence	8	3

associated with risk of repetition, suggesting that such behaviour tends for a while at least to have an element of self-perpetuation. However, it is ill-judged to take on for treatment only those with a well-established history of DSH. It is just as important to concentrate on the 'first evers', the aim being to prevent a repetitive pattern of self-harm from becoming established. In all patients it is worth spending some time discussing ways in which DSH, especially when it is repetitive, produces a hostile reaction in others: many patients appear not to have given this aspect of the problem serious consideration.

Secondary psychiatric intervention must, apart from providing adequate treatment for serious mental illness, avoid falling into the trap of providing positive reward for such behaviour. Self-harm is now a most effective method whereby a distressed individual can ensure an immediate response from both the community and hospital services. Help should not be a process of doing things on behalf of a passive patient, but rather a way of helping him to make his own decisions: it aims to provide support which allows him to face up to life's difficulties in a more constructive manner on the assumption that full responsibility for personal behaviour is retained.

Accepting Suicide Risks
Occasionally a situation arises in which a patient repeatedly self-harms after full psychiatric care, perhaps even including several hospital admissions. In such circumstances when major psychotic illness causes impaired judgement, it may be necessary to insist on psychiatric treatment, if necessary implementing a section of the Mental Health Act. In the majority of such instances, however, DSH is being used as a deliberate strategy in order to coerce others or to avoid intolerable situations. It is here that the clinician may have to tolerate a degree of suicide risk in order to ensure that full responsibility for personal behaviour is retained by the patient, this being a necessary prerequisite for any continuous progress in therapy. In such a situation it is crucial that the therapist does not angrily reject the behaviour as mere manipulative acting out. The majority of such patients are struggling, albeit inappropriately, with major life difficulties, in the face of which they develop serious emotional upset. The therapist should continue to make himself available should the patient want to seek a constructive resolution of the situation.

Primary Prevention

In view of the poor results of secondary intervention, it becomes imperative to examine other approaches to the problem of DSH. The various factors in society which may have contributed to this modern epidemic have already been discussed. Of these, the most relevant to medical practice is the fashion of psychotropic drug prescription by the primary health care team or hospital services. It is a remarkable fact that little is known about either the rate at which such prescriptions are complicated by DSH or the risk factors involved, and further investigation along these lines is urgently needed.

It may be that DSH reflects a major deficiency in present day health care services. Medical practice, rapidly increasing in technological complexity, is ignoring the basic needs of people in distress to share their burden with others who have the basic skill of listening in a constructive way. The general practitioner, no matter how enthusiastic he is, may not have the time to do this and we must therefore look at the primary health care network further. Who can develop the necessary skills and how should these individuals relate to the doctor in his surgery and indeed to the psychiatrist in his clinic? When these questions have been answered, there may be a reduction in the inappropriate use of psychotropic drugs as a panacea for unhappy people struggling with complex life problems and we will have gone some way towards controlling the current epidemic of deliberate self-harm.

References

Aitken, R. C. B., Buglass, D. and Kreitman, N. (1969). The changing pattern of attempted suicide in Edinburgh 1962–1967. *Br. J. prev. soc. Med.*, **23**, 111–115

Bagley, C. (1974). Social policy and the prevention of suicidal behaviour. *Br. J. soc. Work*, **3,** 4

Buglass, D. and Horton, J. (1974). A scale for predicting subsequent suicidal behaviour. *Br. J. Psychiat.*, **124,** 573–579

Chowdhury, N., Hicks, R. and Kreitman, N. (1973). Evaluation of an after-care service for parasuicide patients. *Soc. Psychiat.*, **124,** 573–578

Greer, S. and Bagley, C. (1971). Effect of psychiatric intervention in attempted suicide. *Br. med. J.*, **1,** 310–312

Griffin, N. (1973). A study of hospital staff attitudes to the overdose patient. Elective undergraduate dissertation, Bristol University Medical School

Gull, W. W. (1874). Anorexia nervosa (apepsia hysterica, anorexia hysterica). *Trans. clin. Soc.*, **7,** 22–28

The *Lancet* (1974). Annotation, self-injury, *Lancet*, **ii,** 936–937

Morgan, H. G., Pocock, H. and Pottle, S. (1975a) The urban distribution of non-fatal deliberate self-harm. *Br. J. Psychiat.*, **126,** 319–328

Morgan, H. G., Burns-Cox, C. J., Pocock, H. and Pottle, S. (1975b). Deliberate self-harm: clinical and socio-economic characteristics of 368 patients. *Br. J. Psychiat.*, **127,** 564–574

Morgan, H. G., Barton, J., Pottle, S., Pocock, H. and Burns-Cox, C. J. (1976). Deliberate self-harm: a follow-up study of 279 patients. *Br. J. Psychiat.*, **128,** 361–368

Smith, A. J. (1972). Self-poisoning with drugs—a worsening situation. *Br. med. J.*, **iv,** 157–159

11 Child Abuse

Selwyn M. Smith

Although the phenomenon of child abuse has existed since the dawn of history, it is only in recent decades that changing social values have led to its identification as a widespread medical-social problem that is subject to investigation and solution. It is interesting that among both animals and humans, the instinct to nourish and the impulse to maim and destroy exist side by side. Sigmund Freud, in his paper, 'A Child is Being Beaten', described what he considered the universal unconscious wish to hurt the young. He also commented that his patients were more embarrassed by and more reluctant to talk about their sadistic feelings concerning children than they were about their sexual fantasies.

Child abuse has many facets. Social implications are the co-ordinating link for all professions—medicine, nursing, education, law, and judiciary. It is important to understand the problem in an historical context and this chapter will attempt to review what is known about the problem medically, socially and legally. It will also comment on the extent of the problem, the aetiology, the cultural attitudes, and the various treatment approaches that have been adopted.

Table 11.1 lists the major historical landmarks associated with the child abuse phenomenon. While these developments have been reviewed in depth elsewhere (Smith, 1975), it is nevertheless worthwhile highlighting some points related to these developments.

The early reports of battered children by Ambroise Tardieu and Samuel West antedated the discovery of X-rays in 1895 and could not therefore be confirmed. It is interesting to observe also that legislation against cruelty to animals had preceded legislation against cruelty towards children by a period of 75 years. Indeed, it was against a background of physical harm to a member of the animal kingdom that 'The National Society for the Prevention of Cruelty to Children' was founded in New York State in 1899.

Caffey's description of a new medical syndrome 'comprising multiple fractured long bones in association with recurrent subdural haematomas' initiated the modern period of medical recognition. Silverman, in 1953, a colleague of Caffey's, was the first to suggest that trauma was responsible for Caffey's syndrome, but it remained for two paediatricians, Woolley and Evans (1955) to actually point out that the child's parents were responsible for child abuse. Following a nationwide survey of hospitals, Kempe *et al.* (1962) coined the emotive term, 'Battered Child Syndrome'. The term caught hold and other case descriptions began to be described in the medical literature confirming that child abuse was a worldwide phenomenon.

Table 11.1
Historical survey of child abuse

1860	Ambrose Tardieu	Described the medico-social phenomenon of maltreated children
1888	Samuel West	Described familial periosteal swellings (atypical rickets)
1899	National Society for the Prevention of Cruelty to Children	Founded in New York State
1946	John Caffey	Described a 'new syndrome' of recurrent subdural haematomas in association with fractured long bones
1953	F. Silverman	First to suggest that trauma was responsible for Caffey's Syndrome
1955	Woolley and Evans	First to suggest the parents were responsible for child abuse
1962	Kempe and Colleagues	Coined the emotive term Battered Child Syndrome
1963	Index Medicus	The subject heading, Child Abuse, first appears as an official listing in the source book of medical literature
1966	British Paediatric Association	Issues Warning Memorandum and offers definition and guidelines for treatment
1968	Reporting Laws	U.S.A. and other countries (United Kingdom excepted) pass mandatory reporting legislation
1972	Selwyn Smith and Colleagues	Describe psychiatric, psychological and social characteristics of baby batterers
1973	Tunbridge Wells Study Group	Publishes recommendations for improving management of the problem
1975	Children's Act	New legislation passed in United Kingdom making further provisions for children. Breaks with the concept of 'parenthood means ownership' of the child
1977	J. Densen-Gerber and Colleagues	Bring to the American public's attention the widespread practice of sexual exploitation of children. Responsible for legislation prohibiting pornography involving children

Definition

In 1962, Kempe and his colleagues used the term the Battered Child Syndrome 'to characterize a clinical condition in young children who have received serious physical abuse, generally from a parent or foster parent'. The coining of this dramatic term has proved useful in rivetting the attention of a reluctant public to the hard realities of the situation. For practical purposes the following definitions should also be considered:

(1) *A battered baby* is an infant who shows clinical or radiological evidence

of lesions which are frequently multiple and involve mainly the head, soft tissues or the long bones and thoracic cage, and which cannot be unequivocally explained.

(2) *A neglected child* is one who shows evidence of physical or mental ill-health due primarily to failure on the part of the parents or caretakers to provide adequately for the child's needs.

(3) *A persecuted child* is one who shows evidence of mental ill-health caused by the deliberate infliction of physical or psychological injury which is often continuous.

It is difficult to arrive at a consensus of opinion concerning definition. Child neglect, in the legal sense, constitutes all those conditions listed in law and under which a court may find a child neglected or in need of protection. The term child neglect covers the abused and battered child, as well as the child whose parents are unable or unwilling to adequately care for him.

Child abuse and battering is at the end of a neglect continuum, which ranges from neglect due to ignorance on the part of the parents to deliberate maltreatment, and it is not always possible to distinguish the point at which neglect becomes abuse. Abuse can take the form of a direct physical attack, severe or unusual discipline, the deprivation of basic needs such as food, or any other action that could cause immediate physical or mental damage to a child. The term child battering is usually confined to one type of abuse—direct physical injury to the child, resulting from intentional use of excessive force by an adult.

Child abuse, if broadly defined, would include child neglect, child battering, sexual abuse of children, emotional abuse, failure to thrive children and nutritional abuse. The U.S. Child Abuse Prevention and Treatment Act, passed in April 1975, defines child abuse as 'the physical or mental injury, sexual abuse, negligent treatment or maltreatment of a child under the age of 18, by a person who is responsible for the child's welfare, under circumstances which indicate that the child's health or welfare is harmed or threatened thereby'.

Unfortunately, confusion and lack of definition have limited communication between those working in the field and fostered misunderstanding among those who wish to define the problem more clearly. Many of the terms applied to describe the phenomenon of child abuse are euphemistic expressions that maintain public complacency. In contrast to medical and social definitions, the police classify non-accidental injuries under such headings as murder, attempted murder, manslaughter, infanticide, wounding, assaults and cruelty. Clarity of definition is further hampered by the fact that courts determine the definition. Courts of law are influenced by the public and so the definition will change from time to time and be dependent on the emotional climate in a particular area.

From a practical point of view, the diagnosis is not a difficult one. Child abuse must be considered in any child exhibiting evidence of a fractured bone, subdural haematoma, failure to thrive, soft tissue swelling, skin bruising or sudden infant death. When the degree and type of injury is at variance with the history given concerning the occurrence of the trauma, the child must be considered to be a battered child until proven otherwise. Indeed, any injury other than a road traffic accident to a child under the age of two years must be considered to be an instance of the battered child syndrome (*Lancet*, 1971).

It seems to the author that Silverman's comments written in 1953, are just as cogent today: 'It is not often appreciated that many individuals responsible for the care of infants and children . . . may permit trauma and be unaware of it, may recognize trauma but forget or be reluctant to admit it, or may deliberately injure the child and deny it' (Silverman, 1953).

Types of Injury Resulting from Physical Abuse

The literature describing the clinical manifestations of child abuse is extensive (Helfer and Kempe, 1968; Kempe and Helfer, 1972; Fontana, 1971; Smith, 1975). Bruises, head injuries and fractures are highly suggestive and are often caused by a parent striking a child or using any object that comes to hand. Poisonings and overdoses appear to be more frequently encountered than in the past, and seem to represent a general lack of care on the part of the caretaker. The classic picture comprising signs of repeated injuries—old and new bruises, healing and new skin lesions, fractures at different stages of healing—is pathognomic of the condition. The diagnosis should also be considered when subdural haematomas are associated with fractured long bones (Caffey, 1946). Serial skeletal surveys to observe the progression of suspected fractures should be carried out.

Skin Lesions
Although children bruise easily, the important factor in suspecting child abuse is the distribution of the bruises. Old and new lesions may have a pattern suggesting the implement used—lash, electric cord, belt buckle, cigarette burns, bite marks. Scarring, if present, may be hyper- or hypo-pigmented.

The examiner should be particularly suspicious if full-thickness burns are present. The most frequent presentation is that of burns of the lower extremities, buttocks and perineum caused by 'dunking' in hot liquids.

Bone Injuries
'To the informed clinician, the bones tell a story the child is too young or too frightened to tell' (Cameron, 1970). Repeated pulling and twisting of an infant's long bones results in epiphyseal separation and subperiosteal haemorrhage in the metaphyseal and epiphyseal areas. Such haemorrhage is followed by a healing process resulting in callus formation that is diagnostic (Silverman, 1968). Fractures of ribs at varying stages of healing, a fractured skull and crushed vertebral fractures are frequently seen. Stellate, multiple

fractures particularly of the occipital bone and basket-handle fractures at the junction of the growth plate and metaphyses should be looked for (Genieser and Becker, 1974).

Consultation with a radiologist is essential not only to exclude other rare conditions, but to seek advice concerning the implementation of other radiological aids that will help exclude such associated conditions as a pericardial effusion, a ruptured abdominal viscus or an intramural haematoma in the gastrointestinal tract.

Visceral Injuries
Rupture of the liver and other abdominal viscera usually associated with laceration of the mesentery is common. Intramural haematoma of the duodenum and jejunum, resulting in bowel obstruction, is occasionally observed (Cameron, 1970; McCort and Vaudagna, 1964; Kempe, 1971).

Eye Injuries
Mushin (1971) and Harcourt and Hopkins (1971) have emphasised that permanent visual impairment may occur as a result of physical maltreatment and underlined the necessity for a complete ophthalmic examination in suspicious cases. Injuries to the eyelids (Cameron *et al.*, 1966), posterior subcapsular cataracts (Kiffney, 1964), peripheral choroidoretinal atrophy (Maroteaux and Lamy, 1967) and pre-retinal and retinal haemorrhages (Gilkes and Mann, 1967) may of course result in partial or complete blindness in these children.

Head Injuries
These may result from either blunt injury or shaking the child. Brain contusions, cerebral and subdural haemorrhages, multiple subgaleal haematomas and glial scars (Lindenberg and Freytag, 1969) may result in permanent neurological damage.

Oliver (1978) has collected evidence to also suggest that punctate haemorrhages of the brain resulting from excessive shaking of the baby is an important and frequent cause of intellectual impairment. Varying combinations of malnutrition and psychosocial deprivation superimposed on 'rough handling' by a parent may be a frequent cause of mental subnormality and may preclude school and employment success.

Extent of the Problem

The true extent of child abuse is not known for many cases are not reported, or go unrecognised. In the U.S.A., it has been predicted that between 1973 and 1982 there will be one and a half million reports of child abuse: 50 000 deaths, 300 000 permanent injuries and one million potential abuses. In 1973, the reporting rate in the United States was 350 cases per million population. In

Canada the rate is estimated to be 250 cases per million population (Anderson, 1976). In England, Oliver *et al.* (1974) in a careful study have estimated that the likely rate of severe attacks on children under 5 years of age is 10 per 100 000 population, or 2450 severely battered children per annum.

The major problem in trying to determine the extent of child abuse has been establishing the ratio between the number of actual cases compared to the number of reported cases. The actual number of reported cases depends on the effectiveness of the reporting system in any given area. The report of the New York State Assembly Select Committee on Child Abuse of April, 1972, for example, noted that there were some 400 reported cases of suspected child abuse in that State alone, in 1966. By 1971, when New York's reporting system had become more effective, the annual total had climbed to 3200 cases.

It is the author's view that current statistics underestimate the problem. Improvement could readily be made if child welfare organizations referred a suspected case to experienced medical personnel for confirmation and computer recording of the diagnosis. It is also of interest that in the United States, where mandatory reporting of child abuse cases has been in existence for a number of years, conflicting estimates still occur. Unfortunately, even if reliable statistics were available, it does not necessarily imply that efficient management of the problem would occur. In terms of morbidity and mortality, conservative estimates strongly suggest that child abuse is a problem of major concern to society.

Causation

Although it has been argued that every parent is a potential 'baby basher' (Kempe, 1970), clinical experience suggests that adults responsible for the care of children rarely cross the threshold into violence. Most parents have experienced exasperation by the behaviour of their children, but such exasperation usually stops short of real violence. Indeed, anthropological evidence (Malinowski, 1927; Mead, 1928) has demonstrated that groups of people suffering from extreme stresses, deprivations and frustrations, have not battered and would not injure their children. One can thus only speculate as to an individual's inside mechanisms and surrounding cultural forces that create and maintain a child-abusing situation.

Child abuse has been regarded as a syndrome or a specific variety of violence. It has been the author's experience, however, that baby battering is but a microcosm of violent crime. The same broad factors observed in crime and delinquency in general are therefore to be found. One observes also the same difficulty in determining causative factors and a similar constellation with other inadequacies or deficiencies. The expected wide parental variations with a small malignant hard-core group that are eclipsed by a larger number of cases that are easily helped and who are unlikely to repeat the offence, are observed in practice. Differences in the abuse situation appear to depend upon the family setting, the support of the spouse, and to a certain extent, the characteristics of the child victim. Collusion and domestic secrecy adds to the difficulties in case management.

Violence towards children represents a social derivative of biological, psychological and cultural interaction, and theories as to causation must therefore be framed in terms of these factors. A variety of models have been established to assist in the understanding of child abuse—psychodynamic models, personality or character trait model, social learning model, family structure model, environmental stress model, social-psychological model and a mental illness model (Justice and Justice, 1976). While none of these models is complete in itself, each contains a central core of determinants that have been considered as basic to causation. Space does not allow for a detailed discussion on each of these models, but a brief overview is helpful in providing a summary of existing knowledge concerning causation.

Psychodynamic Model

The Denver school have been the main advocates in suggesting that battering parents are not confined to any particular personality type, intelligence level, or social class, and that 'child abuse is psychodynamically related and has nothing to do with race, colour, sex, creed, income, education, or anything else' (Kempe, 1969). This school regards the lack of 'a mothering imprint' as the basic dynamic of the potential to abuse. An inability to nurture their own children results from the parents being reared in a way that precluded the experience of being mothered. It is combined with a lack of trust in others, a tendency towards isolation, a non-supportive marital relationship, and excessive expectations towards the child. Before the potential to abuse is activated, two other factors must be present: a 'special' child (the abusing parent views him as retarded, hyperactive, or in some other way different) and a crisis involving varying degrees of stress.

Linked to this model is a concept of 'role reversal' put forward by Galdston (1965). This alludes to the expectation that a child must act like an adult and give the parent love and care, rather than vice versa. According to Galdston, role reversal appears as an important ingredient in an abusing situation. Such parents are provoked into battering because they feel unloved, unhappy, and anxious when the child cries or misbehaves.

A lingering concern when attempting to account for child abuse is finding specific reasons why violence is expressed instead of other problem behaviour. Being rejected as a child, developing no trust or close relationships, learning no love, having little tolerance for stress, are all factors that can produce problems with wide-ranging expressions—alcoholism, criminality, personality anomaly, etc. One can only speculate why a background of abnormal rearing expresses itself specifically in child abuse. This theory does not provide the answer.

Personality or Character Trait Model

This model is similar to the psychodynamic model but fails to emphasise the factors that underlie the personality traits of the batterer. Emphasis is placed on labelling—parents who abuse their children are 'immature', 'self-centred', or 'impulse-ridden'. Other descriptions applied to abusive parents include 'chronically aggressive', 'highly frustrated' and 'lonely, suspicious and untrusting people'.

Merrill (1962) has been the main exponent of this model and has suggested that battering parents exhibit three distinct clusters of personality characteristics. Parents in the first group seemed to be beset with continual and pervasive hostility and aggressiveness, sometimes focused and sometimes directed at the world in general. Their angry feelings stemmed from inner conflicts and were often rooted in their early childhood experiences. Merrill's second group were identified by traits of rigidity, compulsiveness, lack of warmth, lack of reasonableness, and lack of pliability in thinking and attitudes. These parents defended their right to batter their child, had marked child-rejection attitudes, exhibited an inability to feel love and protectiveness towards their children and felt that their children were responsible for many of their troubles. The parents in the third group were characterised by strong feelings of passivity and dependence and often competed with their own children for the love and attention of their spouses. These parents were considered immature, moody, unresponsive and generally depressed. Merrill also described a fourth group comprising young fathers who were generally intelligent men with acquired skills who, because of some physical disability, were now fully or partially unable to support their families. In these situations, the mothers worked while the fathers stayed home and cared for the children. Their frustrations led to swift and severe punishment and to angry, rigid discipline.

Although it is important to identify the personality or character traits of an abusing person, one must avoid the tendency to merely label or brand the individual as though that is sufficient explanation for child abuse. This model is useful if considered within the larger context of environmental influences and the part that the child possibly plays in abuse.

Social Learning Model

This model emphasises the failure of child abusers to acquire the skills to function adequately in the home and society. Such parents are regarded as lacking social skills, are frequently ignorant of child development and gain little satisfaction from their role as parents. Steele and Pollock (1968) emphasise that child-rearing patterns encompass a set of attitudes in which children are expected to satisfy many of the parents' emotional needs. Parents have expectations of the child far beyond his chronological years. According to this view, the child abuser has an intense need to turn to the child for affection and if no gratification is received, the parents respond with frustration and anger. Such parents are inclined to utilise physical discipline on their children and recreate in their own child-rearing practices, the methods they themselves experienced as children.

This model is useful in the formulation of intervention and treatment strategies. Methods of teaching child-rearing skills based realistically on the parents' capabilities provide a helpful method of correcting their ineffectual parental care.

Family Structure Model

The alliances, coalitions, enmeshments and disengagements among family members are important factors in leading to child abuse. Of particular importance is the lack of family cohesiveness. Studies have shown that the biological father is frequently absent from the home and that the mothers are living with some other man (Fontana, 1971; Smith, 1975). Disharmony in child-rearing, scapegoating and dissatisfaction with the partner's handling of the child are often observed. Premarital conception, short acquaintances before marriage, lack of kinship support, and other marital adversities suggest that important stabilising forces within the marriage are weak and that a substantial number of battered children will eventually grow up in broken homes. Such children are thus at risk not only of further physical and possibly fatal injury but also will experience social and educational deprivation, deviant behaviour and delinquency.

Environmental Stress Model

Gil (1970) is the leading exponent of this model and reported that baby battering is concentrated among the socio-economically deprived segments of the population. He views child abuse solely as a function of educational, occupational, economic or social stress. Underpinning such stresses is the cultural attitude that permits the use of physical force in child-rearing. According to this view, solutions must therefore rest with a global control of environmental problems. Gil has also recommended educational efforts aimed at gradually changing the cultural attitudes amongst the socio-economically deprived, who heavily rely on the use of physical force in their child-rearing practices. On the national level, he has recommended the establishment of clear-cut prohibitions against the use of physical force and corporal punishment.

One must caution against viewing child abuse as solely due to environmental stress. Psychological factors within the parents themselves seem to be of prime importance in the causation of this phenomenon. Child abuse also appears to stem from a defect in character, leading to lack of inhibition in expressing frustration and other impulsive behaviour. Although socio-economic factors may place added stress on the basic weakness in personality structure, such factors are not of themselves sufficient or necessary causes of child abuse. Gil's efforts, therefore, in attempting to obtain the ultimate objective of reducing violence in society, do not answer the basic question of why some parents batter their children while others under similar stress factors, do not.

Mental Illness Model

Delsordo (1963) has produced a helpful typology of abusive parents, similar to Merrill's categories that have been mentioned above. He identified five types of parents:

(1) Abuse resulting from 'parent's mental illness'.
(2) Abuse as 'an overflow from the parent's aimless way of life'.
(3) 'A non-specific disturbance in the parent, resulting in severe battering of the child'.
(4) Abuse due to 'parent's harshness in disciplining children'.
(5) Abuse due to 'parent's misplaced conflicts'.

Smith and his colleagues (Smith, 1975) have described in detail the psycho-social characteristics of parents who abused 134 battered children. In this study it was found that most parents were young and that abuse was associated with youthful parenthood. The parents were also poorly prepared for taking on the responsibility of rearing a dependent child. There was an infrequent occurrence of battering by older parents with large families, suggesting that child abuse diminished with parental age. Parents were also predominantly from the lower social classes. An important factor, closely paralleling the Family Structure Model mentioned above and underlying baby-battering, was a lack of family cohesiveness. In more than one-third of cases, the biological father was absent from the home and in half the cases, the mother was living with some other man. Half the mothers had married before the age of 20 years and three-quarters had conceived premaritally, such a combination being particularly likely to lead to marital breakdown. Other predictors of divorce included short acquaintance before marriage, disharmony in child-rearing, dissatisfaction with their partner's handling of the child, and neurotic and personality disorders. The evidence strongly suggested that battered children would eventually grow up in broken homes and also be at risk of social and educational maldevelopment. The rates of occurrence of premarital conception and illegitimacy were, respectively, two and three times higher than the general population rates and appeared to be important precursors of child abuse. Smith and his colleagues (1975) found this disturbing and highlighted the fact that this accorded with Resnick's (1969) data that showed that the inconvenience of an unwanted and illegitimate child is the most common motive responsible for child murder. Three-quarters of the mothers and two-thirds of the fathers had abnormal personalities. The less severe types of personality disturbance were more commonly found among the mothers who, in general, had features of emotional immaturity and dependence. Nearly half were of subnormal intelligence. In many cases, child abuse occurred as an ineffectual method of controlling a child's behaviour and techniques of teaching appropriate child-rearing skills based realistically on the mother's low intelligence, need to be applied as a method of correcting such ineffectual parental care. In contrast to the mothers, the fathers were of normal intelligence. One-third of them were psychopaths, a finding that contrasted strikingly with Kempe's (1969) generalisation that psychopathy is a feature in only 2 per cent of battering parents. Nearly one-third of the fathers (and a significant proportion of mothers) had criminal records, usually for larceny. Nine per cent of the fathers had committed crimes of violence and five per cent had been convicted for serious sexual offences. Recidivism was also a striking feature of child abusers. A fact that highlighted the capriciousness of the legal system towards parents who battered babies, was the finding that, although one-fifth of the battered children's siblings had also been previously abused, only one parent had been charged with cruelty or neglect. It appears clear, therefore, that criminality and recidivism, particularly if associated with a psychopathic personality disorder, should caution against an optimistic outcome and invoking a care order is essential if further battering incidents are to be prevented.

Another sub-group among the parents were those with neurotic illness, nearly half the mothers being in this group. The usual symptomatology present was an admixture of depression and anxiety. One-third reported having an unhappy childhood. Such neurotic mothers (in contrast to psychopathic fathers) confessed to harming their children and expressed a willingness to discuss their difficulties further. From a treatment point of view, such mothers will respond to symptomatic relief, combined with a programme of social learning.

Another separate and fortunately small group of parents were those with psychotic illness. These parents tend to inflict bizarre injuries, in keeping with their delusional and hallucinatory experiences, and their management must accordingly differ, and is that of their underlying mental illness.

Management of Child Abuse

The earliest response to child abuse—that followed the 'Mary Ellen case' in 1875 and persisted for some 70 years thereafter—was removal of the child from the home with occasional prosecution of the parents under Criminal Legislation. Over the past few years, however, Kempe and his colleagues introduced an orientation that assumed that baby-batterers were sick people in need of treatment and help, and that social workers, psychiatrists, and helping agencies had the knowledge to treat and cure such sickness. In the review of causative factors, mentioned above, it is clear that not all incidents of child abuse have a single set of aetiological factors and while some parents may indeed be ill, others may be quite normal and may merely follow a culturally acceptable child-rearing pattern—perhaps in a somewhat exaggerated manner because of situational stress. Mistakes occur by not recognising that many parents possess a type of personality deviation that is resistant to known methods of treatment.

Essentially, the aim of management is to ascertain the causes of family malfunction and overcome them. The dual aim underlying treatment is to protect the child and hopefully rehabilitate the parents. The emphasis on management must be to protect the child and accept that these two aims cannot always be reconciled.

Following an abuse incident, the child should be admitted to hospital. Hospitalisation takes the steam out of the situation and provides a safe place for the child. The family and siblings should be encouraged to visit the hospital as this will afford an opportunity to yield important information. Medical, nursing and social work staff involved in the assessment of a child-abuse situation require special understanding, tact, and skills in conducting interviews with the parents. Because of this, the author recommends a specialist hospital-based team, consisting of a paediatrician, a psychiatrist, a nurse, a social worker, and a psychologist, to achieve these aims. An initial confrontation with the parents often results in antagonism and removal of the child from hospital, with a failure to achieve crucial information that will assist in decision-making.

The physician's task is to obtain a detailed history from the parents, focusing on the child's developmental milestones and problem areas in parent–child interaction. The parent's method of child-rearing should be discussed. Injuries should be clearly described and recorded by photographs. It is important to exclude those rare conditions that may occasionally mimic child abuse by requesting haematological and biochemical investigations as well as skeletal surveys and other relevant tests. Information should also be sought from the family practitioner, other hospitals and police. Enquiries should be made from social agencies as to the child's possible previous involvement and whether there have been previous causes for concern. Child Abuse Registers, if available, should be searched for evidence of previous abuse. Serial electroencephalograms are helpful in monitoring the effects of head injury. Psychological testing will not only provide a baseline of the child's behaviour and intelligence level, but will assist in exploring parental claims that their child is 'difficult to handle'. The child's height and weight, accurately measured under standardised conditions, should be plotted on percentile charts.

Most parents, if skilfully handled, gain confidence and understanding of the specialised medical team's approach. When this stage is reached, the parents will relax sufficiently to allow for a detailed explanation of their family, marital and other problems. The psychiatrist, assisted by an experienced social worker, should arrive at a diagnosis with an understanding of the family dynamics, in a space of two or three weeks. Coupled with background information obtained from a variety of sources, immediate long-term management of the child and his family can then be planned. In approximately one-third of cases, a detailed psycho-diagnostic evaluation will establish that the likelihood of parents responding to treatment will be remote. In such cases, strong consideration must be given to permanent removal of the child from his parent's care. The paediatrician or psychiatrist, as leader of the medical team, should notify the Statutory Agency of his opinion and be prepared to provide written or oral evidence to substantiate his opinion. He should not shirk this important duty. Separating an abused child from his family is usually considered a last resort that is harmful to the 'therapeutic situation'. The converse is, however, often the case. Removal from a battering situation is usually beneficial, provided substitute foster care that provides adequately for the child's needs, can be obtained. Efforts should not be made to rehabilitate the parents at the expense of the safety of the child. This unfortunately frequently occurs. Supervision by social workers, whether it is voluntary or by Court Order, does not overcome the inherent difficulty in managing the hard-core group of cases—namely, that no supervisor can be with a child or his family for more than a fraction of the time. One needs to overcome a reluctance by medical and social welfare agencies to inform legal agencies that in their opinion the child should be removed. Such reluctance, which is often coupled with unilateral decision-making by a particular agency, deprives a child of his legal rights of protection.

Child abusers share a striking similarity with other behavioural deviants. If this is accepted, a great deal of disappointment and wasted effort in treating the phenomenon might be saved. Among child abusers there is a small nucleus of individuals who will be difficult or impossible to help. These are overlapped by a larger group, shading into the community as a whole, in which simple methods of treatment and support will be eminently satisfactory. Because there is no universal type of abusing parent, there is, of course, no one common cause or factor that needs to be eradicated. In many cases (approximately two-thirds), and with skilled help, child abusers can be managed by identifying and modifying those factors that cause and release their anger. Apart from the usual professional services—supportive individual or group psychotherapy, social case work and custodial treatments that have been reviewed elsewhere (Smith, 1975)—a number of community organisations have been established to help abusing parents. These include Mothers Anonymous, Homemaker Services, 24-Hour Life-Line Services and Parents' Aid. Such self-help groups, if provided with professional leadership and utilising carefully selected and trained volunteers, will provide an effective means of improving the relationship between the parents and their children, and of parents with each other. Many abusive parents can benefit from therapy, in terms of their own personality, their self-esteem, their capability to adapt to stress, and their ability to utilise people and agencies for their own needs. With support also, the parents' attitudes and behaviour towards their children can be substantially modified.

Prevention

The foregoing review has revealed that the professional approach to child abuse, these last three decades, has roughly followed a crude pattern of initial denial by the helping agencies, followed by a second phase of legal reform, centring around the passage of reporting laws. The third and current phase appears to be an emphasis on protective case work for victimised children and abusive parents. The author has recently detected a gradual awareness among helping professionals, that casework for many abusive parents may not be successful and that legislation is no better than its implementation. Indeed, the forcefulness of the law, which appears satisfactory in many quarters, is hindered in its implementation if the community lacks the appropriate resources.

Emphasis thus remains on treating the abused or neglected child and his parents after the act has occurred. The ideal aim of course, for which no substitute is currently available, is to prevent the initial abuse or neglect. High priority must therefore be given to the planning and creation of specific and imaginative programmes for prevention. Until this is achieved, the following initiatives should be planned for the prevention of child abuse.

(1) Society and parents must accept the responsibility that children have the right to grow and develop normally. Children in our society usually develop optimally as part of the family unit and society's efforts to prevent abuse may lie in the promotion of assisting the family as a whole. Solving society's ills—poverty, fear, loneliness, frustration, and emotional and social disorders—may go some way towards diminishing the tensions and stresses within the family unit. These adversities also give rise to numerous other social problems and unfortunately are not amenable to any easy solution.

There has been an increased emphasis on preventive services in Child Welfare Legislation since the early 1960s. Support services to parents and children including Day Care, Homemaker, Counselling and respite services, as well as encouragement and support of self-help groups have been increasingly developed and are becoming more widely used in different countries. The problem has been, however, one of delivering needed services to children and their families whether it be by government or voluntary agency. There has often been a fragmentation and over-lapping of re-sponsibilities and lack of co-ordination and integration of services. This has prevented substantial progress in the field.

(2) Measures that would result in more effective intervention and possible treatment of the abused child and his family need to be developed. There is a need to strengthen interdisciplinary co-operation and co-ordination in the education of allied health professionals working in this field.

(3) Social Services legislation in most developed countries pays but lip service to the topic of prevention of child abuse. Training in child-rearing, counselling, household management, services that provide relief to parents

when under stress, and emergency child care services in crises are important areas that need to be expanded and supported with funds. Developmental services should provide children with the opportunity to grow intellectually, socially, culturally, and physically and help parents who feel that provision of such services would reduce the likelihood of abuse or neglect. The promotion of community parent groups formed to provide self-help, child care courses, or social and recreational services for parents and/or children, should be encouraged.

(4) Wider dissemination of information to the general public as well as the helping professions needs to be expanded. The mass media might be used as an effective force for publicising and promoting 'good' family life as some television documentaries have already attempted to do.

(5) There needs to be increasing emphasis in our educational system on realistic and practical courses for young children, both male and female, in such subjects as child rearing and child care, family life, marriage, responsibilities of parenthood, homemaking and management of finances.

(6) The development of children's centres, offering health and social services including pre-natal care to pre-school children and their parents, that will provide for prevention, early detection and correction of medical and social problems, should be established.

Conclusion

Essentially, therefore, the diagnosis and treatment of child abuse may be a poor second-best to prevention of the problem. Parenthood and childhood are conditions of extraordinary needfulness and disability. The welfare of the total society depends on appropriate support to parents and children. The statutory agencies should not deal with the child abuser in the same way in which a child abuser deals with his child. The rendering of support services to a child-abusing family should be carried out in a way that does not entail any diminution of human dignity.

The author has sat on many committees and read a number of reports concerned with enquiries into the deaths of battered children. The familiar charge that society as a whole must bear the ultimate blame, has come through. In many cases, however, it is the professionals who have failed. The current political situation, promises of future legislation and improvements, carry little certainty. Because the day-to-day responsibility for children known to be at risk is nowadays generally in the hands of social workers, there needs to be improved communication between the professionals involved in the management of these difficult cases. Social work is a new and young profession and many social workers are recent entrants lacking both experience and confidence. The lesson learned from these unfortunate deaths has been that it is only too easy for an error in assessment to be made by an inexperienced observer, in whatever profession. The problem of the battered child is not solely a problem of welfare: it is a problem of health, welfare, the law, education, and social well-being. Leadership in this area must continue to come from the national level and encouragement to use Government Grants at the local level must be rigorously promoted by those in authority.

References

Anderson, J. (1976). Extent of the problem. In *Child Abuse and Neglect. A Report to the Canadian House of Commons.* Printing and Publishing Supply and Services, Ottawa, Canada

Caffey, J. (1946). Multiple fractures in the long bones of infants suffering from chronic subdural hematoma. *Am. J. Roentg. Rad. Ther. nucl. Med.*, **56**, 163–173

Cameron, J. M. (1970). The battered baby. *Br. J. Hosp. Med.*, **4**, 769–777

Cameron, J. M., Johnson, H. R. M. and Camp, F. I. (1966). The battered child syndrome. *Med. Sci. Law.*, **6**, 2–21

Delsordo, J. (1963). Protective casework for abused children. *Children*, **10**, 213–218

Fontana, V. J. (1971). *The Maltreated Child. The Maltreatment Syndrome in Children.* Charles C. Thomas, Springfield, Illinois

Galdston, R. (1965). Observations of children who have been physically abused and their parents. *Am. J. Psychiat.*, **122**, 440–443

Genieser, N. B. and Becker, M. H. (1974). Head trauma in children. *Radiol. Clinics N. America*, **12**, 333–342

Gil, D. G. (1970). *Violence against Children. Physical Abuse in the United States.* Harvard University Press, Massachusetts

Gilkes, M. J. and Mann, T. P. (1967). Fundi of battered babies. *Lancet*, **ii**, 468–469

Harcourt, B. and Hopkins, D. (1971). Ophthalmic manifestations of the battered baby syndrome. *Br. med. J.*, **III**, 398–401

Helfer, R. E. and Kempe, C. H. (Eds) (1968). *The Battered Child.* University of Chicago Press, Chicago

Justice, B. and Justice, R. (1976). *The Abusing Family.* Human Sciences Press, New York

Kempe, C. H. (1969). The battered child and the hospital. *Hosp. Pract.*, **4**, 44–57

Kempe, C. H. (1970). Quoted in Cameron, J. M. (1970). The battered baby syndrome. *Br. J. Hosp. Med.*, **4**, 769–777

Kempe, C. H. (1971). Pediatric implications of the battered baby syndrome. *Archs Dis. Childh.*, **46**, 28–37

Kempe, C. H. and Helfer, R. E. (Eds) (1972). *Helping the Battered Child and his Family.* J. B. Lippincott, Philadelphia and Toronto

Kempe, C. H., Silverman, F. N., Steele, B. S., Droegemuller, W. and Silver, H. K. (1962). The battered-child syndrome. *J. Am. med. Ass.*, **181**, 17–24

Kiffney, G. T., Jr. (1964). The eye of the battered child. *Archs Ophthal.*, **72**, 231–233

Lancet, (1971). Editorial. Violent parents. *Lancet*, **ii**, 1017–1018

Lindenberg, R. and Freytag, E. (1969). Morphology of brain lesions from blunt trauma in early infancy. *Archs Path.*, **87**, 298–305

Malinowski, B. (1927). *Sex and Repression in Savage Society.* Harcourt, Brace and World, New York

Maroteaux, P. and Lamy, M. (1967). Fundi of battered babies. *Lancet*, **ii**, 829

McCort, J. and Vaudagna, J. (1964). Visceral injuries in battered children. *Radiology*, **82**, 424–428

Mead, M. (1928). *Coming of Age in Samoa.* Morrow, New York

Merrill, E. J. (1962). Physical abuse of children. An agency study. In *Protecting the*

Battered Child (Ed. V. de Francis), Children's Division, American Humane Association, Denver, Colorado

Mushin, A. S. (1971). Ocular damage in the battered baby syndrome. *Br. Med. J.*, **III**, 402–404

Oliver, J. E. (1978). The extent of child abuse. In *Maltreatment of Children*. (Ed. S. M. Smith) Medical and Technical Pub. Co., Lancaster, University Park Press, Baltimore

Oliver, J. E., Cox, J., Taylor, A. and Baldwin, J. A. (1974). *Severely ill-treated young children in North-east Wiltshire*. Research Report No. 4. Oxford Record Linkage Study. Oxford Regional Health Authority

Resnick, P. J. (1969). Murder of the newborn: A psychiatric review of neonaticide. *Am. J. Psychiat.*, **126**, 1414–1420

Silverman, F. N. (1953). The roentgen manifestations of unrecognized skeletal trauma in infants. *Am. J. Roentg. Rad. Ther. nucl. Med.*, **69**, 413–426

Silverman, F. N. (1968). Radiologic aspects of the battered child syndrome. In *The Battered Child* (Ed. E. E. Helfer and C. H. Kempe), University of Chicago Press, Chicago

Smith, S. M. (1975). *The Battered Child Syndrome*. Butterworth, London

Steele, B. F. and Pollock, C. B. (1968). A psychiatric study of parents who abuse infants and small children. In *The Battered Child* (Ed. R. E. Helfer and C. H. Kempe), University of Chicago Press, Chicago

Woolley, P. W. and Evans, W. A. (1955). The significance of skeletal lesions in infants resembling those of traumatic origin, *J. Am. med. Ass.*, **158**, 539–43

12 Tardive Dyskinesia and Problems of Assessment

Thomas Barnes and Tim Kidger

Introduction

1. Background

Tardive dyskinesia (TD) is a movement disorder first described by Schonecker in 1957. Although spontaneous cases do occur it is most frequently a drug-induced phenomenon. The syndrome was slow to be recognised, partly perhaps because of the natural resistance of clinicians to accept any iatrogenic condition (Crane, 1973a). In addition TD was largely confined to psychotic patients in long-stay wards, probably the population attracting the least intensive medical involvement. Superficially the abnormal movements may resemble schizophrenic stereotypies and clinically the condition is easily overlooked especially as patients rarely complain spontaneously (Paulson, 1975).

Following the initial descriptions of the syndrome there was a progressive increase in both the number of cases reported and concern about such a frequent and persistent adverse drug effect (Crane, 1968). TD is now recognised as a valid diagnostic entity and a serious complication of anti-psychotic medication. It is a relatively late side effect, occurring after a minimum of 3–6 months' treatment, and most cases are identified only after at least 2 years' continuous medication (Faurbye *et al.*, 1964; Crane, 1973a). The condition is often exacerbated by neuroleptic withdrawal (Degkwitz *et al.*, 1966; Crane *et al.*, 1969) and was originally described as 'irreversible' (Hunter *et al.*, 1964; Crane, 1971b) but it is now generally accepted that following discontinuation of anti-psychotic drugs gradual improvement may occur in a proportion of patients (Crane, 1973b; Quitkin *et al.*, 1977).

2. Prevalence

Reviewing the literature Jus *et al.* (1976 *a*, *b*) found the reported prevalence of TD varied from 0.5 to 41.3 per cent. This discrepancy can be attributed to important variables in the patient populations studied, including:

(1) diagnosis;

(2) age;

(3) drug dosage and duration of administration; as well as

(4) the different methods used to obtain information; and

(5) difficulties in differentiation from other drug-induced motor disorders such as akathisia.

Perhaps the most important single factor contributing to this variation in incidence is the bias in clinical assessment. The syndrome is relatively ill defined, some workers including only patients with orofacial movements (Brandon *et al.*, 1971), while others employed broader diagnostic criteria. The difficulties we encountered in the development of a rating scale designed to overcome these problems and provide a standardised evaluation are discussed below.

In their own careful epidemiological study of 332 chronic schizophrenic in-patients treated with neuroleptics, Jus *et al.* (1976*a*, *b*) found an over-all prevalence of 56 per cent. They also investigated several of the patient factors previously suggested to be related to the prevalence of this condition such as:

(1) age;

(2) sex;

(3) type of schizophrenia and mode of onset;

(4) the presence or absence of organic syndromes; and

(5) the development of neuroleptic-induced extra-pyramidal syndromes.

They concluded that age was the only significant variable. In their sample, TD was diagnosed in approximately 40 per cent of patients under 49 years of age, 60 per cent of patients between 50 and 70 years of age and 75 per cent of patients over 70 years.

With regard to the role of neuroleptic drugs in high dosage their data led them to conclude that the total amount of neuroleptic administered, the type of neuroleptics and the mean duration of neuroleptic treatment were not directly related to the prevalence of TD. However, their idiosyncratic classification of neuroleptics and the failure to distinguish between depot and oral preparations leaves their findings open to criticism. The main positive finding was that the prevalence of TD is significantly increased when treatment begins at a higher age.

In our own recent epidemiological investigation (Kidger, Barnes, Taylor, unpublished) we studied two patient populations. The prevalence of TD in 65 chronic schizophrenic in-patients was 55 per cent while the corresponding figure for 130 schizophrenic out-patients regularly receiving a depot neuroleptic was 25 per cent.

3. Disability

A vast quantity of literature has been generated in the past few years regarding

TD and this reflects the concern among clinicians. Reasons for this intensive study of the condition include:

(1) the degree of disability to patients;

(2) the fact that, as there is at present no effective alternative to neuroleptic drug treatment for schizophrenia the condition would appear to be unavoidable;

(3) interest in the neurochemical mechanisms implicated, and

(4) the realisation, in America at least, that the development of TD may constitute a case for litigation.

Extreme cases exhibit gross abnormal movements and lack of muscle co-ordination which may lead to dyspnoea and cyanosis (Hunter *et al.*, 1964) and difficulty in swallowing (Schmidt and Jarcho, 1966). Involvement of trunk and limb movements can cause quite serious impairment of mobility. However, much of the disability related to TD is of a more subtle nature. Among the predominantly schizophrenic out-patient population the constant, often grotesque movements of the lips, cheeks, jaw and tongue present an obvious stigma of 'madness' and as such constitute a severe social handicap. The presence of these orofacial movements may, by causing embarrassment to family and friends and apprehension on the part of potential employers, hinder all efforts to improve the ability of these patients to function successfully within the community.

Clinical Features

1. The Classical Triad

Classical advanced TD presents no diagnostic problem. The most common abnormal movements of this syndrome are those of the face, masticating muscles, tongue and cheeks. The triad of cheek, tongue and jaw movements was referred to in early descriptions as the bucco-lingo-masticatory (BLM) syndrome. The movements themselves are referred to as chewing, lip pursing, cheek puffing, tongue protrusion and facial grimacing. The particular combination of movements varies considerably from patient to patient, but the character of the movements is consistent from day to day for each individual.

Although the so-called BLM triad is the most common presentation of TD, it is probably true to say that there is not a single voluntary muscle that cannot be involved in this condition. Hand and finger movements are quite often seen and can be distinguished from Parkinsonian tremor by their greater complexity, lower frequency and more irregular occurrence. Movements of the arm are involved and are commonly of a choreo-athetoid nature, although more sporadic complex movements do occur. Shoulder girdle movements often form part of a more complex intermittent arm-flapping movement involving muscles of the legs, trunk and arms. The neck is sometimes rhythmically flexed and extended in association with orofacial TD, but can be involved with the trunk, in gentle rocking movements. In some subjects the respiratory muscles can be involved, although it is not clear how much this may significantly embarrass respiration. Leg involvement sometimes causes choreo-athetoid movements, rhythmic tapping, or jigging of one or both legs. More complicated repetitive movements of the legs also occur, and are sometimes difficult to distinguish from akathisia. If this differentiation is a problem the correct diagnosis can sometimes be made by noting whether the movement is accompanied by a subjective sense of restlessness. If this is so akathisia is more likely. In addition simple sedation with benzodiazepines often reduces akathisic movements whereas dyskinetic movements are relatively unaffected. Reduction or cessation of neuroleptics characteristically exacerbates TD, but can reverse an akathisia.

2. Other Variants

There is contradictory evidence over the existence of 'sub syndromes' of TD. Jus *et al.* (1976 *a,b*) refer to four types of TD:

(1) choreo-athetoid;
(2) bucco-lingual;
(3) bucco-linguo-masticatory;
(4) 'rabbit syndrome'.

They claim very high inter-judge agreement in the allocation of patients to these categories. However, Brandon *et al.* (1971) considered the orofacial movements the 'core' of the syndrome, and other more peripheral movements, whilst constituting part of the syndrome, are not essential for the diagnosis.

Brandon *et al.* (1971) also commented on the gradation of severity of abnormal movements in TD with no definite 'cut-off' point. Jus *et al.* (1973) were able, by recording electromyographic changes in orofacial muscles, to detect abnormal movements in patients who appeared clinically normal. They claim that their method is: more sensitive; able to pick up obscured tongue movements and able to record the amplitude, frequency, rhythmicity and site of movements simultaneously. Unfortunately the procedure is elaborate and therefore more suitable for the detailed study of small numbers of patients, rather than for routine clinical or epidemiological studies.

Very little work has been reported on the early signs of TD. It is clinically very difficult to decide—for example—whether an infrequent, apparently purposeless lip pursing movement is a manifestation of TD. The threshold for the diagnosis varies from observer to observer, and that may account for some of the discrepancies in results from different workers.

3. Factors Altering the Severity of TD

Although the characteristics of dyskinetic movements tend to be fairly constant from day to day in each individual, the frequency and amplitude of the movements can vary considerably and some exacerbating and relieving factors have now been identified. The most common precipitant of TD is the reduction of dose of neuroleptic in a patient who has been receiving this drug continuously. There is usually a sudden appearance or worsening of movements, followed by a gradual subsidence. The degree of recovery is variable and often incomplete. There is a suggestion (Allen and Stimmel, 1977) that the rate and completeness of recovery is related to the duration of previous neuroleptic treatment. This pattern of exacerbation and then gradual subsidence of signs may account for spurious 'cures' in studies where neuroleptics are discontinued immediately before the study is commenced. A crossover design would seem the obvious method of overcoming this difficulty.

The use of anticholinergic drugs may precipitate, and certainly exacerbates TD. This may be either a drug interaction leading to a lowering of neuroleptic levels in the blood, or a direct effect on dopaminergic – cholinergic balance within the nigrostriatal system.

Substances other than neuroleptics have been reported to cause TD. Among them are tricyclic antidepressants (Fann et al., 1976) and anticonvulsants (Chadwick et al., 1976).

As will be discussed later, if the dosage of neuroleptic is increased, the signs of TD will diminish. Lowering the dose of anticholinergics has the same effect.

Several psychological factors have been observed to modify the severity of the dyskinetic movements. These are more pronounced when the patient is anxious, concentrating or moving another body part. Brandon et al. (1971) reported a marked increase in movements during the phase of clouded consciousness soon after waking to the extent that in some cases this clarified a doubtful diagnosis. The movements stop completely during REM sleep (Jus et al.,1973).

Problems of Assessment

When assessing a patient one usually requires to discover two things. First, if the disease is present; and secondly, if it is, how severe it is.

1. Diagnosis

The assessment of infrequent minor movements in patients at risk is difficult. There has been little research on how much seemingly purposeless movement occurs in normal individuals. Patients receiving neuroleptics may move more than normals because of Parkinsonian tremor, acute dystonia, akathisia or

TD. Tremor is easily distinguished (see above) and acute dystonias are usually recognisable by their more dramatic nature and rapid response to anticholinergic medication. Akathisia may produce diagnostic difficulties and methods of overcoming these are also outlined above. In our recent investigation we videotaped both patients who have been exposed to neuroleptics and control patients matched for age and sex. We found that the normals made very few apparently purposeless movements in our standardised situation and that even small infrequent movements were much commoner in our neuroleptic-exposed group. This leads us to believe that, in the standardised situation to be described below, small, infrequent, apparently purposeless movements may be considered as abnormal.

2. Assessment of Severity

When a diagnosis of TD has been made the problem of assessing improvement or worsening of the movements over a period arises. This is of particular importance when a possible treatment for TD is being evaluated.

Several rating scales for TD have been quoted—almost one for each research team. Most of them record the amplitude, frequency and site of each movement during a standard time interval. This can be assessed visually and recorded on videotape, or via EMG recording apparatus attached to the affected muscles. In addition one patient's jaw movements were recorded via a pressure transducer attached to a balloon within the mouth. Very sophisticated techniques have recently been reported by Fann *et al.* (1977) involving complex computer assisted analysis of vocal function and arm movements. The complexity of apparatus, however, makes these techniques only suitable for highly specialised research departments.

3. The Problems of Rating Scales

Most of these methods produce an accurate, fairly detailed record of the movements and it is usually easy to 'eye ball' gross changes in the severity of the movements. However, difficulties arise when patients have to be compared as this requires the extraction of a TD score for each individual, and the validity of various techniques, for example adding frequency scores for movements in separate sites, is questionable. We are at present attempting a factor analysis of three rater assessments of 190 videotaped patients to determine how a total TD score might be determined. The rating scale used is similar to those of other workers and gives measures of amplitude and frequency of movements in nine body sites, each on a four-point scale. Tremor in each site is assessed separately (table 12.1).

4. Controlling Variables that Alter TD

As the severity of TD is so sensitive to the current pharmacological status of

Table 12.1
System for recording movements in tardive dyskinesia

	Lips	Cheeks	Tongue	Jaw	Neck	Trunk	Arms	Hands	Legs
Frequency									
Amplitude									
Tremor									

Amplitude 0 = Absent
             1 = Movement just perceptible at that site
             2 = Moderate movement at that site
             3 = Maximum movement possible at that site

Frequency 0 = Less than 3 movements per minute
             1 = 3 or more movements per minute but movement present less than
                 half of time
             2 = Movement present more than half of time
             3 = Continuous movement

All apparently purposeless movements should be rated. Tremor should be rated
separately at each site:
             0 = Absent
             1 = Fine
             2 = Medium
             3 = Coarse

the patient it is important that this be taken into account during the
assessment. One would predict that as blood levels of neuroleptics and
anticholinergics vary the severity of TD will vary also. This is of particular
importance in patients receiving depot neuroleptics as a patient reassessed 4
days after a monthly injection may have fewer movements than at an
assessment immediately before the injection merely because neuroleptic levels
are higher and the disorder therefore suppressed. The exacerbation and then
gradual improvement which occurs when neuroleptics are withdrawn may
simulate a satisfactory response to a potential treatment substituted after
stopping neuroleptic medication. It is therefore essential, if involved in an
investigation, to ensure that neuroleptic and anticholinergic dosages have not
been recently changed. There is evidence that a change of either can upset the
equilibrium of blood neuroleptic levels for at least 12 weeks (Jus *et al.*, 1977).

As has already been mentioned the patient's mental set, degree of
concentration, physical activity and level of consciousness all affect the
severity of TD. To overcome this we have devised a standardised assessment
procedure. This is quick, simple and requires no special apparatus. The
patient sits in a straight-backed chair. Hands and mouth must be empty and
the patient is asked if he is wearing dentures. A sample of standard prose
(Schonnell No. R2) is supported on a stand in front of the patient in such a
way as not to obscure any part of the body. The patient is asked to read
through the prose to himself and warned that he will be asked some questions
about it afterwards. The patient is assessed for 1 minute—either by a rater

present at the time, or by videotape in a standardised manner (30 seconds close-up head and neck and then 30 seconds whole body). All movements that have no apparent purpose that occur during this time are recorded in the manner outlined above. We have found that a normal population move very little during this procedure relative to a neuroleptic-exposed population. We disregarded the answers to the questions asked after the standard reading period.

We have found that this method makes close scrutiny of patients possible while controlling mental set, degree of concentration, level of consciousness and physical activity as far as possible. We believe that discrimination between normal and abnormal movements is very much easier in this setting (Kidger, Barnes, Taylor—material in preparation).

Neurochemical Mechanisms

1. Dopaminergic Theory

TD is thought to be related to dopaminergic mechanisms by analogy with both Huntington's chorea and L-dopa induced dyskinesias in patients with Parkinson's disease. In addition the condition may be directly observed in association with long-term neuroleptic therapy.

Antipsychotic drugs, comprising predominantly members of the phenothiazine, butyrophenone and diphenylbutylpiperidine groups are known to increase intracerebral dopamine turnover. This phenomenon is considered to be a compensatory mechanism to the postsynaptic dopamine receptor blocking action of these drugs. This receptor blockade is effectively a chemical denervation. It is postulated that prolonged denervation, within the nigro-striatal system at least, leads to postsynaptic receptor hypersensitivity (Klawans, 1973 a). These sensitised receptors may then respond abnormally to small amounts of dopamine that reach them. TD is thought to be the motor manifestation of this abnormal response.

There is indirect evidence to support this hypothesis. For patients receiving long-term neuroleptic therapy, withdrawal of the drug may precipitate or worsen the condition (Degkwitz et al., 1966). This may be understood as an intense response of the hypersensitive receptor when exposed to normal levels of dopamine by removal of the receptor blockade. Conversely increasing the dose of neuroleptic may temporarily improve the movement disorder by preventing any stimulation of the receptor. This produces a paradoxical situation whereby a drug found to ameliorate the disorder is the same or pharmacologically similar to that which led to its development. However, it seems that the increased blockade induces further receptor hypersensitivity and the condition recurs (Kazamatsuri et al., 1972b). Increasing the dose of neuroleptic is therefore not considered appropriate therapy as it tends to lead to an escalating dosage situation.

Further evidence that TD reflects dopaminergic hyperactivity is the observation that administration of the dopamine precursor L-dopa worsens the condition, while α-methyl-p-tyrosine (AMPT) which reduces catecholamine synthesis, produces a marked improvement (Gerlach et al., 1974). In addition the dyskinetic movements produced by L-dopa in patients with Parkinson's disease are similar to those of TD. It has been suggested that these movements may also be related to the development of denervation hypersensitivity of striatal dopaminergic receptors. In this case the hypersensitivity follows nigrostriatal pathway degeneration rather than chemical denervation. Klawans (1973b) argues that a significant dopamine receptor denervation and subsequent hypersensitivity must occur before dyskinesias are induced by L-dopa. Nigrostriatal degeneration is known to accompany the ageing process and this fact may help to account for the observation that, in response to neuroleptic therapy, the older brain seems to be more susceptible to the development of TD; the young brain being apparently more susceptible to the development of acute dystonic reactions.

2. Dopaminergic – Cholinergic Balance

It is known that manipulation of the cholinergic system influences these movement disorders and, increasingly, emphasis has been put on the state of balance between the dopaminergic and cholinergic systems as highly relevant to their emergence (Klawans and Rubovits, 1974; Gerlach et al., 1974, Tamminga et al., 1977). Thus reduced cholinergic activity as well as increased dopaminergic activity may result in the relative dopaminergic dominance with which TD is associated. In this respect TD may be thought of as reciprocal in pathophysiology to Parkinson's disease, in which there is a functional dopamine deficiency and thus a relative cholinergic dominance within the nigrostriatal system and basal ganglia. The two conditions have been reported to co-exist in three patients (Fann and Lake, 1974). It was found that the symptoms of TD were exacerbated by treatment of their Parkinson's disease and vice versa.

Logical application of these ideas has led to therapeutic attempts with various drugs. Physostigmine, a centrally acting anticholinesterase known to increase brain acetylcholine concentration, has been shown to produce improvement in some patients with TD (Fann et al., 1974; Gerlach et al.,1974). There have also been reports of beneficial effects with administration of deanol, an agent also assumed to increase the amount of brain acetylcholine (Tamminga et al., 1977). Choline, the physiological precursor of acetylcholine, has also been tried with some limited therapeutic success (Growdon et al., 1977; Davis et al., 1976) although, unfortunately, the patients developed a strong 'fishy' odour which may mean that this treatment would merely succeed in substituting one social disadvantage for another.

It is generally agreed that anticholinergic drugs worsen or even induce tardive dyskinesia (Crane, 1968; Klawans, 1973a) and orofacial dyskinesia has been reported in association with anticholinergic drugs alone (Birket-Smith,1974). At least two anticholinergic drugs, biperiden and scopolamine, have been shown to aggravate TD movements (Klawans and Rubovits, 1974; Gerlach *et al.*, 1974).

Treatment Approaches

1. Prevention and Early Detection

There are several simple ways in which it is hoped TD can be either prevented or detected at an early stage. The risks of long-term neuroleptic drug use must be weighed against the benefits. The relatively high risk of TD must bring into question the use of neuroleptics in the treatment of neurotic disorders.

No studies to date have been able to demonstrate conclusively that duration, dosage, or identity of a neuroleptic is directly related to the appearance of TD. However, it seems advisable, on common-sense grounds, to keep the dose of neuroleptic to a minimum when it is necessary to give it on a long-term basis, especially in the aged who have been shown to be more susceptible to this disorder.

It is now well established that there is no place for the *routine* administration of antiparkinsonian drugs with long-term neuroleptic therapy. It has been suggested that these drugs should only be initiated if signs of parkinsonism or dystonia occur, and that they should be reassessed after 3 months. It has been found that about 90 per cent of patients receiving routine anticholinergics on a long-term basis can safely be withdrawn from them (Klett *et al.*, 1972). As anticholinergic drugs can both cause and exacerbate TD, the withdrawal of these drugs in patients who show signs of TD seems particularly necessary.

One of the easiest methods of ensuring early detection and possible prevention of some cases of TD is the so-called 'drug holiday' (American College of Neuropsychopharmacology—Food and Drug Administration Task Force, 1973; Crane, 1973a). This entails cessation of all neuroleptic drugs for 1–2 months. This is, hopefully, too short a time for psychotic relapse to occur and if TD is developing the movements will become more noticeable aiding the diagnosis of early cases. It is also hoped that by re-establishing stimulation of the dopamine receptor this may prevent, or reverse, developing denervation hypersensitivity.

2. Drug Therapy of Tardive Dyskinesia

There is no satisfactory method of treating TD. The dopaminergic de-nervation hypersensitivity hypothesis has proved heurisitic, and many drugs that alter the cholinergic–dopaminergic balance have been investigated in this disorder. There are also a large number of substances that do not directly alter either cholinergic or dopaminergic function that have been tried in some patients.

(i) Drugs Affecting Dopaminergic Function

It is now accepted that drugs that reduce stimulation of the dopaminergic postsynaptic receptor diminish the signs of TD. Some authors have recommended this as a means of treatment (Degkwitz and Wenzel,1976; Kennedy, 1969; Roxburgh, 1970; Carruthers, 1971; Haddenbrock, 1964). However, this approach is only suppressive and not curative. The movements tend to eventually reappear, necessitating further dosage increases until a ceiling is reached when further dosage increments fail to suppress movements. This can be compared to treating delirium tremens with alcohol!

Drugs that deplete striatal dopamine have the same effects as dopamine receptor blockade in this disease. They are subject to the same criticism of being suppressive rather than curative. These include: reserpine, tetrabenazine, oxypertine and α-methyldopa. (table 12.2).

Table 12.2
Dopamine depletors used in the treatment of tardive dyskinesia

Name	Reference
Reserpine	Schmidt and Jarcho (1966)
	Villeneuve and Böszörmenyi (1970a)
	Sato et al. (1971)
	Carroll et al. (1977)
Tetrabenazine	Brandrup (1961)
	McCallum (1970)
	Godwin-Austin and Clark (1971)
	Kazamatsuri et al. (1972a)
	Pakkenberg and Fog (1974)
Oxypertine	Eckmann (1968)
α-Methyldopa	Villeneuve and Böszörmenyi (1970a)
	Villeneuve (1970b)
	Viukari and Linnoila (1975)
	Kazamatsuri et al. (1972c)

Some neuroleptic drugs have been singled out for assessment in the suppression of TD. The efficacy of each drug probably only reflects its relative dopamine blocking potency and intrinsic anticholinergic activity. Drugs in this group include: pimozide, thioproperazine, haloperidol, clozapine, thioridazine, and papaverine (table 12.3).

More recently a paradoxical improvement in TD was noticed in patients given the dopamine agonists apomorphine and L-dopa. This curious finding may be due to stimulation of dopaminergic presynaptic receptors which inhibit dopamine release (Carroll et al., 1977). If this effect is replicated this may open an avenue of research into the treatment of TD.

(ii) Drugs Affecting Cholinergic Function

As commented on above, anticholinergic drugs worsen TD and should therefore be reconsidered and if possible, stopped in patients with this disorder.

Table 12.3
Dopamine receptor blockers used in the treatment of tardive dyskinesia

Name	References
Pimozide	Pakkenberg and Fog (1974)
	Claveria *et al.* (1975)
Thiopropazate	Singer and Cheng (1971)
and /or Perphenazine	Schmidt and Jarcho (1966)
	Roxburgh (1970)
	Kazamatsuri *et al.* (1972*b*)
	Rosin and Exton-Smith (1965)
	Carruthers (1971)
	Uhrbrand and Faurbye (1960)
	Wertheimer (1965)
Thioproperazine	Bourgeois and Hébert (1970)
Chlorpromazine	Kennedy (1969)
Haloperidol	Kazamatsuri *et al.* (1972*b*)
	Kazamatsuri *et al.* (1973)
	Gilbert (1969)
Clozapine	Simpson and Varga (1974)
	Carroll *et al.* (1977)
Thioridazine	Kobayashi (1976)
	Linden (1977)
	Carroll *et al.* (1977)
Papaverine	Gardos *et al.* (1976)

Several workers have recently investigated substances for cholinergic enhancing activity. As TD is considered to be a disease of relative dopaminergic dominance with cholinergic hypofunction, the augmentation of cholinergic activity should redress the balance and diminish dyskinetic movements. This has been found to be the case.

Physostigmine, a central acetylcholinesterase inhibitor, has been given to patients with beneficial results (Klawans and Rubovits, 1974; Gerlach *et al.*, 1974; Tarsy *et al.*, 1974; Tamminga *et al.*, 1977; Fann *et al.*, 1974). However, as this drug has to be given intravenously, it is unsuitable for clinical use.

Deanol, a possible precursor of acetylcholine has been used in patients with TD. After some initial enthusiasm it now seems likely that any improvement produced by this substance is probably short-lived (Widroe and Heisler, 1976; Bockenheimer and Lucius, 1976; Kumar, 1976; Mehta *et al.*, 1976; Casey and Denney, 1975; Casey, 1977; Davis *et al.*, 1977; DeSilva and Huang, 1975; Miller, 1974; Escobar and Kemp, 1975; Crane, 1975; Carroll *et al.*, 1977; Tamminga *et al.*, 1977).

More recently, choline, an acetylcholine precursor, has shown encouraging results in some trials (Davis *et al.*, 1975; Tamminga *et al.*, 1977; Hirsch *et al.*, 1977). Wurtman *et al.* (1977) have found that serum-free choline levels can be more efficiently raised with oral lecithin, and this substance may therefore warrant further investigation.

(iii) Other Drugs Investigated in the Treatment of TD

The variety of drugs that have been given to treat TD is bewildering. Space does not permit an analysis of the merits of each one, but it is probably fair to say that none has proved to have effects superior to those of the preparations already mentioned.

The list of non-dopaminergic–cholinergic drugs so far investigated includes: manganese and niacin, cyproheptadine, diazepam, amantidine, pyridoxine, penicillamine, 5-hydroxytryptophan, L-tryptophan, MAOIs, AMPT, lithium, melanocyte stimulating hormone release inhibiting factor I, clonazepam, valproate and lioresal (table 12.4).

Table 12.4
Miscellaneous drugs used in the treatment of tardive dyskinesia

Name	References
Manganese and niacin	Kunin (1976)
Cyproheptadine	Goldman (1976)
Diazepam	Singh (1976)
Amantidine	Merren (1972)
	Pearce (1971)
	Dynes (1970)
	Crane (1971*a*)
	Vale and Espejel (1971)
	Decker *et al.* (1971)
Pyridoxine	Paulson (1971)
	Dynes (1970)
	Crane *et al.* (1970)
Penicillamine	Greenblatt *et al.* (1970)
5-Hydroxytryptophan	Guilleminault *et al.* (1973)
L-Tryptophan	Prange *et al.* (1973)
MAOIs	Bucci (1971)
α -Methyl-*p*-tyrosine (AMPT)	Gerlach *et al.* (1974)
Lithium	Reda *et al.* (1974)
	Dalen (1973)
	Simpson *et al.* (1976)
Melanocyte stimulating hormone release inhibiting factor I	Ehrensing *et al.* (1977)
Clonazepam	O'Flanagan (1975)
	Sedman (1976)
Valproate	Linnoila *et al.* (1976)
Lioresal	Korsgaard (1976)

2. Treatments Not Involving Additional Pharmacological Agents

The earliest and most obvious treatment attempted for TD was the withdrawal of the neuroleptic drug being administered. As mentioned above this causes an exacerbation of the dyskinetic movements and then a gradual improvement. The recovery is often incomplete; however, at present this is the only hope of truly 'curing' TD (Ayd, 1970).

It is now accepted that anticholinergic agents worsen TD as mentioned above and these agents should be withdrawn if possible.

It has been noticed that patients with TD tend to be more often edentulous than unaffected individuals (Pryce and Edwards, 1966), and it has been suggested that lack of dentures may enhance the abnormal movements (Joyston-Bechal, 1965). Ill-fitting dentures have even been thought to cause dyskinetic movements in some patients not receiving neuroleptics (Sutcher *et al.*, 1971). It seems sensible therefore to provide well-fitting dentures to affected patients whenever possible, although Brandon *et al.* (1971) have suggested that the movements may prevent the retention of dentures and that this may account for the high proportion of edentulous patients seen in the TD population.

Electromyographic feedback techniques have been reported to improve orofacial dyskinesia (Farrar, 1976) but this needs further evaluation.

Neurosurgical measures have helped some patients (Nashold, 1969), but this must be considered a treatment for severely afflicted patients who have not responded to other forms of therapy.

Summary

(1) Patients receiving long-term neuroleptic therapy run a high risk of developing TD.

(2) This condition may produce both physical and social handicap.

(3) Anticholinergic drugs are known to cause exacerbation of TD and their routine use is thought to be associated with its development.

(4) There is no satisfactory treatment for this movement disorder; however, the introduction of 'drug holidays' should aid early detection and may have some prophylactic value.

(5) Assessment of TD is difficult and the patient's recent drug therapy, mental set and the circumstances of the assessment should all be taken into account.

References

Alien, R. E. and Stimmel, G. L. (1977). Neuroleptic dosage, duration and T.D. *Dis. Nerv. Syst.*, **38**, 385–387

American College of Neuropsychopharmacology – Food and Drug Administration Task Force (1973). Neurologic syndromes associated with anti-psychotic drug use. *New Engl. J. Med.*, **289**, 20–23

Ayd, F. J., Jr. (1970). Prevention of recurrence (maintenance therapy). *Clinical Handbook of Psychopharmacology* (Ed. A. DiMascio and R. I. Schader), Science House, New York, pp. 297–310

Birket-Smith, E. (1974). Abnormal involuntary movements induced by anticholinergic therapy. *Acta neurol. scand.*, **50**, 801–811

Bockenheimer, S. and Lucius, G. (1976). Zer Therapie mit Dimethyl Aminoethanol (Deanol) bei Neuroleptikain Duzierten Extrapyramidalen Hyperkinesen. *Arch. Psychiat.*, **222**, 69–75

Bourgeois, M. and Herbert, A. (1970). Les Dyskinesies Tardives des Neuroleptiques. *Bord. Med.*, **3**, 345–352

Brandon, S., McClelland, H. A. and Protheroe, C. (1971). A study of facial dyskinesia in a mental hospital population. *Br. J. Psychiat.*, **118**, 171–184

Brandrup, E. (1961). Tetrabenazine treatment in persisting dyskinesia caused by psychopharmaca. *Am. J. Psychiat.*, **118**, 551–552

Bucci, L. (1971). The dyskinesias: a new therapeutic approach. *Dis. Nerv. Syst.*, **32**, 324–327

Carroll, B. J., Curtis, G. C. and Kokmen, E. (1977). Paradoxical response to dopamine agonists in tardive dyskinesia. *Am. J. Psychiat.*, **134**(7), 785–789

Carruthers, S. G. (1971). Persistent tardive dyskinesia. *Br. Med. J.*, **3**, 572

Casey, D. E. (1977). Deanol: a survey of opinions by experts. *Convulsive Ther. Bull.*, **2**(3), 50–51

Casey, D. E. and Denney, D. (1975). Deanol in the treatment of T.D. *Am. J. Psychiat.*, **132**, 8

Chadwick, D., Reynolds, E. H. and Marsden, C. D. (1976). Anticonvulsant induced dyskinesias: a comparison with dyskinesias induced by neuroleptics. *J. Neurol. Neurosurg. Psychiat.*, **39**, 1210–1218

Claveria, L. E., Teychenne, P. F., Caine, D. B. *et al.* (1975). Tardive dyskinesia treated with pimozide *J. neurol. Sci.*, **24**, 393–401

Crane, G. E. (1968). T.D. in patients treated with major neuroleptics. *Am. J. Psych.*, **124** (Suppl.), 40–48

Crane, G. E. (1971*a*). More on amantidine in tardive dyskinesia. *New Engl. J. Med.*, **285**, 1150–1151

Crane, G. E. (1971*b*). Persistence of neurological symptoms due to neuroleptic drugs. *Am. J. Psychiat.*, **127**, 1407–1410

Crane, G. E. (1973*a*). Persistent dyskinesia. *Br. J. Psychiat.*, **122**, 395–405

Crane, G. E. (1973*b*). Rapid reversal of tardive dyskinesia. *Am. J. Psychiat.*, **130**, 1159

Crane, G. E. (1975). Deanol for tardive dyskinesia. *New Engl. J. Med.*, **292**, 926–928

Crane, G. E., Ruiz, P., Kernohan, W. J., *et al.* (1969). Effects of drug withdrawal in tardive dyskinesia. *Activitas nerv. sup.*, **11**, 30–35

Crane, G. E., Turek, I. S. and Kurland, A. A. (1970). Failure of pyridoxine to reduce drug-induced dyskinesias. *J. Neurol. Neurosurg. Psychiat.*, **33**, 511–512

Dalen, P. (1973). Lithium therapy in Huntington's chorea and tardive dyskinesia. *Lancet*, **i**, 107–108

Davis, K. L., Berger, P. A. and Hollister, L. E. (1975). Choline for tardive dyskinesia. *New Engl. J. Med.*, **293**, 152

Davis, K. L., Berger, P. A. and Hollister, L. E. (1977). Deanol in tardive dyskinesia. *Am. J. Psychiat.*, **134**, 807

Davis, K. L., Hollister, L. E., Barchas, J. D., *et al.* (1976). Choline in T.D. and Huntington's disease. *Life Sci.*, **19**, 1507–1516

Decker, B. L., Davis, J. M., Janowsky, D. S., *et al.* (1971). Amantidine hydrochloride treatment of tardive dyskinesia. *New Engl. J. Med.*, **285**, 860

Degkwitz, R. and Wenzel, W. (1976). Persistent extrapyramidal side effects after long term application of neuroleptics. *Neuropsychopharmacology* (International Congress series 129)

Degkwitz, R., Wenzel, W., Binsack, K. F., Herkert, H. and Luxenburger, O. (1966). Zum Probleme Der Terminalen Extrapyramidalen Hyperkinesen an Hand von 1600 Langfristig mit Neuroleptica Behandelten. *Artzneimittel Forschung*, **16**, 276–278

DeSilva, L. and Huang, C. Y. (1975). Deanol in tardive dyskinesia. *Br. med. J.*, **3**, 466

Dynes, J. B. (1970). Oral dyskinesias, occurrence and treatment. *Dis. Nerv. Syst.*, **31**, 854–859

Eckmann, F. (1968). Zur Problematik von Dauerschaden nach neuroleptischer langzeit Behandelung. *Ther. Ggw.*, **107**, 316–323

Ehrensing, R. H., Kastin, A. H., Larsons, P. F. and Bishop, G. A. (1977). Melanocyte-stimulating-hormone-release-inhibiting-factor I and tardive dyskinesia. *Dis. Nerv. Syst.*, **38**(4), 303–307

Escobar, J. I. and Kemp, K. F. (1975). Dimethylaminoethanol for tardive dyskinesia. *New Engl. J. Med.*, **292**, 317–318

Fann, W. and Lake, C. R. (1974). On the coexistence of parkinsonism and tardive dyskinesia. *Dis. Nerv. Syst.*, **35**, 324–326

Fann, W., Lake, C. R., Gerber, C. J. *et al.* (1974). Cholinergic suppression of tardive dyskinesia. *Psychopharmacologia*, **37**, 101–107

Fann, W., Lake, C. R. and McKenzie, G. M. (1974). Proceedings: adrenergic and cholinergic factors in extrapyramidal disorders. *Psychopharmac. Bull.*, **10**(3), 52–53

Fann, W., Stafford, J. R., Malone, R. L., Frost, J. D. and Richman, B. W. (1977). Clinical research techniques in tardive dyskinesia. *Am. J. Psychiat.*, **134**(7), 759–762

Fann, W. E., Sullivan, J. L. and Richman, B. W. (1976). Dyskinesias associated with tricyclic antidepressants. *Br. J. Psychiat.*, **128**, 490–493

Farrar, W. B. (1976). Using electromyographic biofeedback in treating orofacial dyskinesia. *J. Prosthet. Dent.*, **35**, 384–387

Faurbye, A., Rasch, P. J., Peterson, P. B., Brandborg, G. and Pakkenberg, H. (1964). Neurological symptoms in pharmacotherapy of psychoses. *Acta psychiat. scand.*, **40**, 10–27

Gardos, G., Cove, J. O. and Sniffen, C. (1976). An evaluation of papaverine in tardive dyskinesia. *J. clin. Pharmac.*, **16**, 304–310

Gerlach, J., Reisby, N. and Randup, A. (1974). Dopaminergic hypersensitivity and cholinergic hypofunction in the pathophysiology of tardive dyskinesia. *Psychopharmacologia (Berl.)*, **34**, 21–35

Gilbert, M. M. (1969). Haloperidol in severe facial dyskinesia. *Dis. Nerv. Syst.*, **30**, 481–482

Godwin-Austin, R. B. and Clark, T. (1971). Persistent phenothiazine dyskinesia treated with tetrabenazine. *Br. med. J.*, **4**, 25–26

Goldman, D. (1976). Treatment of phenothiazine-induced dyskinesia. *Psychopharmacology*, **47**, 271–272

Greenblatt, D. L., Shader, R. I. and DiMascio, A. (1970). Extra-pyramidal effects. In *Psychotropic Drug Side Effects* (Ed. R. I. Shader and A. DiMascio) Williams and Wilkins Co., Baltimore, pp. 92–106

Growden, J. H., Hirsch, M. J., Wurtman, R. J. and Wiener, W. (1977). Oral choline administration to patients with tardive dyskinesia. *New Engl. J. Med.*, **297**, 524–527

Guilleminault, C., Tharp, B. R. and Cousin, D. (1973). HVA + 5HIAA CSF measurements and 5HTP trials in some patients with involuntary movements. *J. neurol. Sci.*, **18**, 435–441

Haddenbrock, S. (1964). Hyperkinetische Dauersyndrome nach hochdosierter und lang Streckerbehandlung mit Neuroleptika. In *Begreiterscheinungen und Misserfolge der Psychiatrischen Pharmakotherapie* (Ed. H. Kranz and K. Heinrich), Georg Thieme, Stuttgart, pp. 54–63

Hirsch, M. J., Growdon, J. H. and Wurtman, R. J. (1977). Oral choline administration to patients with tardive dyskinesia. *Meeting of American Academy of Neurology*

Hunter, R., Earl, C. J. and Thornicroft, S. (1964). An apparently irreversible syndrome of abnormal movements following phenothiazine medication. *Proc. R. Soc. Med.*, **57**, 758–762

Joyston-Bechal, M. P. (1965). Persistent oral dyskinesia in treatment with phenothiazine derivatives. *Lancet*, i, 600–601

Jus, A., Pineau, R., Lachance, R., Pelchat, G., Jus, K., Pires, P. and Villeneuve, R. (1976*a*). Epidemiology of tardive dyskinesia, Part I. *Dis. Nerv. Syst.*, May, 210–214

Jus, A., Pineau, R., Lachance, R., Pelchat, G., Jus, K., Pires, P. and Villeneuve, R. (1976*b*). Epidemiology of tardive dyskinesia, Part II. *Dis. Nerv. Syst.*, May, 257–261

Jus, A., Gautier, J., Villeneuve, A., Jus, K., Pires, P. and Gagnon-Binette, M. (1977). Chronology of combined neuroleptic and antiparkinsonian administration. *Am. J. Psychiat.*, **134**, 1157

Jus, K., Jus, A. and Villeneuve, A. (1973). Polygraphic profile of oral tardive dyskinesia and of rabbit syndrome for quantitative and qualitative evaluation. *Dis. Nerv. Syst.*, **34**, 27–32

Kazamatsuri, H., Chien, C. and Cole, J. O. (1972a). Treatment of tardive dyskinesia I. Clinical efficacy of a dopamine depleting agent tetrabenazine. *Archs gen. Psychiat.*, **27**, 95–99

Kazamatsuri, H., Chien, C. and Cole, J. O. (1972b). Treatment of tardive dyskinesia II. Short term efficacy of dopamine-blocking agents haloperidol and thiopropazate. *Archs gen. Psychiat.*, **27**, 100–103

Kazamatsuri, H., Chien, C. and Cole, J. O. (1972c). Treatment of tardive dyskinesia III. Clinical efficacy of a dopamine competing agent, methyl dopa. *Archs gen. Psychiat.*, **27**, 824–827

Kazamatsuri, H., Chien, C. and Cole, J. O. (1973). Long-term treatment of tardive dyskinesia with haloperidol and tetrabenazine. *Am. J. Psychiat.*, **130**, 479–483

Kennedy, P. F. (1969). Chorea and phenothiazines. *Br. J. Psychiat.*, **115**, 103–104

Klawans, H. L. Jr. (1973a). The pharmacology of tardive dyskinesias. *Am. J. Psychiat.*, **130**, 82–86

Klawans, H. L. Jr. (1973b). The pharmacology of extrapyramidal movement disorders. *Monogr. neurol. Sci.*, **2**, 1–136

Klawans, H. L. and Rubovits, R. (1974). Effect of cholinergic and anticholinergic agents on tardive dyskinesia. *J. Neurol. Neurosurg. Psychiat.*, **37**, 941–947

Klett, C. J., Point, P. and Caffrey, E. (1972). Evaluating the long term need for antiparkinson drugs by chronic schizophrenics. *Archs gen. Psychiat.*, **26**, 374–379

Kobayashi, R. M. (1976). Orofacial dyskinesia–clinical features, mechanisms and drug therapy. *West J. Med.*, **125**, 277–288

Korsgaard, S. (1976). Baclofen (Lioresal) in the treatment of neuroleptic induced tardive dyskinesia. *Acta psychiat. scand.*, **54**, 17–24

Kumar, B. B. (1976). Treatment of tardive dyskinesia with deanol. *Am. J. Psychiat.*, **133**, 978

Kunin, R. A. (1976). Manganese and niacin in the treatment of drug-induced dyskinesias. *J. Orthnomoleculat. Psychiat.*, **5**, 4–27

Linden, D. (1977). Treatment of dyskinesia. *New Engl. J. Med.*, **296**(17), 1004–1005

Linnoila, M., Viukari, M. and Hietala, O. (1976). Effect of sodium valproate on TD. *Br. J. Psychiat.*, **129**, 114–119

McCallum, W. A. G. (1970). Tetrabenazine for extra-pyramidal movement disorders. *Br. J. Med.*, **1**, 760

Mehta, D., Mehta, S. and Mathew, P. (1976). Failure of deanol in treating tardive dyskinesia. *Am. J. Psychiat.*, **133**, 1467

Merren, M. D. (1972). Amantidine in tardive dyskinesia. *New Engl. J. Med.*, **286**, 268

Miller, E. M. (1974). Deanol: a solution for tardive dyskinesia. *New Engl. J. Med.*, **291**, 796–797

Nashold, B. S. (1969). The effects of central tegmental lesions on tardive dyskinesia. In *Psychotropic Drugs and Dysfunctions of the Basal Ganglia* (Ed. Crane and Gardner Jr.), Public Health Service Publication, Washington D.C., pp. 111–113

O'Flanagan, P. M. (1975). Clonazepam in the treatment of drug induced dyskinesia. *Br. Med. J.*, **1**, 269–270

Pakkenberg, H. and Fog, R. (1974). Spontaneous oral dyskinesia: results of treatment with tetrabenazine, pimozide, or both. *Archs Neurol.*, **31**, 352–353

Paulson, G. W. (1971). Use of pyridoxine in chorea. *Am. J. Psychiat.*, **127**, 1091

Paulson, G. W. (1975). Tardive dyskinesia. *A. Rev. Med.*, **26**, 75–81

Pearce, J. (1971). Mechanism of action of amantidine. *Br. med. J.*, **3**, 529

Prange, A. J., Wilson, I. C., Morris, C. E. (1973). Preliminary experience with tryptophan and lithium in the treatment of tardive dyskinesia. *Psychopharmac. Bull.*, **9**, 36–37

Pryce, I. J. and Edwards, H. (1966). Persistent oral dyskinesia in female mental hospital patients. *Br. J. Psychiat.*, **112**, 983–987

Quitkin, F., Rifkin, A., Gochfeld, L. and Klein, D. F. (1977). Tardive dyskinesia: are the first signs reversible? *Am. J. Psychiat.*, **134**(1), 84–87

Reda, F. A., Scanlan, J. M., Kemp, K. and Escobar, J. I. (1974). Treatment of tardive dyskinesia with lithium carbonate. *New Engl. J. Med.*, **291**, 850

Rosin, A. J. and Exton-Smith, A. M. (1965). Persistent oral dyskinesia in treatment with phenothiazine derivatives. *Lancet*, **i**, 651

Roxburgh, P. A. (1970). Treatment of persistent phenothiazine induced oral dyskinesia. *Br. J. Psychiat.*, **116**, 277–280

Sato, S., Daly, R. and Peters, H. (1971). Reserpine therapy of phenothiazine induced dyskinesia. *Dis. Nerv. Syst.*, **32**, 680–685

Schmidt, W. R. and Jarcho, L. W. (1966). Persistent dyskinesia following phenothiazine therapy. *Archs Neurol.*, **14**, 369–377

Schonecker, M. (1957). Ein eigentumliches Syndrom in ovalen Bereich bei Megaphen Applikation. *Nervenarzt*, **28**, 35–42

Sedman, G. (1976). Clonazepam in treatment of tardive oral dyskinesia. *Br. med. J.*, **2**, 583

Simpson, G. M., Branchey, M. H., Lee, J. H. *et al.* (1976). Lithium in tardive dyskinesia. *Pharmakopsychologis*, **9**, 76–80

Simpson, G. M. and Varga, E. (1974). Clozapine— a new antipsychotic agent. *Curr. ther. Res.*, **16**, 679–686

Singer, R. and Cheng, M. N. (1971). Thiopropazate hydrochloride in persistent dyskinesia. *Br. med. J.*, **4**, 22–25

Singh, M. M. (1976). Diazepam in the treatment of tardive dyskinesia. *Int. Pharmaco-Psychiat.*, **11**, 232–234

Sutcher, H. D., Underwood, R. B., Beatty, R. A. *et al*, (1971). Orofacial dyskinesia, a dental dimension. *J. Am. med. Ass.*, **216**, 1459–1463

Tamminga, C. A., Smith, R. C., Ericksen, S. E., Chang, S., Davis, J. M. (1977). Cholinergic influences in tardive dyskinesia. *Am. J. Psychiat.*, **134**(7), 769–774

Tarsy, D., Leopold, N. and Sax, D. S. (1974). Physostigmine in choreiform movement disorders. *Neurology*, **24**, 28–33

Uhrbrand, L. and Faurbye, A. (1960). Reversible and irreversible dyskinesia after treatment with perphenazine, chlorpromazine, reserpine and ECT. *Psychopharmacologia*, **1**, 408–418

Vale, S. and Espejel, M. A. (1971). Amantidine for dyskinesia tarda. *New Engl. J. Med.*, **284**, 673

Villeneuve, A. and Böszörmenyi, Z. (1970a). Treatment of drug induced dyskinesias. *Lancet*, **i**, 353–354

Villeneuve, A., Böszörmenyi, Z., Dechambault, M., *et al.* (1970b). Tentative de traitment de dyskinesia post-neuroleptique de type permanent. *Laval Med.*, **41**, 923–933

Vinkari, M. and Linnoila, M. (1975). Effect of methyl dopa on tardive dyskinesia in psychogeriatric patients. *Curr. ther. Res.*, **18**(3), 417–424

Wertheimer, J. (1965). Syndromes extra-pyramidaux permanents consecutifs a l'administration prolongée de neuroleptiques. *Schweiz. Arch. Neurol. Neurochir. Psychiat.*, **95**, 120–173

Widroe, H. J. and Heisler, S. (1976). Treatment of tardive dyskinesia. *Dis. Nerv. Syst.*, March, 162–164

Wurtman, R. J., Hirsch, M. J. and Growdon, J. H. (1977). Lecithin consumption raises serum free choline levels. *Lancet*, **ii**, 68–69

SECTION 3
BEHAVIOURAL
APPROACHES

13 Behaviour Therapy as Self-Control

M. G. Gelder

Many psychiatric patients would like to help themselves. The spate of popular books which describe how to relieve tension, or dispel phobias, headaches and other nervous disorders bears witness to this. Despite this, psychiatrists have until recently done rather little to encourage such interests among their patients. It is true that there are information booklets which explain the nature of mental disorders. However, they are usually designed to encourage people in distress to seek expert help or intended to give relatives a better understanding of a patient's problems. It is also true that patients are usually encouraged to take steps to help themselves but these efforts are usually thought of as ancillary to the main thrust of treatment which is seen to come from the therapist, whether this is a psychiatrist, a social worker, a psychologist or a nurse.

Much the same applies in general practice, where most neurotic patients are treated. Here they are most often treated with drugs. Surveys of prescribing by family doctors (e.g. Skegg *et al.*, 1977) show how widely psychotropic drugs are used. Of all the prescriptions written in the five group practices studied, 17 per cent were for psychotropic drugs. Looked at in another way, of nearly 40 000 people on these practice lists, 10 per cent of the men and 20 per cent of the women received at least one prescription for a psychotropic drug in the course of a single year. And in the age group 45–59, 25 per cent of women received a prescription for a sedative or hypnotic, 7.5 per cent for a major tranquilliser and 11 per cent for an antidepressant at least once in the year. There must be few patients with psychological symptoms who leave the surgery without a prescription. Of course, the prescription is usually accompanied by advice about the changes which the patient should try to bring about in his life, but we know how little patients remember of even simple instructions of this kind.

Behaviour therapy has potential as a form of self-help but it has not developed mainly in this way either in Great Britain or in the United States. In this country, Wolpe's desensitisation method has been influential (Wolpe, 1969). Wolpe developed this by adapting the findings of experiments with animals to clinical practice, and in doing so he chose the model of the psychotherapy session. Patients attended for treatment usually once a week, the sessions typically lasted about as long as those of brief psychotherapy, and the patient came to the out-patient clinic or consulting room. Moreover, although the therapist often gave 'homework' to practise between sessions, this was usually seen as an adjunct to the main treatment which was being carried out at the clinic—just as homework is a supplement to instruction in school. In the United States, the operant model was, and still is, more influential. Here great emphasis is put on effecting changes in the patient's everyday life rather than the events taking place at the out-patient clinic. However, this is done mainly by rearranging the environment of the patient who is seen as responding passively to changes in the world around him.

There are good reasons for thinking that behaviour therapy can and should move further towards a position in which it is a form of instruction in self-control. Before we come to the reasons for this, there are two practical considerations which must be noted. The first has been referred to already. Psychotropic drugs are almost certainly overprescribed to neurotic patients. There are therefore good practical reasons for developing alternatives suitable for use in general practice. The second point concerns professional manpower. The shortage of resources for professional staff in the Health Services is likely to continue in this country and most others. It is not realistic to think that the majority of neurotic patients could ever be treated with procedures which require substantial time from psychiatrists or family doctors. This applies as much to most forms of behaviour therapy as it does to psychotherapy. Trained clinical psychologists and social workers are also likely to be a scarce resource. In developing countries such considerations are even more important. Unless they can be developed in a way that requires the minimum of time from skilled people, behaviour therapy methods can have little to contribute to the solution of their health problems.

It is true, of course, that there are already some moves in this direction. Several enterprising psychologists, in this country and the United States, have produced and are marketing tape recordings which give instruction in procedures which purport to control fears or relieve headaches, bodily tension, etc. But these developments are largely taking place outside the mainstreams of medical practice and psychological research. General practitioners do not, as a rule, prescribe these tapes and research workers have not subjected them to the sort of systematic scrutiny which is given to a new drug. We shall see that there are some indications that this approach is practical and may be as effective as some of the clinic based behavioural treatment which has become accepted in the past two decades.

Existing Behavioural Methods of Self-control

The importance of self-control in behaviour modification has been emphasised for nearly a decade, notably by Bandura (1969) and by Kanfer (1970). Bandura pointed out that notions of self-control are essential when we consider how the changes brought about by behavioural treatment persist after that treatment ends. Writing on the stabilisation of behaviour changes (p. 619) he said: 'by far the most important but most neglected aspect of behavioural change processes is the appropriate generalisation of established patterns of behaviour to new situations and their persistence after the original controlling situations have been discontinued. The generalisation and persistence of behaviour can be facilitated by three different means. These include transfer of training, alteration of reinforcement practices of the social environment and the establishment of self-regulatory functions'. This emphasis on self-regulation foreshadowed the recent interest in cognitive aspects of behaviour therapy. It also indicates clearly how self-regulation must logically be a component of any behavioural method which is successful. Despite this wide importance, the actual application of self-control procedures has, however, been surprisingly narrow. Indeed it has almost wholly been concerned with excessive smoking, drinking and drug taking on the one hand; and on the other, with deficits in social and sexual behaviour. Why has the practice been so limited when the promise is so great? To answer this we need first to look in more detail at the ideas behind the self-control procedures which have been used.

The usual model of self-control owes much to the ideas of Kanfer (1970) and to a lesser extent to Meichenbaum (1975). Self-control can be divided into three stages. Self-monitoring, self-evaluation and self-reinforcement. Self-monitoring, in its turn, has two stages. The first consists of systematic observation of the behaviour which is to be changed. A heavy smoker records the number of cigarettes which he smokes, the anxious person notes the frequency, type and severity of his symptoms, and so on. Mahoney and Arnkoff (1978) have reviewed this topic comprehensively. They concluded that most people are not accurate observers of their own behaviour; they can however be trained to do this more accurately. In practice this is usually by the simple expedient of asking them to keep hour to hour written records of their behaviour. These authors also conclude that the effects of this procedure, used alone, are not powerful enough to be of much therapeutic value and that the further stages are required.

The second aspect of self-monitoring is the establishment of links between the behaviour to be changed and events in the world around the patient or within him. Thus the smoker must observe in what circumstances he smokes most (whether alone or in company, etc.) and what internal states such as anxiety or craving for nicotine are associated with smoking. Similarly the anxious person notes the circumstances which appear to provoke his symptoms and any thoughts which regularly precede them. Self-monitoring of this kind logically leads to some action to reduce symptoms. The simplest is to avoid the situations. There may also be more positive actions to be taken such as self-distraction to reduce thoughts which provoke anxiety. It is, however, one of the weaknesses of self-control theory that it has rather little to say about the actions to be taken. It relies, on the whole, upon simple measures which are intuitively plausible. Those who adopt these ideas have not set out to determine in a systematic way what behaviours are most effective. This is one reason why its range of application is so limited.

The second of the three stages of self-control is self-evaluation. The extent of the abnormal behaviour is assessed and so is the effectiveness of any counter measures. It also implies that the patient has to set some criterion for success, and in this way it merges with the next stage.

The third stage is self-reward. Psychological studies such as those reported by Bandura (1969) and Kanfer (1970) have shown that subjects can reward or punish themselves, with silent verbal praise or reproof or by using tangible rewards, and that this modifies their subsequent behaviour. These findings are largely concerned with normal behaviour, particularly that of children. It is a limitation, at least to the clinician, that the studies of self-monitoring in which abnormal behaviour has been observed have been concerned, for the most part, either with behaviour in the classroom (for example Glynn, Thomas and Shee, 1973; McReynolds and Church, 1973; Felixbrook and O'Leary, 1973; Santogrossi *et al.*, 1973) or with the control of body weight (for example Bellack *et al.*, 1976; Gulanick *et al.*, 1975; Mahoney, 1974). Such studies have shown rather convincingly that covert praise and reproof are important elements in social learning. They have not, however, demonstrated that they are able to exert effects which are strong enough to counter the powerful motivating forces which maintain the behaviour of anxiety prone patients.

Bandura (1976) has pointed out that the usual analysis of self-reinforcement is unduly simple. Two aspects have to be considered. If a person is to reinforce himself, the reinforcers must be freely available to him whether they are material rewards or self-praise. Therefore the first question is why he chooses to withhold the reinforcements most of the time and only give them to himself when he has reached the required standard. The second problem is how he sets standards for himself.

These issues are particular relevant to clinical problems but for reasons which are very different to those which apply to normal subjects. With the latter, the problem is why subjects do not deny themselves reinforcements and set sufficiently high criteria for success. With patients it is more often why they do not reward themselves enough and why they set such high standards for themselves. Beck (1976) has suggested convincingly that depressed subjects have distorted attitudes which make them withhold reinforcement from themselves and fail to be pleased by reasonable performance, partly because they dismiss successes as the results of chance rather than their own efforts. Clinical observations suggest that these problems are widespread in patients with neuroses in which anxiety and depression occur together. If this analysis is correct, it suggests that special measures would be needed with neurotic patients to supplement the effects of self-reinforcement. Accounts of social learning usually emphasise the motivating forces of the peer group. For the young person with behavioural problems this is indeed appropriate but for adult neurotic patients the most powerful effects are within the family. We shall see later that there are other reasons for seeking social reinforcement in the family but first we must consider another set of procedures.

Biofeedback as Self-control

Biofeedback can also be viewed as a self-control procedure. Indeed the great and rather surprising popularity of the method in the United States relates to just this issue. A passage in a popular book on biofeedback puts this point of view clearly:

> The value of biofeedback training lies not simply in its power to alter behaviour. Much of what it accomplishes can also be achieved through drugs, surgery, operant conditioning and electrical stimulation of the brain. Biofeedback training is important because it places the power of change and control in the hands of the individual, not with an external authority. Of all the technologies for altering behaviour, this is the first to rely on the individual's ability to guide his own destiny (Karlins and Andrews, 1975).

The reality is rather different. There is no convincing evidence that simple biofeedback methods, which patients can use themselves, are powerful therapeutic agents. Indeed there is little to indicate that they have effects greater than those which instructions to relax can exert on the same bodily functions. Unfortunately, few clinical reports have controlled adequately for the non-specific elements in biofeedback. When adequate controls have been used the specific effects of feedback have been found to be quite small. For example Steptoe (1976) showed that blood pressure feedback over four sessions leads to improvement of less than 5 mmHg more than that obtained from simple instructions to relax given over the same period. Steptoe's experiments were carried out in resting conditions in a quiet laboratory and there is some evidence (Steptoe, 1978) that the effects of feedback may be greater when the subject is doing mental work. Even so the effects are too small to account convincingly for the changes reported after clinical applications of biofeedback. It must be concluded that a large part of these changes are due to factors in the treatment other than the specific effects of feedback.

Similar conclusions were reached by Blanchard and Young (1974) in their comprehensive review of the literature about the clinical applications of biofeedback. They considered that most of the published studies have methodological flaws, and they suggested that good evidence exists only for specific effects of EMG feedback in muscle retraining and in the reduction of tension headaches. However, even this limited conclusion is probably too optimistic for work by Mathews and Martin (1978) throws serious doubt on the value of EMG feedback for tension headaches. The most convincing report of clinical uses of biofeedback, which has appeared since Blanchard and Young's review, is by Patel who studied the control of blood pressure (Patel, 1977). It is, however, of a rather different kind.

Although Patel used biofeedback, it was not information about blood pressure which was given to the patient but information about the GSR. This was used as an adjunct to a form of relaxation training and it helped the patient to monitor the degree of tension reduction during the relaxation sessions. The patient did not know his blood pressure either during these sessions or, more importantly, in the course of daily life. With this procedure Patel obtained striking changes in blood pressure in subjects with hypertension (Patel and North, 1975). Good relaxation may not, of course, be the only therapeutic factor in Patel's treatment. It is possible that the particular relaxation procedure, which was based on Yoga, brought about changes in patients' general approach to life's stresses and problems.

Despite Patel's good results, the general conclusion must be that biofeedback is not a powerful means of self-control. However, there is a further conclusion to be drawn. Biofeedback experiments are not as a rule conceptualised in terms of the stages of a process of self-control, despite the obvious relevance of this schema and even though this is the aspect which has interested the lay public. We shall see in a later section that such a framework helps to understand the potential value of biofeedback. For example, it helps by pointing to the important distinction between feedback as a way of teaching self-monitoring, and feedback as a way of teaching a specific response which can counter disordered autonomic function. However, before we consider this distinction further, there are some lessons to be drawn from the treatment of agoraphobia.

Lessons from the Treatment of Agoraphobia

In Oxford we have taken agoraphobia as a representative neurotic disorder against which we could test different methods of behaviour therapy. The result of this work has been a clearer understanding of the kind of simple behavioural procedure which is useful in agoraphobia. It turns out that this is a form of self-treatment and that it is of a form which can be applied in a general way to neurosis. It differs, however, in important ways from the self-control methods we have discussed so far.

The work to be described took many years but the findings can be summarised quite briefly. We first studied systematically the conditions under which exposure to phobic situations leads to improvement in phobias. There are three main variables: the level of anxiety at which exposure takes place, the duration of the exposure, and its form, that is whether it takes place in reality or is merely imagined. We found that anxiety should not be kept at the very high levels characteristic of flooding treatment but at a lower level (Mathews and Shaw, 1973; Johnston and Gath, 1973). At the same time Stern and Marks (1973) demonstrated that exposure is not most effective when it is very brief as in desensitisation; it should last for much longer, probably an hour or more. Finally we and other workers found that exposure to real situations is more effective than imagery (Mathews *et al.*, 1976; Crowe *et al.*, 1972; Emmelkamp and Wessels, 1975).

Up to this point we had assumed that the main therapeutic changes in behavioural therapy for phobic states take place during treatment sessions and that any practice which the patient does at home is subsidiary to this. A further investigation (Mathews *et al.*, 1976) changed this view. This compared the effects of three methods of exposure treatment given to agoraphobic patients. The design of the experiment was a little complicated but the essential comparisons were: exposure in the situations which provoked anxiety, 'exposure in imagination' and a combination of the two. Contrary to expectation, the results of the three were the same when measured at the end of a series of treatment sessions. This finding appeared to contradict other reports (Stern and Marks, 1973; Watson *et al.*, 1973) that exposure to real situations is more effective than merely imagining them. However, the conflict was resolved when we examined measures taken at the end of each session. These confirmed that more immediate change occurred after exposure to real situations. Now all three groups had been encouraged to practise exposure to real situations frequently between treatment sessions. The results could best be explained by assuming that the cumulative effect of this practice at home, which was common to all treatments, outweighed the different effects of the procedures gone through in the out-patient sessions. Once arrived at, this conclusion is quite persuasive; it does seem likely that the final effect of many hours of practice at home should be greater than that of an hour a week of treatment, unless the latter is very powerful indeed. An important point follows from this: it is likely to be more useful to make the daily practice at home more efficient, rather than attempt to improve further the effects of the brief weekly intervention at the clinic. We shall see later how this was done, but before that there is another problem to consider.

Although there are many studies which show that agoraphobia improves in the course of behavioural treatment, there was until recently no adequately controlled study that reported improvement, which continued after treatment sessions had stopped (Gelder, 1977). And yet improvement should go on. Once patients have learnt how to go out to meet the situations which they fear, they should be able to continue to do this on their own. If they do this, their fears should recede further. There are several reasons why this continuing improvement might not come about but two seem particularly important. The first is that the patients may not understand clearly enough what they have to do. The second is that they may not be motivated adequately to do it. Both are obvious but both have been neglected.

It is surprising that behaviour therapists have paid so little attention to the problem of ensuring that their patients understand what behaviours they are to carry out. It is, after all, well known that patients remember little of even quite simple instructions given to them by their doctors. The phobic patient, if he is to treat himself, must learn a complicated set of behaviours. Moreover he has to learn not mere set pieces of behaviour but strategies which enable him to adapt what he does to changing, and often unexpected, circumstances. As long as we think of the behaviour which patients practise between their visits to the therapist as mere homework carried out between the all important treatment sessions, these questions may not seem very important. However, once it is accepted that the few hours of treatment can have only a small effect when compared with opportunities for relearning in the long hours between and following these sessions, then the role of instructions is seen to be important.

Mathews, working in Oxford, was the first to see this point clearly and to introduce an instruction manual for agoraphobic patients (Mathews *et al.*, 1977). This manual can be read and re-read and discussed with the therapist until it is certain the patient has sufficient knowledge of the principles and details of the procedures to be able to carry them out himself. The effects of the manual cannot be separated completely from those of the other components of treatment in this trial but experience in its use and the reports of patients strongly suggest that it was an important element in the good results which Mathews and his colleagues obtained.

We have noted already that understanding is of little value unless the patient also has the motivation to carry out the procedures he has learnt. And clinical experience with neurotic patients suggests that poor motivation is indeed a frequent reason for lack of continuing progress after treatment ends. It is important therefore to consider where the patient can acquire the necessary motivation.

In behaviour therapy as in other forms of psychological treatment, we try to select patients who are well motivated from the start. The therapist often tries to enhance this intrinsic motivation as treatment progresses with the expectation that, when treatment ends, it will be sufficient to keep the patient working at his problems. Why this sometimes fails can be seen if we consider the predicament of an agoraphobic patient who is told to continue to practise going out to overcome his fears. Going out repeatedly into frightening situations is not rewarding in itself. There is some satisfaction from doing the task well but really strong motivation only comes when the patient can travel easily enough to enjoy visits to friends and relatives, or to feel at ease in places of entertainment. Unless treatment is rather lengthy, the patient has seldom reached this stage completely when it ends. It might be said that there is a 'motivation gap' between the period of treatment during which the patient has the rewards of pleasing the therapist each week and the time when improvement is sufficient to bring its own rewards. Marks and his colleagues recognised this problem and tried to enhance and prolong motivation by treating patients in groups, using the powerful motivating forces of group cohesion (Hand *et al.*, 1974). In Oxford, Teasdale *et al.* (1977) attempted to replicate Hand *et al.*'s finding that treatment in a socially cohesive group leads to improvement which continues after the treatment sessions end. However, although they obtained almost exactly the same amount of improvement in phobias during the period of treatment, they did not find the continuing improvement after the sessions stopped which Hand *et al.* reported. This may have been because the groups were less 'cohesive' than those of Hand *et al.*, or it may have been because Teasdale *et al.* achieved a more complete follow-up of their patients.

It seemed, in any case, that rather than use group processes it might be better to attempt to increase motivation from within the family. After years of living with agoraphobia, family members have often ceased to respond positively to the patient's small successes. Instead they often show more concern and attention on those occasions when the patient is most distressed. In doing this they are reinforcing 'illness behaviour'. It seems appropriate therefore to teach relatives to reinforce counter-neurotic behaviour and to praise and reward improvement. Mathews *et al.* (1977) therefore enlisted the help of the patient's spouse who was instructed in the principles of social reinforcement and made responsible with the patient for planning the programme of counter-neurotic behaviour. At the same time the therapist's role changed to become that of a teacher who helps patient and spouse to reach an understanding which allows them to continue with treatment when he no longer sees them.

It is difficult to test the value of these measures directly and our attempt to do so is so far inconclusive. This is because Mathews *et al.* combined, in one treatment, measures to improve both instructions about the required be-haviour and work with the husband to improve the social reinforcement of this behaviour. Moreover the study was in the form of a preliminary enquiry; it did not use random allocation between the new treatment and the old but re-lied on established knowledge about the effects of the old with similar patients.

With these reservations, we can summarise Mathews *et al.*'s procedure and their main findings. There were eight sessions of treatment, each conducted at the patient's home. The agoraphobic patient and her spouse received an instruction booklet which described in a simple way the rationale of exposure treatment for phobias and added advice about the best way of coping with symptoms of anxiety. The therapist then taught the patient and spouse how to set graduated goals and how to adapt their plans to new or unexpected circumstances. The spouse was encouraged strongly to reinforce the patient's efforts at practice and any evidence of improvement. At the end of the 8 sessions of treatment the change in phobic symptoms was only slightly less than that achieved after 16 sessions of a similar form of behaviour therapy given in weekly out-patient sessions. However, the more important finding was that improvement continued after treatment sessions with the couple came to an end. A second study is now being carried out to determine whether these findings are repeated in a controlled clinical trial with 'blind' ratings. However, even before the results of this trial become available, there does seem good reason to conclude that instructions and motivation are issues which require considerable emphasis in any form of self-treatment.

Self-treatment: A Synthesis

We have now examined three aspects of our subject and it is time to attempt to put them together. When considering the self-control therapies we saw the value of thinking of stages of self-monitoring, self-evaluation and self-reinforcement. We noted that there is evidence that these processes are important in regulating the behaviour of normal children. However, when we turned to abnormal behaviour we saw that, although the ideas still appear to have explanatory powers, they have not led to treatment methods which have wide utility. Indeed, even in the narrow range of disorders for which they have been used they have not produced striking results. In part this may be due to an unduly simplistic approach to the kind of behaviour which the patient should practise in order to control the abnormal behaviours. However, we identified another problem as well. Self-reinforcement can only be effective if the patient makes rewards available to himself appropriately. With normal people the problem is to teach them to withhold reinforcements which are readily available until an appropriate criterion has been reached. With patients who show any degree of depression—and this includes most of those with long-standing neuroses—the problem is the reverse. They do not reward themselves enough for good performance. Beck's cognitive therapy may eventually be shown to deal with these problems effectively, but until then the therapist must try to circumvent the problem. The studies of agoraphobia indicate that this can be done effectively by using external reinforcement drawn from the source of the patient's most intense relationships—the family.

Biofeedback experiments illustrate two issues. The first is that special measures have to be used to teach the subject the response which is to be used to control his behaviour. Two approaches have been used. Patel employed a response (relaxation training) which can largely be taught through words. She used feedback information to improve performance, but the task can be learnt without it. Most other biofeedback experiments assume tacitly that the procedure cannot be imparted through verbal means: feedback is then essential for the subject to discover through trial and error a response which cannot be described in words. This approach is attractive but so far it has not yielded powerful therapeutic effects.

The second issue concerns self-monitoring. Feedback experiments indicate that, for some functions at least, subjects have to be helped in special ways before they can monitor their own performance effectively. This help may take the form of additional information from physiological instruments. Alternatively subjects may be trained to become more aware of visceral sensations—an approach which has been less fully exploited than the first. These experiments point to the inadequate attention which is given to training in self-monitoring.

When we examined the findings of research on the phobic states, it became apparent how the original formulation of self-control needs to be modified if it is to have more general clinical utility. We saw the need to identify in a very specific way the counter-neurotic behaviour which is effective and at the same time simple enough for the patient to carry out on his own. In the case of phobic states this behaviour turns out to be repeated practice in entering and remaining in situations which provoke anxiety. This is best carried out with anxiety levels kept at a rather low level and it must be prolonged. In the case of obsessional disorders with rituals, work by Levy and Meyer (1971) and by Marks and his colleagues (Marks et al., 1975) indicates that the effective counter behaviour is the prevention of rituals in the presence of environmental stimuli which normally provoke them. Again it is important that the patient should practise this behaviour conscientiously for long periods. Essentially similar findings were reported by Mills et al. (1973). It is less certain whether there is any behaviour which can effectively counter obsessional ruminations. Thought stopping has been proposed but one controlled investigation found it to have no more effect than simple distraction (Hackman and McLean, 1975). The same doubt is present about the best behaviour for the control of intrusive anxious thoughts which are a frequent component of anxiety syndromes. Mathews and Shaw (1978) compared the effects of thought stopping and a desensitisation procedure and found no difference. The mainstay of treatment of anxiety states of all kinds remains the use of relaxation procedures. While these reduce physiological levels of arousal, there is still no good evidence that any one method of relaxation training is more effective than the others. Indeed one investigation of a brief relaxation technique showed that although it led to a fall in skin conductance as compared with a control procedure, muscle tension did not fall (Mathews and Gelder, 1969). This is consistent with clinical impressions that methods which emphasise muscle relaxation and meditational techniques produce similar effects. It is clear that we have some way to go before other counter-neurotic behaviours can be specified as clearly as those which have been identified for phobic states. Nevertheless the direction for research is clear.

The final shortcoming of the original formulation of self-control lies in its handling of the problem of motivation. It is not enough to consider self-reinforcement. Nor is it enough to extend this, as Bandura has done, in a rather general way to the social environment. Anxiety is a powerful motivating force and patients must be able to draw on equally powerful sources of motivation if they are to overcome anxiety related symptoms. Our work suggests that this can be obtained from the place in which emotional ties are strongest: the spouse or another person in a similar close relationship to the patient.

The revised model has four stages. The first is self-monitoring, which includes the identification of environmental factors which provoke symptoms as well as judging the severity of the symptoms themselves. The second is to teach a carefully selected counter-neurotic behaviour. The third is self-evaluation of the effects of the therapeutic behaviour. The last, but arguably the most important is the arrangement of an effective system of motivation to carry this counter-neurotic behaviour through until there is suffucient improvement to make achievement rewarding in itself.

This model of self-treatment can be illustrated by considering a patient with tension symptoms. The first step is to teach the patient how to monitor his symptoms accurately. For this purpose it is best to use a simple record made on cards which can be carried about and filled in hour by hour. A retrospective account of the whole day is usually much less accurate. The patient should record not only the symptoms he complains of but also any anxious or depressive thoughts which occur. Most people need a period of supervised practice before they can do this effectively. At the same time he has to learn to identify and note down the circumstances in which the symptoms and intrusive thoughts appear. When sufficient records have been compiled, he must find out how to look for the common features of these events and decide whether any can be avoided or modified. The therapist then decides the appropriate counter-neurotic behaviour for this patient. For a tension state, one component will almost certainly be relaxation training. This can be carried out in several ways. It might seem plausible to suggest that methods which emphasise physical relaxation would be more useful for patients who complain of physical tension while meditational procedures might be more appropriate for those with mainly psychological symptoms. There is, however, no definite evidence that this is so. In the present state of knowledge it is therefore reasonable to allow the patient to learn the method which he finds most convincing. It is also uncertain whether feedback of autonomic activity is generally useful. Some patients say that it is helpful, others relax more easily without it. Until the question has been investigated systematically, it is best to offer feedback only to patients who do not relax quickly without it.

The second part of the counter-neurotic behaviour consists of a means of controlling thoughts which increase anxiety. While much has been written about cognitive therapy, there is little solid evidence which allows the therapist to choose between procedures. Mathews and Shaw's (1978) results suggest that a common feature may be simple distraction. This is certainly the easiest method for the patient to learn and it is reasonable to begin with it before attempting more complicated things.

Careful attention must be given to the best way to teach these behaviours. It is useful to employ an instruction booklet which gives reasons for the treatment and explains what has to be learnt about monitoring abnormal behaviour, identifying its antecedents and learning to control it. The patient should not only read this and answer questions about it, but re-read it until he is thoroughly familiar with its contents and has discussed it several times with his spouse. The actual relaxation technique can usually be learnt from tape recorded instructions.

From the start, the therapist must ensure that everything is being done to produce lasting motivation to carry out these behaviours. The spouse should play an active part from an early stage; if he is not eager to help then joint interviews may help to resolve the problem. Patient and spouse should decide how best to arrange pleasurable consequences both for diligent practice and for success in reaching behavioural goals.

This approach gives patients the best chance of helping themselves. It seems to provide something which they desire and it brings behaviour therapy nearer to the stage when it is economical enough to be available more freely than it is now. No doubt there will be changes as knowledge grows, but I believe that it is the right direction for progress.

References

Bandura, A. (1969). *Principles of Behaviour Modification*. Holt, Rinehart and Winston, London

Bandura, A. (1976). Self reinforcement: theoretical and methodological considerations. *Behaviorism*, **4**, 135–155

Beck, A. T. (1976). *Cognitive Therapy and Emotional Disorder*. International Universities Press, New York

Bellack, A. S., Glanz, L. M. and Simon, R. (1976). Self reinforcement styles and covert imagery in the treatment of obesity. *J. consult. clin. Psychol.*, **44**, 490–491

Blanchard, E. B. and Young, L. D. (1974). Clinical applications of biofeedback training. *Archs gen. Psychiat.*, **30**, 573–589

Crowe, M. J., Marks, I. M., Agras, W. S. and Leitenberg, H. (1972). Time limited desensitisation, implosion and shaping for phobic patients. *Behav. Res. Ther.*, **10**, 319–328

Emmelkamp, P. M. G. and Wessels, H. (1975). Flooding in imagination vs. flooding *in vivo*: a comparison with agoraphobics. *Behav. Res. Ther.*, **13**, 7–15

Felixbrook, J. J. and O'Leary, K. D. (1973). Effects of reinforcement on children's academic behaviour as a function of self determined and externally imposed contingencies. *J. appl. behav. Anal.*, **6**, 241–250

Gelder, M. G. (1977). Behavioural treatment of agoraphobia: some factors which restrict change after treatment. In *Phobias and Obsessions* (Ed. J. Boulogouris and A. Rabavilas), Pergamon Press, Oxford

Gelder, M. G. Bancroft, J. H. J., Gath, D. H., Johnston, D. W., Mathews, A. M. and Shaw, P. M. (1973). Specific and non-specific factors in behaviour therapy. *Br. J. Psychiat*, **123**, 445–62

Gulanick, N., Woodburn, L. T. and Rimm, D. C. (1975). Weight gain through self control procedures. *J. consult. clin. Psychol.*, **43**, 536–539

Glynn, E. L., Thomas, J. D. and Shee, S. M. (1973). Behavioural self control of on-task behaviour in an elementary classroom. *J. appl. behav. Anal.*, **6**, 105–113.

Hackman, A. and McLean, C. (1975). A comparison of flooding and thought stopping in the treatment of obsessional neurosis. *Behav. Res. Ther.*, **13**, 263–269

Hand, I., Lamontagne, Y. and Marks, I. M. (1974). Group exposure (flooding) *in vivo* for agoraphobics. *Br. J. Psychiat.*, **124**, 588–602

Johnston, D. W. and Gath, D. (1973). Arousal levels and attribution effects in diazepam assisted flooding. *Br. J. Psychiat.*, **123**, 463–466

Kanfer, F. H. (1970). Self regulation: research, issues and speculation. In *Behaviour Modification in Clinical Psychology* (Ed. C. Noufinger and J. L. Michael), Appleton-Century-Crofts, New York

Karlins, M. and Andrews, L. M. (1975). *Biofeedback Turning on the Power of Your Mind*, Sphere Books, London

Levy, R. and Meyer, V. (1971). Ritual prevention in obsessional patients. *Proc. R. Soc. Med.*, **64**, 1115

McReynolds, W. T. and Church, A. (1973). Self control, study skills development, and counselling approaches to the improvement of study behaviour. *Behav. Res. Ther.*, **11**, 233–235

Mahoney, M. J. (1972). Research issues in self management. *Behav. Ther.*, **3**, 45–63

Mahoney, M. J. (1974). *Cognition and Behaviour Modification*, Ballinger, Cambridge, Mass.

Mahoney, M. J. and Arukoff, D. (1978). Cognitive and self control therapies. In *Handbook of Psychotherapy and Behaviour Change*, 2nd edition (Ed. A. Bergin and S. Garfield), Wiley, New York

Marks, I. M., Hodgson, R. and Rachman, S. (1975). Treatment of chronic obsessive compulsive neurosis by *in vivo* exposure: a two year follow up and issues in treatment. *Br. J. Psychiat.*, **127**, 349–364

Mathews, A. M. and Gelder, M. G. (1969). Psychophysiological investigations of brief relaxation training. *J. psychosom. Res.*, **13**, 1–12

Mathews, A. M., Johnston, D. W., Lancashire, M., Munby, M., Shaw, P. M. and Gelder, M. G. (1976). Imaginal flooding and exposure to real phobic situations: treatment outcome with agoraphobic patients. *Br. J. Psychiat.*, **129**, 362–371

Mathews, A. M. and Martin, P. (1978). *J. psychosom. Res.* (in press)

Mathews, A. M. and Shaw, P. M. (1973). Emotional arousal and persuasion effects in flooding. *Behav. Res. Ther.*, **11**, 587–98

Mathews, A. M. and Shaw, P. M. (1978). Cognitions related to anxiety: a pilot study of treatment. *Behav. Ther.*, **8**, 915–24

Mathews, A. M., Teasdale, J., Munby, M., Johnston, D. W. and Shaw, P. M. (1977). A home based treatment programme for agoraphobia. *Behav. Ther.* (in press)

Meichenbaum, D. (1975). A self instructional approach to stress management. In *Stress and Anxiety*, Vol. 2 (Ed. I. Sarason and C. D. Spielberger) Wiley, New York

Mills, H. L., Agras, W. S., Barlow, D. H. and Mills, J. R. (1973). Compulsive rituals treated by response prevention. *Archs gen. Psychiat.*, **28**, 324–329

Patel, C. H. (1977). Biofeedback aided relaxation and meditation in the management of hypertension. *Biofeedback and Selfregulation*, **2**, 1–41

Patel, C. H. and North, W. R. S. (1975). Randomised controlled trial of yoga and biofeedback in management of hypertension *Lancet*, **2**, 93–95

Santogrossi, D. A., O'Leary, K. D., Romanczyk, R. G. and Kaufmann, K. F. (1973). Self evaluation by adolescents in a psychiatric school token programme. *J. appl. behav. Anal.*, **6**, 277–287

Skegg, D. G., Doll, R. and Perry, J. (1977). Use of medicines in general practice. *Br. med. J.*, **1**, 1561–1563

Steptoe, A. (1976). Blood pressure control: a comparison of feedback and instructions using pulse wave velocity measurements. *Psychophysiology*, **13**, 528–535

Steptoe, A. (1978). To be published

Steptoe, A. and Johnston, D. W. (1976). The control of blood pressure using pulse-wave velocity feedback. *J. psychosom. Res.*, **20**, 417–424

Stern, R. S. and Marks, I. M. (1973). Brief and prolonged flooding: a comparison in agoraphobic patients. *Archs gen. Psychiat.*, **28**, 270–276

Stuart, R. B. (1967). Behavioural control of overeating. *Behav. Res. Ther.*, **5**, 357–365

Stunkard, A. J. and Mahoney, M. J. (1976). Behavioural treatment of eating disorders. In Leitenberg, H. *Handbook of Behaviour Modification*, Appleton-Century-Crofts, New York

Teasdale, J. D., Walsh, P. A., Lancashire, M. and Mathews, A. M. (1978). Group exposure for agoraphobia: a replication. *Br. J. Psychiat.*, **130**, 186–93

Thorensen, C. E. and Mahoney, M. J. (1974). *Behavioural Self Control*. Holt, Rinehart and Winston, New York

Watson, J. P., Mullett, G. E. and Pillay, H. (1973). The effects of prolonged exposure on agoraphobic patients treated in groups. *Behav. Res. Ther.*, **11**, 531–545

Wolpe, J. (1969). *The Practice of Behaviour Therapy*. Pergamon Press, Oxford

14 Behaviour Therapy and Depression: A Review of Some Aspects of Aetiology and Treatment

R. McAuley

Any integrated theory of depression must include places for genetic, biochemical, psychosocial and intrapsychic factors, and it is only during the past 7–8 years that behaviour therapists have made serious attempts to contribute to our understanding.

Some Behavioural Characteristics of the Depressed Individual

The symptoms and signs of depression are numerous and varied. However, in the more common depressive disorders most authorities would agree that the symptoms can be summarised under three major headings which are: performance deficits; verbal statements or complaints made by the patient; and lastly physical and emotional changes.

Performance Deficits

Generally the depressive is less active in all motor spheres than when he was well. He is slower on psychomotor tasks (Martin and Rees, 1966), and has greater difficulty with intellectual activities. On intelligence testing he will perform less well. Seligman (1975) describes a case in which a depressed but previously successful businessman was advised on the basis of aptitude testing, to seek employment on an assembly line. This unfortunate advice was offered at a time when the client was functioning far below his potential. Measures of motivation, memory and intellectual ability will probably show deficits in all but the mildest of depressions. Depressives also show reduction in social interaction. Eye-contact is reduced (Hinchcliffe *et al.*, 1971), voice intonation is dull and monotonous (Beck, 1967), and there is a reduction in non-verbal communicative hand gestures (Ekman and Friesen, 1974). These researchers have reported that each of these non-verbal components improves as the depression diminishes. In a series of studies Lewinsohn and co-workers

(Lewinsohn *et al.*, 1970, 1973; Libet and Lewinsohn, 1973; Lewinsohn and Graf, 1973), have been examining the social interactions of depressed college students. They have demonstrated that these individuals have fewer people in their interactional field and that they engage in fewer activities which were previously regarded as pleasant. In the majority of cases the previously pleasant activities had been social in nature. These researchers have carefully explored some of the fine-grain interactions of the depressed students. In interactional situations the depressives elicited less behaviour from peers, they emitted fewer positive social reinforcements, and showed a greater response latency than did non-depressed students. In other words the depressives received less talk, gave out fewer positive statements and took longer to respond than the normals. While most of the depressive's behaviour did not appear aversive in kind, in a few clinical incidents Lewinsohn has observed that depressed subjects may additionally emit aversive behaviours such as criticism, which serve to further reduce the amount of behaviour directed towards them. In summary of this work Libet and Lewinsohn (1973) stress that it is the depressive's response capability rather than his response performance which was most at fault. It must be remembered, however, that the subjects in these studies were depressed college students who were selected from an undergraduate population on the basis of various inventories. In more severely depressed subjects it is likely that a decrement in response performance would be of greater importance. Seligman (1975) notes that many depressives show a reduction in aggressive behaviour, which he defines as being the ability to direct hostility towards others. This behaviour is not so far removed from the lowered assertiveness which Wolpe (1971) notes characterises many depressives. In view of Lewinsohn and his colleagues' findings the lowered assertiveness is not surprising.

Verbal Complaints

Commonly depressives make negative value judgements about themselves, their present circumstances, and their view of the future. Respectively, these will often involve statements of guilt, self-reproach, self-debasement, of inability to act, and of gloomy expectations for the future. These distortions about self, current circumstances and the future have been referred to by Beck (1967) as the cognitive triad, principally because he believes that they are central to the problems of the depressive as is discussed below. These statements which represent the individual's feelings of hopelessness or helplessness, are also held central to the theories of Seligman (1975) and Melges and Bowlby (1969), which are discussed below.

Physical and Emotional Symptoms

The most common physical symptoms of depression include loss of appetite, loss of libido and loss of sleep, while the common emotional ones include crying, dysphoria, anxiety and loss of feeling. It is perhaps wrong to separate these two sets of symptoms since they probably have similar mechanisms. Recent researchers, Beck (1967) and Seligman (1975), have questioned the relative importance of these symptoms. The fact that depression has frequently been classified as an affective disorder suggests that some authorities have considered mood to be of central importance. On the basis of clinical observation Beck (1967) suggests that mood improves only when the cognitive distortions improve. This claim is supported by Schachter (1964) whose work suggests that emotions are to a large degree shaped by cognitions. Observations by Lewinsohn (1975) add further support. He records that mood fluctuates directly with the depressive's engagement in pleasant activities (positively reinforcing events). Of course physiological or biological disturbances can also result in emotional changes. However in these instances cognitive changes will also occur. Seligman (1975) suggests that confusion about cognitive and emotional disturbances is perhaps as much a failure of our language as it is of our understanding.

Behavioural Theories of Depression

Ferster (1966) suggests on the basis of experimental results from animal research, that the following factors may all play a significant part in the aetiology of depression:

(1) Sudden environmental changes which may involve significant losses of reinforcement.

(2) Aversive stimuli. Seligman (1975) reports on the basis of extensive animal and human experimental research, that in many depressives loss of reinforcement control is a significant factor. In other words the depressive's experience has been such that he now views environmental reinforcers as beyond his control—he feels helpless. Most persons who experience loss or unpleasant events do not become severely depressed or in the long term feel helpless. For instance, the major symptoms following loss of a spouse usually subside within approximately 6 weeks (Parkes, 1972a). Thus any theory which devotes its attention to psychosocial aspects must consider not only current life events, but also the person's past history and ability to deal with unpleasant circumstances. In the following section the ideas put forward by Ferster and Seligman are discussed as they relate to the individual's behavioural style and life history.

Loss of Reinforcement and Changes in Reinforcement Contingencies

Loss of a spouse (Parkes, 1964) loss of a limb (Parkes, 1972b) and onset of a serious physical illness are all serious events which are frequently associated with the onset of depression. Following the occurrence of any of these events an individual loses a wide range of potential reinforcers. For instance, with the onset of heart disease an individual's physical activity may be restricted, or following the loss of a spouse the potential for many shared and reinforcing activities is lost. Some parts of the individual's behavioural repertoire may extinguish unless he can in other ways engineer the same reinforcers or turn to other activities with reinforcing properties. The ability to do so is obviously an important social skill which may protect the individual from developing a depressive disorder. Rippere (1977) has referred to this skill as anti-depressive behaviour.

The losses mentioned above are all large and their significance would probably be readily assessed in most first interviews. However, the majority of depressives presenting at an out-patient clinic do not present with such obvious precipitant histories. Both Paykel et al. (1969) and Brown et al. (1973) have demonstrated the importance of common life events, especially those of an 'exit' nature in the precipitation of depression. Brown et al. (1973) note that in the year preceding the onset of depression there is a significant increase in the number of these events. Such events may involve losses which are threatened, real or imagined, the most notable being separations. The painstaking methods which these researchers have adopted suggest that many areas of reinforcement loss may be difficult to assess. It is likely that several of these apparently small events interact to result in depression. McLean (1976) notes that many married women exist in an environment of chronically low positive reinforcement. It is not hard to envisage how further small losses might precipitate a depressive illness. As another example of reinforcement loss, Liberman and Raskin (1971) have mentioned success depression. Promotions may be associated with significant losses in reinforcement. For instance, a newly appointed top executive may lose much reinforcement for successful work simply because there is now no one in authority to supply this.

The impact of any event associated with loss of reinforcement must be assessed in relation to the individual's social repertoire. In persons who have wide and varied social repertoires it is unlikely that even large losses will result in serious depression. On the other hand, individuals whose repertoires are restricted are more at risk. For instance a wife who is dependent on her husband to stimulate social activities, to take decisions and to help at home, may suffer more with his loss, since much of her social behaviour is under his reinforcement control. Similarly, a successful concert pianist who develops arthritis may become depressed because such a wide and important area of his behaviour is curtailed.

Aversive Events

The occurrence of loss or life events of an exit nature (as discussed above) have aversive properties (Azrin and Holz, 1966). While many writers have discussed the social reinforcement model in depth, few have concentrated on the role of aversive stimuli in the precipitation and maintenance of depressive behaviours. This is somewhat surprising since many of the common symptoms and signs of depression such as reduction in social behaviours, unpleasant emotions, cognitions such as denials of illness (which are avoidance behaviours), and expressions of helplessness, might all be equally well understood as a result of aversive stimuli. Wolpe (1971) suggests that anxiety is an important component in the maintenance of some depressive behaviours. He speculates that the unpleasant emotions and cognitions simply serve to motivate avoidance behaviours and thus encapsulate the depressive illness. For instance in social situations the individual may feel anxious, dull and uninteresting. On this basis he may avoid social encounters. In this case the depression is like a phobic illness and as such desensitisation will be a prime component of treatment. The importance of Wolpe's ideas receives further support in the finding that many depressed persons experience further aversive events as relatively more unpleasant than normal people (Lewinsohn et al., 1973).

Aversive events can have a variety of effects. These will depend to some degree on the parameters of the aversive stimuli (Church, 1969), and also the individual's history in relation to the handling of unpleasant life circumstances. Intense aversive stimuli will bring about more suppression of behaviour and more emotionality than less intense ones. However, the magnitude of effects is also governed by the contingency of the aversive event. Generally aversive stimuli which are non-contingent (unrelated to ongoing behaviour) are associated with suppression of a wider range of behaviours and more emotionality, than are ones which are contingent on behaviour. The latter instance which is one of punishment, is usually associated with suppression of only that behaviour which is followed by the aversive stimuli. Of course when punishment is used very frequently many behaviours may be suppressed. However, loss of reinforcement is frequently non-contingent and unrelated to the individual's behaviour. For example, loss of a spouse or redundancy are non-contingent.

These latter events are also often unexpected: the relative expectancy of loss is important and has been commented on by Parkes (1972a). Young widows seem to suffer more with intense grief reactions than do older widows. Death in the former instance is less expected than in the latter. The individual's life history is important in that most persons fairly rapidly overcome the effects of non-contingent aversive events. Normally following the loss of a spouse many stimuli which were associated with the spouse such as parts of the home, clothing, social activities, will all for a time elicit depressive behaviours. These have become conditioned stimuli, much in the same way as the sounding of a bell as a signal for food did in the experiments described by Pavlov. However, since for the bereaved these conditioned aversive stimuli do not now signal any further traumatic events, the associated grieving behaviour should gradually undergo extinction. In many chronically depressed persons this does not seem to happen. Some appear to have become sensitised to painful events (Church, 1969), others avoid the conditioned aversive stimuli and thus prevent extinction, and others become helpless. Some aspects of the aetiology of these patterns is discussed in the next two sections.

Some Aspects of Past History and Social Skills

Libet and Lewinsohn (1973) have emphasised the importance of deficiencies in social skills in depressed persons. Much of Lewinsohn's work was summarised in an earlier section. It has been suggested (Patterson and Rosenberry, 1969; McLean, 1976; Libet and Lewinsohn, 1973) that these social skill deficits exist as chronic problems in many persons who are prone to frequent episodes of neurotic depression. During each episode the deficits are intensified. In this chronic state of low interpersonal success and failure to control interpersonal situations, the individual is highly susceptible to mild changes in his environment. He will view himself as powerless and will hold his efforts to change events in low regard. In contrast, persons who are unlikely to become depressed will exhibit more confidence in their own ability to shape and modify their environment. When confronted with unpleasant events these latter persons will often engage in activities which will restore their confidence. As mentioned above Rippere (1977) has referred to this as anti-depressive behaviour. Thus in understanding the patient's current illness it is crucial that we gain some knowledge of their interpersonal efficiency and its development, and that we ascertain how they have handled unpleasant life events in the past. This information will partly dictate the treatment required. Females who are either married, separated, or divorced, and who have children are at a high risk of becoming depressed, see McLean (1976). This suggests that some factors within family relationships are important in the development of later depression. Patterson et al., (1976) has described how the habitual use of aversive behaviours to control a spouse (coercion) can lead to decreases in the frequency of positive interchanges and generalised marital dissatisfaction. Most frequently it is the wife who (in the role of the victim) submits to further avoid her husband's negative behaviours. In marriages typified by coercion most of the associated behaviours such as poor problem solving skills, will remain specific to that marital interaction (Vincent, 1972). Many of the couples will display quite normal skills in alternative social interactions. It is only when the dissatisfaction and reduction of positive behaviours become generalised that depression will develop. However, negative marital relationships must set the spouse at risk.

Many of the roots of poor social skills and susceptibility to depression will lie in childhood. McLean (1976) suggests two simple mechanisms. One of the first complaints of many depressed parents is inability to manage their children (McLean et al., 1973). Thus, prolonged illness may result in chronic child mismanagement, which may be associated with an increased likelihood of psychiatric disturbance in the child, either now or later as an adult. However, lack of effective control of behaviour in childhood will not necessarily specify the type of disorder experienced except that in males there may be a greater tendency to sociopathic disorders, while in females neurotic disorders may be more common. The second mechanism involves the modelling of the parent depressive behaviours by the child. For instance the low self-esteem, the hopelessness, poor problem solving skills and poor social reinforcement performance may all be learnt by the child. The amount learnt in this way may, however, depend on how much reinforcement the depressed parent receives, since modelling depends partly on the amount of reinforcement the model receives. We are less likely to model a person who stands on the fringe of a group avoiding conversation than a person who is in the 'thick of things' and is receiving a high level of social reinforcement. Thus, if a variety of adult models are frequently available to the child it is likely that the child will model the adult whose behaviour appears to be most frequently reinforced. Unfortunately, families experiencing frequent psychiatric illness often tend to exist in cultural isolation (Tonge et al., 1975) and thus multiple models often may not be available.

Liberman and Raskin (1971) describe how depressive behaviours may be learnt directly as a result of reinforcement. In some persons depressive behaviours may be viewed as a deviant skill used to gain attention and approval. In most bereavements for example , it is common enough for much sympathy and attention to be focused on the depressive behaviours in the initial stages. After a few weeks there is a tendency for others to stop attending to these behaviours (Parkes, 1972a). Normally the bereaved person has a range of skills which will gain reinforcement without the continued use of depressive behaviours to achieve this end. In neurotic persons this range is frequently narrower and thus a highly reinforced behaviour such as depressive symptoms, is more likely to be learnt and used in the future, see Burgess (1969). It is important to recognise this form of learnt depression since treatment in this type may differ from treatment in other types. For instance, in cases of chronic bereavement in which the depressive and grieving behaviours are analysed as manipulative, satiation techniques may be appropriate, whereas in other grief reactions desensitisation techniques are most appropriate (McAuley and Quinn, 1975). The way in. which people handle unpleasant life events will help us predict the probable effect of future losses. Parkes (1972a) notes that many persons with chronic bereavement have exhibited severe grief reactions following past bereavements. Maddison and Walker (1967) suggest that a poor response to unpleasant life events which preceded the bereavement may dictate outcome. In a series of careful animal experiments Church (1969) has examined the effects of differing intensities of non-contingent electric shock on animals' ongoing behaviour. Animals exposed to initial intense shock show a marked reduction in ongoing social behaviour. In later experiments (with the same animals) when the shock level was reduced the animal still exhibited a marked reduction in ongoing behaviour. Church suggested that the animal had become sensitised to shock. When the experiments with naive animals were conducted starting with low levels of shock, the animals appeared to adapt to shock in that their ongoing behaviour was not seriously disrupted by more intense shocks later. Of course it is difficult to make generalisations from animal to human behaviour and from the one variable experimental situation to the natural environment. However, as already mentioned there is evidence that sensitisation might be important, though it only remains as one possible variable among many.

Learned Helplessness

Learned helplessness is perhaps one of the most exciting models of depression to have been developed over the last decade. As a model it offers some important explanations for the frequent depressive behaviours of hopelessness and helplessness. The initial experimental work was conducted by Maier *et al.* (1969) on dogs. They demonstrated that many dogs who were exposed to uncontrollable shock while restricted in a harness failed to learn escape behaviours in a shuttle box when this latter task was conducted within 24 hours of the initial shocks. The reversal of this failure was frequently in the initial stages only brought about by physically forcing the animals to perform escape behaviours. However, in later days it was generally found that this 'maladaptive' behaviour gradually wore off. The researchers, after exhausting several hypotheses, concluded that these dogs had learned helplessness. Further studies have reported similar findings in other animals and more recently in man, see Seligman (1975). Interestingly, some other authorities from apparently unrelated fields have also emphasised the importance of the learning of helpless and hopeless behaviours in depressed patients (Beck, 1971; Melges and Bowlby, 1969).

In discussing how learned helplessness might apply to depression Seligman (1975) has carefully compared the symptoms and signs observed in helpless animals and humans to those observed in depressed humans. There appear to be a number of similarities. (1) Both exhibit motivational defects in that they perform less well on a variety of tasks and show deficits in the response initiation. (2) They have difficulty in learning that their own efforts have any effect. Often humans will state for example, that there is no use trying because it is hopeless. (3) Both helpless subjects and depressed individuals frequently exhibit lowered aggression. (4) Learned helplessness and depression are similar in that they frequently dissipate over time. (5) There are many similarities between the somatic upsets of the helpless animal and the depressed subjects, which include loss of appetite and loss or reduction in sexual responsiveness. Seligman (1975) is however careful to emphasise that similarities in behaviour do not provide proof of similarities in aetiology. Further he emphasises that only some depressions may result from learned helplessness. While more research is required, perhaps one of the most interesting questions which remains to be answered relates to how helplessness generalises from one situation to many. For instance most of us would be helpless when confronted with a broken radio, however this does not generalise to our ability to drive our cars or to do our work. Under what circumstances do these discriminations break down as they would appear to have done in many depressives?

This examination of behavioural theories of depression is by no means exhaustive, however it does illustrate some of the complexities involved in the aetiology of neurotic depression. Whilst Moss and Boren (1972) emphasise the importance of low rates of reinforcement, Seligman (1975) emphasises loss of controllability (following loss or aversive events), Libet and Lewinsohn (1973) stress the importance of social skills, and Wolpe (1971) emphasises the role of anxiety in the genesis of neurotic depression. Clearly the important psychosocial elements in this disorder are multiple, and it is possible that each of the models mentioned here has some validity.

Assessment

Frequently psychiatric assessment has been based on: (1) What the patient or client tells us; (2) the use of various standardised psychometric instruments; (3) a few relatively short clinical interviews. The verbal behaviours of depressed persons are frequently unreliable. The clients often perceive the world, themselves and the future as negative and thus many of their verbal behaviours do not reflect what is happening in reality. This is not to say that how the client sees the world is unimportant. We do require a knowledge of both. Many psychometric instruments and especially personality inventories have little value, since they do not usually throw any light on aetiology. Mischel (1968) has contested much of the writings on trait theory. He has made the important point that behaviour is not determined by traits but by situational factors. Further, when used carelessly psychometric instruments may result in erroneous advice as was suggested earlier in this article. Treatment should not begin until there is a reasonable understanding or hypothesis about the depression and its aetiology. It is unlikely that the average neurotic depression can be understood on the basis of one or two interviews. It is arrogant to believe that we can adequately understand an individual's problem and how this relates to his life history in such a short time. For instance, the information which is required in order to understand just one behaviour is complex, see figure 14.1.

Traditionally, in assessing psychological problems behaviour therapists have favoured the use of naturalistic observation as an adjunct to history taking, because such observation facilitates objective quantification of the problem, allows a fine grain analysis of its components and provides baseline data against which treatment progress can be judged. Patterson and Rosenberry (1969), Lewinsohn and Shaffer (1971), and McLean (1976), have found home observation of the depressed person and his family to be a promising technique. Generally observations are conducted at times when all members of the family are likely to be present, for example teatime. Libet and Lewinsohn (1973) assess the interaction in terms of the amount of behaviour,

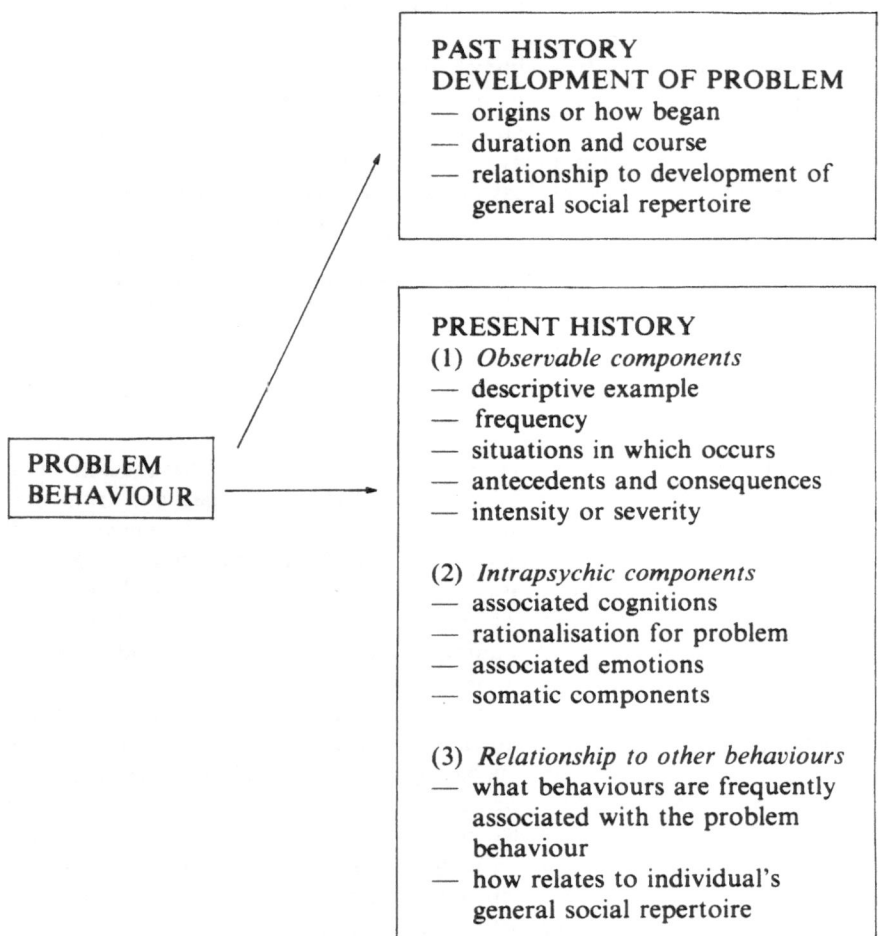

Figure 14.1   The assessment dimensions of a problem behaviour

the use of positive and negative behaviours, and the range of interaction and interpersonal efficiency, that is the amount of verbal reciprocity between persons. In this way a clear knowledge of both appropriate and inappropriate behaviours can be gained. McLean (1976) in one family assessment noted that a wife's depressive behaviours appeared to be maintained not only by her husband's negative behaviours and his lack of positive reinforcement, but also by attention for depressed behaviours from her children. When the mother was well her children tended to ignore her. The treatment implications of this example are obvious. Observations of this type (and others discussed below) are associated with problems of observer reactivity, and these are similar in many ways to the response sets which are encountered in interview settings.

For instance Johnson and Lobitz (1974) have demonstrated that parents can make their children look better or worse, by varying instructions given to the parents prior to the observation. McLean (1976) has attempted to circumvent some of these issues by using sound recordings of family interactions when observers are not present. For a full discussion on some of these observational issues see Johnson and Bolstad (1973). Perhaps the most important advantages of family observation include: (1) An assessment of the families' motivation and willingness to become involved in treatment. (2) The provision of concrete examples of behaviour which may require to be increased or decreased. (3) An emphasis on the fact that family relationships might be important in the target person's depression. (4) The fact that observation is frequently conducted in the prime treatment situation. For instance if marital social skills or child management skills are deficient then training in these areas can begin in the home following several observations. Lewinsohn *et al.* (1970) have also employed a peer group observational technique. Noticing that many depressed college students had few interpersonal relationships, they found it necessary to form a group of depressed students in order that each member's interactional behaviours could be studied. In this group, observation and treatment were closely interwoven. Perhaps the most frequently employed observational strategy is one which involves patient self-observation, see Patterson and Rosenberry (1969), Lewinsohn *et al.* (1969), and McLean (1976). Typically the patient is asked to record predefined activities and rate the amount of associated pleasure or interest. From these records (providing they are reasonably reliable), one can pinpoint accurately areas of deficiency (for example avoidance of social activities), and also identify events which may be potentially reinforcing. Information of this type emphasises the importance of patient involvement in treatment and provides concrete examples which the therapist can discuss. More importantly, the records represent the beginning of treatment in that they provide the patient with relatively more accurate feedback about his behaviour. When patients can apply this skill of self-observation they can then pinpoint problems and examine the behavioural antecedents and consequences.

Treatment

A wide variety of behavioural techniques have been sucessfully used in the treatment of depression. These reflect both the viewpoint of the therapist and the diversity of ways in which the depressive can present. In many case studies several different techniques have been used in managing the same patient. For instance Ramsay (1975) successfully treated a young bereaved patient by using a technique which contained elements of systematic desensitisation, *in vivo* assignments and assertive training. This type of approach is heartening because it demonstrates that each patient's treatment has been carefully tailored on the basis of a meticulous assessment. In the section below the common techniques are examined in turn. This does not imply that any of these are mutually exclusive.

Reinstating Reinforcement and Contingency Management

The most common problem in the depressive is his/her lack of engagement in positively reinforcing activities. Many therapeutic reports have focused on the correction of this deficit. When loss of reinforcers has been aetiologically important in the precipitation of depression then the primary focus of therapy is in that area.

Burgess (1969) describes a case in which a 'bright' student became depressed following his marriage. The history revealed that he was having considerable difficulty in grasping academic concepts. Since his marriage the student had been spending much less time in academic discussion with friends. Following therapist instructions to engage in more regular meetings and academic discussions with college mates the student's depression and conceptual ability improved considerably. Lazarus (1968) reports the use of a time-projection technique in re-establishing lost reinforcers. Under light hypnosis a depressed girl was asked to imagine herself increasingly over time, becoming involved in activities which she had enjoyed prior to her recently broken romance. After two sessions the girl had improved considerably.

In many depressive illnesses it may not be possible to either reinstate lost reinforcers (for example after the loss of a spouse), or to identify specific areas of lost reinforcement. In these circumstances Burgess (1969) and Lewinsohn *et al.* (1969) focus on increasing a variety of reinforcing activities which have decreased since the depression began. In several cases Burgess (1969) constructed a hierarchy of behaviours which were to be completed from session to session (for instance, mowing the lawn, making a date and fixing a car). On the basis of an inventory—the Pleasant Events Schedule—Lewinsohn (1974) first identifies those events which have been enjoyed in the past and which now appear to be correlated with mood. Following this a therapeutic goal of increased involvement in these activities is constructed. Lewinsohn's work emphasises the importance of demonstrating that events are mood sensitive (or positively reinforcing). In other words the completion of tasks must be associated with satisfaction. For instance, there is little point in advising a patient to take a holiday in the sun if this is not associated with pleasure. In some circumstances such advice may enhance a sense of failure.

In many cases instruction alone may be insufficient to bring about an increase in reinforcing activity. Lazarus (1976) suggests that in the initial stages of therapy it may often be essential to push or directly guide the patients into these activities. This advice has interesting parallels with the work of Ayllon and Azrin (1968). In devising token economies in institutional settings these researchers found it necessary to persuade patients to sample reinforcers before they would begin to exchange their tokens for the same reinforcers.

Lazarus (1968) has also suggested that a period of sensory deprivation (for instance an enforced period of bedrest), may help to enhance the reinforcement value of events. This type of approach has its parallels in Morita Therapy (Kora, 1965). The author is unaware of any behaviour therapy reports which have examined the efficacy of this technique.

The utility of the Premack Principle in increasing the patient's activity level has been demonstrated by Lewinsohn et al. (1969). This principle states that the occurrence of a high-rate behaviour (a frequently occurring one), can be used to reinforce the occurrence of a low rate behaviour. Depressed persons' high-rate behaviours will include verbalisations about their problems, feelings of hopelessness and unpleasant affect. In therapy these behaviours can be used to reinforce talk and discussion about infrequently occurring adaptive behaviours, such as task completion or planning activities. Practically this will involve the therapist applying rules which state that depressive talk will be encouraged after a discussion about a prerequisite amount of predefined adaptive behaviour.

Most therapists have emphasised the importance of therapist social reinforcement for completed tasks coupled with therapist withdrawal of attention for depressive talk (Burgess, 1969; Liberman and Raskin, 1971). Lewinsohn (1974) reported a successful study in which the amount of therapy time was made contingent upon the number of completed patient assignments. This approach in common with the Premack Principle, assumes rightly or wrongly that therapists and therapeutic time are reinforcing. Further, if the therapy is confined to a consulting room, reinforcement focuses on and is consequent on the patient's verbal behaviour, which may be unreliable or unrepresentative of his behaviour elsewhere. Liberman and Raskin (1971), Patterson and Rosenberry (1969) and McLean et al. (1973) have trained significant people in the patient's interactional field to reinforce constructive task-orientated behaviour and to ignore depressive behaviours. This approach has two important advantages. (1) In the past the majority of therapists have relied on people in the patient's environment to provide reinforcement for increased activity, without, as part of the therapeutic plan, ensuring that they have the skills to do so. (2) As mentioned above the patient's improved verbal behaviour in the consulting room may not have generalised to other settings. Training the spouse as contingency manager helps to overcome this problem of generalisation. In the following section there is further discussion on the training of spouses in interactional skills.

Social Skills Training and Desensitisation

The lack of variety of interactional skills in the depressive has been noted by Libet and Lewinsohn (1973). Social skills training may be useful in the treatment of many depressives. However, Burgess (1969) suggests that it may not be essential in all cases. In this study she noted that improvements in depressed patients were frequently associated with increases in assertive behaviours although no attempts had been made to teach these patients assertive behaviours. This would seem to suggest that social skills training is most appropriately employed in those cases in which skill deficits are instrumental in the onset of the depression rather than being a symptom of the disorder. However, Lazarus (1968) notes that training in affective expression may sometimes be useful in treating the affective symptoms of depression. He states that affects such as anger, amusement, or affection are frequently absent and also incompatible with depression. Lazarus discusses several brief examples of how assertive affects might 'break-up' a depressive cycle.

Lewinsohn et al. (1969) reported the teaching of social skills to a group of depressed students. Each student was taught: (1) to observe and pinpoint his (and other subjects') behaviour problems. The areas of importance such as low rates of positive reinforcement, long response latencies, etc., have been mentioned previously; (2) to define goals and set up assignments for behaviour change; and (3) how to change his behaviour in the group setting. This involved constant feedback and practice during assigned group discussions.

The recognition that many depressives have marital problems has led to a focus on social skills training in this area (Lewinsohn and Shaffer, 1971; Patterson and Rosenberry, 1969; McLean et al., 1973). The treatment strategies adopted by each of these researchers have been rather similar. The main emphasis has been on training couples to increase positive and reduce negative behaviours and on teaching problem solving skills which aim at contractual solutions. Patterson et al. (1976) videotape their couples discussing problem areas. Feedback and corrective suggestions on positive and negative behaviours are made during replay and then discussion sequences are repeated. At a problem solving level the couple are taught listening, expressive, descriptive and agreeing skills. Directly supervised sessions of this nature are enhanced by home assignments.

Wolpe (1971) has stressed the role which anxiety might play in the genesis of some depressive disorders. He suggests that anxiety may inhibit the individual's social skills and he asserts that desensitisation coupled with social skills training may be required in some cases. Unfortunately no case examples are provided. Ramsay (1975) reports a case in which the approach is similar to that suggested by Wolpe. In this example a depressed young man was taught under relaxation to express aggression initially towards peers and later towards his own father, who appeared to be the cause of his inhibition. Improvement in his depression occurred at a stage when he was able to comfortably talk about his father in both positive and negative terms.

Resolution of grief can sometimes be brought about using systematic desensitisation. Often the anxiety or unpleasant affects which are common in severe or chronic grief may motivate avoidance behaviours, which prevent the extinction of these affects. Under relaxation it may be possible for the therapist to guide the patient towards the unpleasant experience and extinguish the associated affects. Frequently a gentle desensitising approach is difficult, and Ramsay (1975) suggests that the process of extinction of emotions in chronic or severe grief is often more akin to flooding than desensitisation. However, the process can be made less painful for the patient by using a drug assisted desensitisation. McAuley and Quinn (1971) reported a case in which a suicidally bereaved patient was successfully treated using the technique Declining Drug Dose Desensitisation (McCormick and O'Gorman, 1971).

Cognitive Therapy and Techniques for Enhancing Self-control

Treatment techniques which have been developed by Beck (see Beck, 1967) over the past 15 years, focus on altering the negative and frequently unrealistic cognitions which are so common in depression. While his techniques may be useful in interrupting the downward spiral of depressive illnesses, he suggests that the techniques used either on their own or as therapeutic adjuncts, are most useful after the low point in each depressive illness has been reached. The therapy is divided into four stages. After taking a history which focuses particularly on the patient's attitude to himself and his environment, the therapist explains the rationale of the procedure. For instance the patient is informed how attitudes such as 'I'm a failure' can shape behaviour and emotion. At the second stage the patient is taught to accurately pinpoint the negative cognitions, to track the situations in which they occur and to identify the effects which these have on his emotions. The keeping of diary descriptions and records is encouraged. In the next stage the patient is taught to apply logic and reality to the cognitions. For instance if a patient has been ignored by a friend, rather than taking this as a personal slight, the patient is taught to examine various reasons why his friend might not have spoken to him. As a final stage the patient is encouraged to extend and practise challenging these negative cognitions, either *in vivo* or in fantasy, until the associated unpleasant moods have disappeared. Beck suggests that it is important to ensure that patients continue to use the techniques so that core attitudes such as frequent self-criticisms, can be modified. While case studies using cognitive therapy have been reported (Beck, 1967) this author knows of only one attempt to examine the effectiveness of this approach against other techniques. In this one study Beck and Kovacs (1977) report that cognitive therapy was found more successful than antidepressant drug therapy in a randomly selected sample of 40 depressed patients. However, details about the depressed subjects were not supplied.

Behaviour therapists have in the past few years shown increasing interest in the process of self-control (Thorensen and Mahoney, 1974). Therapies for increasing self-control have evolved and have been applied to a large number of problems (for instance smoking, eating and sexual disorders). These techniques bear a remarkable similarity to Beck's cognitive therapy in that they focus on self-observation, self-evaluation and self-reinforcement or punishment. Fuchs and Rehm (1977) examined the utility of self-control techniques in a small sample of mildly depressed patients. After six weeks' therapy and at six weeks follow-up, the twelve patients treated using self-control techniques showed a greater improvement than non-specific therapy and waiting-list control groups.

Management of Learned Helplessness

The treatment techniques already discussed have largely referred to correcting reinforcement deficits, social skill deficits and cognitive abnormalities. Most of these techniques are also applicable to cases in which learned helplessness is thought to be important. For instance the re-establishment of positive reinforcement, training in social skills and corrections in cognitive abnormalities should all enhance a patient's feeling of controllability of himself in his environment. However, the main therapeutic obstacle is how one is to initiate responses in patients who say 'It's useless, there's no point in me trying.' There are a number of ways in which response initiation might be achieved. (1) The patient may be cajoled into task completion (Lazarus, 1976) or into making an assertive response. Taulbee and Wright (1971) have described an antide-pressant programme in which the first major aim of therapy is to evoke an assertive response. The patient is given menial and monotonous tasks to complete, and is kept working on these until an assertive response (such as refusal to complete further work) is emitted. These responses are encouraged. Each time the depressive symptoms intensify the patient is returned to the menial tasks until further assertive responses are emitted. (2) Initial tasks which are simple and easily completed may help to begin the process of controllability. Seligman (1975) has demonstrated that early experience of success is often crucial in the reversal of both depression and learned helplessness. (3) Manipulations to avoid the helplessness cognitive set can be of value. For instance the patient might be asked to complete a potentially reinforcing task in a novel manner or under novel circumstances. The issuing of paradoxical injunctions (instructions which are contrary to the patient's therapeutic expectations) may also be useful. For a further description of this family therapy technique see Walrond-Skinner (1976).

Summary

A large number of the treatment reports reviewed here have been in the form of preliminary case studies. A number of general criticisms can be made about them. Often clinical details are sparse, the follow-up periods are too short and the fact that depression often has a limited time course is not considered. It is the author's opinion that many of the successfully treated depressive disorders are mild and not typical or representative of the neurotic depressions which are commonly seen at psychiatric out-patient clinics. Thus while there is no doubt that many of the techniques have proved useful in some cases, their general clinical utility has yet to be demonstrated. The author had access to only two reports which have attempted to empirically assess the effectiveness of the behaviour therapists' contribution to the management of depression. McLean *et al.* (1973) demonstrated that a strategy composed of training in social learning principles, in interactional skills and in initiating behavioural contracts, was more successful than therapy conducted using antidepressant drugs and supportive psychotherapy. However, this study was small and the follow-up period was short (3 months). Additionally the changes in both groups were less at follow-up than at the end of the treatment phase. This might imply that either the supportive form of treatment took longer to show its benefits, or that the depressive illnesses were in the process of remission. In the study reported by Fuchs and Rehm (1977) the numbers of subjects were small and the follow-up period was short. However, these studies are important in that they represent the beginnings of an attempt to evaluate the use of behaviour therapy in depression.

References

Ayllon, T. and Azrin, N. H. (1968). *The Token Economy: A Motivational System for Therapy and Rehabilitation.* Appleton-Century-Crofts, New York

Azrin, N. H. and Holz, W. C. (1966). Punishment. In *Operant Behavior: Areas of Research and Application.* (Ed. W. K. Honig), Appleton-Century-Crofts, New York

Beck, A. T. (1967). *Depression: Clinical, Experimental and Theoretical Aspects.* Hoeber, New York

Beck, A. T. (1971). Cognition, affect and psychopathology. *Archs gen. Psychiat.*, **24**, 495–500

Beck, A. and Kovacs, M. (1977). A new way to cure depression. *Psychology Today*, **3**, 6, 32–35

Brown, G. W., Harris, T. O. and Peto, J. (1973). Life events and psychiatric disorders. Part 2: Nature and causal link. *Psychol. Med.*, **3**, 159–176

Burgess, E. P. (1969). The modification of depressive behaviors. In *Advances in Behavior Therapy, 1968*, (Ed. R. D. Rubin and C. M. Franks) Academic Press, New York

Church, R. M. (1969). Response suppression. In *Punishment and Aversive Behavior.* (Ed. B. A. Campbell and R. M. Church), Appleton-Century-Crofts, New York

Ekman, P. and Friesen, W. V. (1974). Non-verbal behavior in psychopathology. In *The Psychology of Depression: Contemporary Theory and Research* (Ed. R. J. Friedman and M. M. Katz), Winston-Wiley, Washington

Ferster, C. B. (1966) Animal behavior and mental illness. *Psychol. Rec.*, **16**, 345–356

Fuchs, C. Z. and Rehm, L. P. (1977). A self control behavior therapy programme for depression. *J. consult. clin. Psychol.*, **45**, 206–215

Hinchcliffe, M. K., Lancashire, M. and Roberts, F. J. (1971). A study of eye-contact changes in depressed and recovered patients. *Br. J. Psychiat.*, **119**, 213–215

Johnson, S. M. and Bolstad, O. D. (1973). Methodological issues in naturalistic observations. In *Behavior Change: Methodology, Concepts and Change* (Ed. L. A. Hamerlynck, L. C. Handy and E. J. Mash), Research Press, Champaign, Ill.

Johnson, S. M. and Lobitz, G. K. (1974). Parental manipulation of child behavior in home observations. *J. appl. behav. Anal.*, **7**, 23–31

Kora, T. (1965). Morita Therapy. *Int. J. Psychiat.*,**1**, 611–640

Lazarus, A. A. (1968). Learning theory and the treatment of depression. *Behav. Res. Ther.*, **6**, 83–89

Lazarus, A. A. (1976). Multimodal behavioral treatment of depression. In *Multimodal Behavior Therapy* (Ed. A. A. Lazarus), Springer, New York

Lewinsohn, P. M. (1974). A behavioral approach to depression. In *The Psychology of Depression: Contemporary Theory and Research* (Ed. R. M. Friedman and M. M. Katz), Wiley, New York

Lewinsohn, P. M. (1975). Engagement in pleasant activities and depression level. *J. abnorm. Psychol.*, **84**, 729–731

Lewinsohn, P. M. and Shaffer, M. (1971). The use of home observations as an integral part of the treatment of depression: Preliminary report and case studies. *J. consult. clin. Psychol.*, **37**, 87–94

Lewinsohn, P. M. and Graf, M. (1973). Pleasant activities and depression. *J. consult. clin. Psychol.*, **41**, 261–268

Lewinsohn, P. M., Weinstein, M. S. and Shaw, D. A. (1969). Depression: A clinical-research approach. In *Advances in Behavior Therapy, 1968* (Ed. D. A. Rubin and C. M. Franks), Academic Press, New York

Lewinsohn, P. M., Weinstein, M. S. and Alper, T. A. (1970). A behaviorally orientated approach to the group treatment of depressed persons: a methodological contribution. *J. clin. Psychol.*, **26**, 525–532

Lewinsohn, P. M., Lobitz, W. C. and Wilson C. (1973). Sensitivity of depressed individuals to aversive stimuli. *J. abnorm. Psychol.*, **81**, 259–263

Liberman, R. P. and Raskin, D. E. (1971). Depression: a behavioral formulation. *Archs gen. Psychiat.*, **24**, 515–523

Libet, J. and Lewinsohn, P. M. (1973). The concept of social skill with special reference to the behavior of depressed persons. *J. consult. clin. Psychol.*, **40**, 304–312

McAuley, R. R. and Quinn, J. T. (1971). Behavioural analysis, treatment and theoretical implications of a case of depression. Paper presented at the Third Annual Conference of the Behavioural Engineering Association, Wexford, Ireland

McAuley, R. R. and Quinn, J. T. (1975). Behavioural models of depression. In *Progress in Behaviour Therapy*, (Ed.-in-chief J. C. Brengelman), Springer-Verlag, Berlin

McCormick, W. O. and O'Gorman, E. C. (1971). Declining-dose-drug-desensitization for phobias. *Psychol. Med.*, **1**, 339–342

McLean, P. D., Ogston, K. and Graner, L. (1973). A behavioral approach to the treatment of depression. *J. Behav. Ther. exp. Psychiat.*, **4**, 323–330

McLean, P. D. (1976). Parental depression: incompatible with effective parenting. In *Behavior Modification Approaches to Parenting* (Ed. E. J. Mash, L. C. Handy and L. A. Hamerlynck), Brunner/Mazel, New York

Maddison, D. and Walker, W. L. (1967). Factors affecting the outcome of conjugal bereavement. *Br. J. Psychiat.*, **113**, 1057–1067

Maier, S. F., Seligman, M. E. P. and Solomon, R. L. (1969). Pavlovian fear conditioning and learned helplessness. In *Punishment and Aversive Behavior* (Ed. B. A. Campbell and R. M. Church), Appleton-Century-Crofts, New York

Martin, I. and Rees, L. (1966). Recreation times and somatic reactivity in depressed patients. *J. psychosom. Res.*, **9**, 375–382

Melges, F. T. and Bowlby, J. (1969). Types of hopelessness in psychopathological process. *Archs gen. Psychiat.*, **20**, 690–699

Mischel, W. (1968). *Personality and Assessment.* Wiley New York

Moss, G. R. and Boren, J. J. (1972). Depression as a model for behavioral analysis. *Compreh. Psychiat.*, **13**, 581–590

Parkes, C. M. (1964). Recent bereavement as a cause of mental illness. *Br. J. Psychiat.*, **110**, 198

Parkes, C. M. (1972a). *Bereavement: Studies of Grief in Adult Life.* International Universities Press, New York

Parkes, C. M. (1972b). Components of the reaction to loss of a limb, spouse or home. *J. psychosom. Res.*, **16**, 343

Patterson, G. R. and Rosenberry, C. (1969). A social learning formulation of depression. Paper presented at the International Conference on Behaviour Modification, Banff/Alberta

Patterson, G. R., Weiss, R. L. and Hops, H. (1976). Training of marital skills: some problems and concepts. In *Handbook of Behavior Modification and Behavior Therapy* (Ed. H. Leitenberg), Prentice-Hall, Englewood Cliffs, New Jersey

Paykel, E. S., Myers, J. K., Dienelt, M. N., Klerman, G. L. Lindenthal, J. J. and Pepper, M. P. (1969). Life events and depression. *Archs gen. Psychiat.*, **21**, 753–760

Ramsay, R. W. (1975). The stress of bereavement: components and treatment. Paper presented at the conference on Dimensions of Anxiety and Stress, Oslo, Norway

Rippere, V. (1977). Some cognitive dimensions of anti-depressive behaviour. *Behav. Res. Ther.*, **15**, 57–63

Schachter, S. (1964). The interaction of cognitive and physiological determinants of emotional state. *Adv. exp. soc. Psychol.*, **1**, 49–80

Seligman, M. E. P. (1975). *Helplessness.* W. H. Freeman, San Francisco

Taulbee, E. S. and Wright, H. W. (1971). A psycho-social-behavioral model for therapeutic intervention. In *Current Topics in Clinical and Community Psychology, Vol. 3* (Ed. C. D. Spielberger), Academic Press, New York

Thorensen, C. E. and Mahoney, M. J. (1974). *Behavioral Self-Control.* Holt, Rinehart and Winston, New York

Tonge, W. L., James, D. S. and Hillam, S. M. (1975). Families without hope: a controlled study of 33 problem families. *Br. J. Psychiat. Special Publication No. 11.* Headley Brothers, Ashford, Kent

Vincent, J. P. (1972). Problem solving behavior in distressed and non-distressed marriage and stranger dyads. Unpublished doctoral dissertation. University of Oregon, Eugene

Walrond-Skinner, S. (1976). *Family Therapy.* Routledge and Kegan Paul, London

Wolpe, J. (1971). Neurotic depression: experimental analog, clinical syndromes and treatment. *Am. J. Psychother.*, **25**, 362–368

15 The Treatment of Social Phobia

P. Shaw

Although this chapter is mainly about treatment, it is appropriate to begin with clinical description. This is necessary because there is still confusion in the use of the terms social phobia and agoraphobia. Moreover certain other diagnostic entities can be mistaken for these phobic states, and at times a patient may have more than one condition, in which case it is necessary to have an agreed way of deciding which is primary. Having considered these issues, the paper will go on to describe the treatment of social phobia, both by psychological means and with drug treatment.

The Clinical Syndromes

Agoraphobia

In this section and those which follow, information is drawn from a recent and, so far, unpublished survey of 144 phobic patients carried out in Oxford. The other important sources of information are summarised by Marks (1969). The term agoraphobia is used to denote a syndrome whose most prominent feature is a fear of being away either from home, or from other places in which the patient feels safe. Fear is usually greater in places which cannot be left easily—theatres, supermarkets—and in crowded surroundings. The experience of fear is almost invariably accompanied by somatic symptoms of anxiety. Fear may be very intense, amounting to panic, especially when the patient feels cut off from 'safety'. As well as intense fear in these situations, the patient may experience other sudden attacks of anxiety (often called panic attacks) which appear unpredictably in places which are 'safe', for example in the home. When these are present it is usually found that the patient also shows increased anxiety throughout the waking day. The whole range of anxiety symptoms may be experienced but in the Oxford survey two were found to occur rather specifically in agoraphobia and were found much less often in association with social phobias. These were weakness in the legs and breathlessness. In addition to these somatic symptoms, most agoraphobics have anxious thoughts, typically about personal catastrophes such as a heart attack or collapse in the street. Patients are also almost invariably afraid of falling. These particular anxious thoughts were seldom described by patients in the survey who had social phobia. Many people whose main complaints are part of the agoraphobic syndrome also describe fears of social situations. As we shall see, the reverse is not found at all frequently.

Agoraphobia begins suddenly in at least half the patients. There are two peak ages of onset: in the early twenties and in the early thirties. Among agoraphobic patients there are about six women to every man. The balance of evidence suggests that agoraphobia is a discrete syndrome and not merely the extreme of a continuum of symptoms which are found in the normal population.

Social Phobia

This term denotes an exaggerated fear of situations in which the patient has to meet other people. The symptoms may appear when he enters a room where there are other people, asks for things in a shop, has to write or do manual tasks in front of other people, eats a meal in company or takes part in a meeting. Patients complain of all kinds of anxiety symptoms but blushing and trembling are reported far more frequently by social phobics than by agoraphobics. The anxious thoughts of a patient with social phobia are invariably that he will attract criticism or ridicule to himself. Unlike agoraphobic patients, social phobics do not experience panic attacks when they are away from phobic situations, even though they too may be generally anxious people. Moreover, very few people who complain of social phobia also have agoraphobic symptoms.

The disorder usually begins in adolescence and, as a rule, it does so gradually. However, subjects often say that they have had some problems in meeting other people for much longer than this. There is, therefore, no definite peak age of onset, but the modal age appears to be around 17 or 18. Men and women are about equally represented with perhaps a slight male predominance.

In dealing with socially phobic patients it is important to remember that they are suffering from a cognitive disturbance as well as from anxiety symptoms. This cognitive disturbance takes the form of a misinterpretation of other people's actions as well as unwarranted expectations about their likely response to the patient. Patients may also misperceive their own behaviour, supposing that their actions and conversational gambits are less acceptable and less appropriate than they really are. In addition, symptoms of anxiety may cause further embarrassment if they become severe. Patients who fear that they may lose control of their bladder, and those who fear that they may vomit may take elaborate precautions to make sure they are never out of reach of a lavatory. As a result some may fear being out in the street and in this way come to resemble agoraphobics. Patients who believe that they sweat excessively may fear that they smell and try to arrange every interpersonal encounter in the open air. Those whose anxiety results in shaking hands may find it impossible to raise a cup or glass to the lips. Others are unable to fill in a form or write a cheque while being watched. Those whose work has to be carried out under the eyes of a foreman, may find themselves totally incapacitated. People who blush excessively come to fear every new encounter and may even fear opening the front door of their house.

There is a special point about those social phobics who are frightened of vomiting. Some of these patients fear not only that they will vomit but that other people may do so. They go to extraordinary lengths to avoid any situation where there is even a remote chance that anyone might be sick. I believe that these patients have obsessional symptoms rather than social phobia. The latter are usually unconcerned if another person is sick. They are aware of sensations of nausea and anxious thoughts about vomiting which appear to be part of their pattern of anxiety just as palpitations or trembling may be.

Many of the problems of social phobics are similar to those experienced by adolescents in the course of normal development. Many of those who present for treatment in their early twenties, have expected to grow out of the symptoms but have found to their dismay that unlike their contemporaries they have not. This is confirmed by the finding that there is a high incidence of social anxiety among a student population (Bryant and Trower, 1974). It is also supported by the results of a fear survey schedule given to normal subjects which indicate that many normal people experience social anxieties to some degree. It is likely, therefore, that there is a continuous variation between the normal population and those who present for treatment of social phobias. For this reason the incidence of social phobias in the population is difficult to determine but it is probable that severe social phobia is much more common than it has been supposed to be. Thus, an unexpectedly large number of people presented for treatment when the facilities were made available and general practitioners were made more aware of the problem.

Social Inadequacy

Michael Argyle, and his co-workers, coined this term as a behavioural description which takes into account gaze, facial expression, posture, gesture, voice, appropriateness of vocalisations and verbalisations. These workers distinguish between primary and secondary social inadequacy. Those who suffer from the primary condition have never learnt normal social skills; those who are described as suffering from the secondary condition have acquired a full repertoire of social skills but are inhibited from using them fully by anxiety or some other problem (Argyle, 1969). The chapter by Trower and Bryant in this volume considers primary social inadequacy in more detail. For my purposes it is necessary to indicate the relationship between this description of behaviour and the diagnosis of social phobia. In a recent treatment trial in Oxford, subjects were selected who had a primary diagnosis of social phobia but who were also rated on measures of social inadequacy. Only 30 per cent of these socially phobic patients were rated socially inadequate and for the most part the disorder was small, usually disappearing when anxiety was relieved. It appears, therefore, that the majority of subjects who complain primarily of the symptoms which are classified by psychiatrists as social phobia have adequate social skills. Their problem is rather that they lack confidence and find difficulty in making full use of the skills they possess.

Some Diagnostic Conventions

Patients with general anxiety states often experience severe attacks of anxiety similar in content to those of agoraphobic patients but not arising in any particular situation. When these symptoms accompany agoraphobia it is conventional to give precedence to the latter diagnosis. Social phobics are often generally anxious and in this case also the phobic diagnosis is conventionally given priority. Social phobics and agoraphobics both suffer at times from symptoms of depression. When these appear after phobic anxiety symptoms and are less intense they are not usually diagnosed separately. Primary depression is, however, quite frequent among agoraphobic patients. In this case, a course of antidepressants, either tricyclics or monoamine oxidase inhibitors, is often beneficial and should be tried before psychological treatment. There is, however, no evidence that antidepressants are useful in treating the majority of patients with social phobia.

The diagnosis of alcoholism may arise in the context of phobias. It is well known that some agoraphobic patients take alcohol to control anxiety before going out shopping. Few become alcoholics. Some social phobics also drink to lessen anxiety and they seem more likely to develop secondary alcoholism. For example, one business man used regularly to drink half a bottle of whisky to alleviate anxiety before board meetings; without this he was quite unable to attend. Drug abuse must also be enquired about in phobic patients.

Personality Problems

The survey in Oxford of phobic patients, from which results have already been quoted, indicated that phobic patients are, in general, unusually conscientious, have many obsessional but few hysterical traits. For the most part these patients showed surprising tenacity in keeping jobs often in the face of crippling symptoms. In this survey agoraphobics tended to be somewhat more introverted than the normal population, while social phobics were significantly more introverted than agoraphobics. This finding has a bearing on treatment and I shall return to it.

Treatment

Non-specific Psychological Treatment

No-one has done more than Jerome Frank to emphasise the importance, in psychological treatment, of factors which are generally regarded as non-specific and often ignored or taken for granted (Frank, 1961). In the treatment of phobias, these non-specific factors are often of great significance. The first and, in some ways, most important, is the therapist's act of taking the patient's complaint seriously. This so often contrasts with previous experience of ridicule, based on ignorance, from relatives and friends and even, at times, from doctors. The discussion of symptoms and reassurance that there is no physical or mental illness is also helpful, especially for patients who fear organic disease. Many patients fear that they may become addicted to drugs or alcohol. They can be assured they are unlikely to have this problem once the phobic anxiety symptoms have improved. It is also reassuring for the patient to learn that other people have the same difficulties, and that it is sufficiently common for it to be likely that he has met others who have social fears and yet hide them. By the very nature of the complaint socially phobic people are the last to admit their disability to others, sometimes even to the spouse.

A number of treatments for social phobias are now available and it is comforting for a patient to learn that these have helped others and may help him. It is appropriate, providing that the therapy is easily available, to discuss with the patient what type of treatment he or she would find most congenial, for, as we shall see, there is some reason to think that the approach which makes most sense to the patient is most likely to help him. Whichever technique is chosen, there is a non-specific benefit from treatment in which he is seen regularly for a clearly defined course of treatment and then followed up at increasing intervals. Phobic patients, more than most others, are often worried about the ending of treatment. For this reason, it is sometimes appropriate to avoid a final discharge date by telling the patient that he can get in touch with the therapist if he should have trouble again. When this offer is made, it is unusual for a patient to ask for further help.

Whatever the nature of the phobic disorder, it is, of course, necessary to consider the personality of the patient. This is especially important for social phobics, for the following reasons. We have seen that social phobics are in general more introverted than agoraphobics (who in turn are more introverted than normal subjects). Now introverts do not enjoy social gatherings nor are they as gregarious as are extroverted people. In their everyday life, however, pressure is brought upon them both by the media and by public opinion to join social groups, to attend parties, and to go to dances and discos. The person who does not join in is often made to feel a social failure by his peers. It is essential, therefore, to point out to social phobics that there is no reason why everyone should enjoy these activities. Many normal, happy people go through life seeing only one or two close friends or members of their immediate family. At the same time it is important, as treatment proceeds, to establish with the patient what level of social activity he or she actually aspires to.

While these non-specific procedures are important and helpful, most patients will also require specific behavioural or psychotherapeutic measures as well. It is these which we shall now review.

The Behaviour Therapies

There are now several behavioural techniques which can be used in the treatment of phobias. In general, however, few differences have been found between the outcome of patients treated by different methods. Thus desensitisation and flooding give identical results with agoraphobic patients although both were more effective than a non-specific treatment (Gelder *et al.*, 1973).

The only trial concerned specifically with social phobias had similar findings (Shaw, to be published). No difference was found between imaginal flooding, imaginal desensitisation and social skills training, three very different types of behavioural approach. With all three treatments patients improved between the beginning and end of treatment but there were no significant differences between them in any outcome measure. An interesting finding was that patients who received flooding worsened at first, as judged by their scores on the semantic differentials. As the final result was no better than that of the other treatments, this finding, if confirmed, suggests that flooding is not the method of choice.

We have seen that social phobics have cognitive distortions. Many are also less assertive than other people. It is difficult for them to complain about faulty goods, to insist on the right change, or to take the lead in similar everyday matters. This problem must also be taken into account when planning treatment.

The most important component of behavioural treatment of phobias appears to be a graded re-entry into the situations which provoke fear. Whether this begins by imagining the situations or actually going to them, a hierarchy of items relevant to the individual's problems must be constructed. This requires careful discussion of the patient's present and desired life style; he must consider what things he is now avoiding, either wholly or in part, and what he would like to be able to do again. In hierarchy construction, between ten and fifteen items are identified and then arranged in a stepwise progression, starting with that which provokes least anxiety and ending with one which is extreme. The intervals between these items should be as equal as possible. The second essential element in the treatment of phobias is practice. It is likely that the reason why no differences have been found between different treatments in clinical trials is that improvement ultimately depends on the extent to which the patient is prepared to practise overcoming his fears. If this is so, it follows that any procedure which motivates the patient to practise will be effective. Equally, it is possible that all patients will not be equally well motivated by the same treatments: each will respond best to that which he believes in most. If this is so, it follows that it is appropriate to describe the available treatments to each patient and then allow him to choose the type which he prefers. Viewed in this way, the therapist's primary tasks, whatever the form of treatment, are goal setting and encouragement of practice between treatment sessions. It must be emphasised repeatedly to the patient that he is ultimately responsible for his own improvement; the therapist can only facilitate it.

Goal Setting and Home Practice

Some patients wish to overcome the phobia themselves with as little help as possible. They do not want formal treatment sessions though they usually find it useful to report progress regularly. The therapist's task is then merely to help the patient construct a hierarchy of items, and to discuss with him how best to tackle each one, starting with the easiest. He should also explain simple steps which the patient can take to reduce anxiety when he is in the situations which provoke his phobias. Tranquillisers taken three-quarters of an hour before he has to enter the feared situation are useful to begin with by making possible first steps which could not be taken without them. As the patient moves up the hierarchy he should cease to use the anxiolytics for the lower items. At the same time, anxiety provoked by fearful thoughts can often be controlled by directing attention to activities or people in the environment. The optimal form of distraction is an individual matter to be worked out with each patient.

Finally, the therapist decides how often he should see his patient. A few need return only monthly to report progress, but most need to be seen more frequently at first, though they are usually content to extend the intervals as they make progress. In a busy outpatient clinic these simple methods are always worth trying first, except in severe cases or when there is much generalised anxiety.

Imaginal Desensitisation

This is the oldest and best tried method of behaviour therapy and there is no need to describe it here. It has proved consistently effective in the treatment of phobias of many kinds although there is some problem of later relapses. For social phobias, however, desensitisation is seldom appropriate by itself but should be used in conjunction with the goal setting and practice which has just been described. In other words, desensitisation should no longer be regarded as a procedure to be administered to the patient. Instead the therapist should be a teacher who, having demonstrated progressive relaxation, encourages the patient to use it in the circumstances of his daily life. He will also teach methods of thought distraction and explain how to take drugs in the most appropriate way. The aim is no longer that something should be done for the patient but rather that he should be taught ways of helping himself.

Imaginal Flooding

There are now no sound reasons for the use of this treatment in its original form, that is by the recital of the patient's worst fears with the intention of creating extreme anxiety. There is no evidence that such a procedure is any more effective than prolonged contact with feared situations in the absence of high levels of anxiety. Such low anxiety flooding treatment is less unpleasant for patient and therapist. It is possible that flooding treatment, whether at high or low anxiety, acts mainly by motivating the patient to practice on his own. This leads to an extinction of fear responses and to a change in the various fearful cognitions. Some therapists add coping instructions but it is not yet certain whether this is effective. Nevertheless, whether these have any specific effect or not, they often give patients confidence that they can deal more effectively with fearful situations.

Assertive Training

This is usually part of social skills training but it can be used alone when the patient is markedly lacking in assertion but not otherwise deficient in social skills. The techniques, which are well known, involve role playing of situations which are representative of those which the patient fears. Assertive training has the advantage that it can readily be carried out in a group with a consequent saving of the time of trained personnel. It is also possible to pair patients to role play situations each taking his turn to adopt the assertive role.

Social Skills Training

This treatment was designed by Argyle and his co-workers for patients who lack primary social skills (Argyle, 1967). They are taught the skills required for listening and for conversation, usually with the help of video feedback. Over the course of weeks they are helped to build up the skills required for brief inter-personal interchanges, such as greetings, together with ways of beginning and ending conversations. As we have noted, the social phobic does not usually lack these skills but he too often benefits from role playing of feared situations with video feedback. Such feedback can, of course, be emotionally painful to a patient who lacks self confidence and must be introduced gradually and with care. Social skills training was one of the treatments assessed in a trial of treatment for social phobias carried out in Oxford (Shaw, 1977). It was found to be equally effective with desensitisation and flooding. However, because it requires more time from skilled therapists as well as more specialised equipment than the other two, it cannot be justified as a general means of treatment. It is, however, an interesting technique for describing and putting right deficits in social skills and should be investigated further.

This cannot be an exhaustive list of behavioural therapies, but it does contain those which are most generally useful for social phobias. The method which is chosen will depend in part on the availability of skilled personnel and of equipment and other facilities. The experience of the Oxford trial suggests strongly that the various approaches which are available are more or less equivalent and it is probably best to describe each to the patient and determine his preference before treatment is started. Many patients will opt for the simple goal setting, advice and reporting back which was described in the first part of this section. Others will ask for more specific help. Of these, some accept treatment in a group, for others this would cause an impossible degree of anxiety. Social skills training, though generally useful, is also terrifying for some patients. For the most timorous, desensitisation (with the adjuncts I have described) is probably the best treatment. A few are attracted to the idea of overcoming severe feelings of anxiety and opt for flooding, and they should receive it.

Other Forms of Psychological Treatment

Group Psychotherapy

Although dynamic or insight psychotherapy in groups is justified for patients with problems of social relationships, I do not consider that it has any important place in the treatment of social phobia. In the Oxford sample, the majority of social phobics did not have grossly disorganised personal relationships. When their specific anxiety could be overcome they were usually able to lead satisfying lives. Group psychotherapy requires a commitment to a minimum period of treatment, usually not less than six months. Behaviour therapy is usually shorter.

Individual Psychotherapy

I believe that there is a definite place for individual therapy on brief or focal lines in selected cases. Indeed, it can be argued that behaviour therapy may produce some of its effects by focusing on patients' problems in a structured manner. The case of a young woman in the Oxford survey is instructive. She presented with severe social phobia and also with marked inhibition in the sexual relationship with her boy-friend. It seemed clear that the two were linked but she found it difficult to talk about either in the way that would have been required in psychotherapy. After a course of desensitisation all her symptoms improved dramatically. However, she remained discontented, saying that she had not got to the bottom of her problems. Like some other patients whom I have treated, she wanted to understand why her problems began, and for this behaviour therapy had no answer. At the end of the follow-up period this girl took part in a few sessions of focal psychotherapy, which were centred on what was clearly the pathological focus—the relationship between herself and her father during adolescence. His jealous, irritable and critical behaviour had almost certainly contributed both to her sexual inhibitions and the social phobia. These sessions of psychotherapy were followed by further improvement in her symptoms but, more importantly, by a new feeling of satisfaction in the patient. In another case in the same series, a successful middle-aged man whose career was threatened by his social phobia became convinced in the course of desensitisation that his real fear was of older men of a particular kind. He was quick to identify as the source of this fear, his father who was a withdrawn and critical man. With this discovery, his symptoms began to improve dramatically. In his case, this insight might have been arrived at through psychotherapy alone and it is possible that this would have been equally effective in changing his symptoms. More work is required on the relationship between individual psychotherapy and behaviour therapy.

Drug Treatment

Drugs, given alone, have no place in the treatment of social phobics. They are, however, a valuable adjunct to any form of goal setting therapy. As described already, they are best given shortly before the patient enters a phobic situation. As a rule a mild tranquilliser is sufficient. Sometimes for patients who suffer acute anxiety on waking, a tranquilliser taken at night is more effective than a morning dose. Only when there is a continuous anxiety is a regular dosage necessary, otherwise it should be taken for specified purposes only. This continuous anxiety often improves simply by virtue of the decrease in social phobia, so that prolonged treatment can be avoided.

Prognosis

Since there have been so few clinical trials including social phobics, there are few sound data on the long-term outcome of any form of treatment. From the evidence of the Oxford trial, short-term outcome is good in that three-quarters of patients have improved. In those followed up for two years there have been very few relapses. This compares favourably with the published reports of trials of treatment of agoraphobia in which fewer patients improved and there were more relapses.

In conclusion, there are several treatments that are effective for social phobias, with nothing at the moment to suggest that one treatment is generally better than the rest. The choice will therefore depend on the facilities which are available and on the patient's own preferences.

References

Argyle, M. (1967). *The Psychology of Interpersonal Behaviour*. Penguin, Harmondsworth

Argyle, M. (1969). *Social Interaction*. Methuen, London

Bryant, B. and Trower, P. E. (1974). Social difficulty in a student sample. *Br. J. educ. Psychol.*, **44**, 13−21

Frank, J. (1961). *Persuasion and Healing*. John Hopkins Press, Baltimore

Gelder, M. G., Bancroft, J. H. J., Gath, D. H., Johnston, D. W., Mathews, A. M. and Shaw, P. M. (1973). Specific and non-specific factors in behaviour therapy. *Br. J. Psychiat.*, **123**, 445−462

Marks, I. M. (1969). *Fears and Phobias*. Heinemann, London

Shaw, P. M. (1977). A comparison of three behaviour therapies in the treatment of social phobia. Unpublished paper to the Annual Conference of the British Association of Behavioural Psychotherapy

16 Social Inadequacy

P. Trower and B. Bryant

Normal social interaction involves competence in the use of systems of verbal and non-verbal communication which are highly complex (Argyle, 1978), and it is not surprising that many individuals will be found lacking in such skills. In a survey by the authors and others at the Elms Clinic, Banbury (Bryant *et al.*, 1976), no less than 27 per cent of a sample of patients with neuroses and personality disorders ($N = 92$) were judged to be socially inadequate. This makes it a problem at least as common as other more traditional psychiatric disorders, and much more common than, for instance, addictions and phobias.

Assessment

In the Elms study, which excluded psychotic conditions, the main criteria used in identifying patients were social isolation and difficulty in forming relationships, feelings of incompetence and observed inadequate social behaviour. A group of such patients were selected by four judges—two psychiatrists and two psychologists—and then compared with another group judged to be socially adequate (though they had, of course, other psychiatric problems) and found to have the following characteristics.

1. Sex and Marital Status
Nearly half (46 per cent) of the male out-patients in the sample ($N = 35$) were judged by at least three of the four judges to be socially inadequate, while only 16 per cent of the women were so judged ($N = 53$). More than 60 per cent of the socially unskilled men were also single. These facts are undoubtedly related to the sex role stereotypes in society, in which men are required to take more initiative than women, especially in courtship, and in which, conversely, women who are dependent and accommodating are considered feminine and desirable.

2. Personality
On psychometric tests the unskilled group were found to be introverted, and lacking in dominance, sociability, self-acceptance, and capacity for status (defined as personal capabilities and attributes such as ambitiousness, effectiveness in communication which underlie and lead to status).

3. Behaviour
On behaviour ratings of their performance in a laboratory conversation task

the unskilled group were judged to speak too softly, slowly and indistinctly and in a dull, monotonous tone. They made little use of face and body to express feelings and tended to avert their gaze. Their speech was brief and punctuated by pauses, and was not spontaneously produced but had to be elicited. The topics they chose tended to be either stereotyped and boring or inappropriate to the situation and they were rather poor at synchronising their conversation with the other. Finally, they tended to allow personal problems and mood to intrude inappropriately into the conversation. On more global dimensions they were seen as rather cold, unassertive, anxious, sad, unrewarding and not in control of the situation.

4. Diagnosis
There was no over-all relationship between diagnosis and inadequacy and in particular no relationship between the diagnosis 'personality disorder, inadequate type' and the present definition of social inadequacy. There was a weak correlation of inadequacy and reactive depression in men.

5. Family and Social Class
There were no statistically significant correlations, but the unskilled patients tended to come from social classes IV and V and from smaller families.

6. History
Nearly all the unskilled group had social difficulties which preceded their 'illness', for example during adolescence had difficulty in mixing with others and dating the opposite sex.

7. Current Social Difficulty
Compared to the adequate group, the unskilled patients experienced more intense difficulty in many more social situations. The worst situations were making the first approach to others, going out with someone of the opposite sex, being with comparative strangers, being in an opposite sex group, going to parties and keeping a conversation going.

Specific Behavioural Deficits

In addition to the general characteristics outlined above, we required for the purposes of social skills training to identify more specifically the performance deficits of unskilled patients and more information on normal skills. In a recent study (Trower, 1976) new samples of skilled ($N = 23$) and unskilled ($N = 37$) patients were selected with the method used in the Elms study, and their performances compared during another 12-minute conversation task with two 'stranger' role-partners. Behaviour was measured objectively and reliably from video recordings, using electronic timers and counters. In the first phase of the conversation, patients were asked to talk about themselves and take responsibility for keeping the conversation going (speaking phase), while in the second part the woman role-partner was asked to talk while the others mainly listened (listening phase). The third phase of the conversation was 'free', but, unknown to the patient, the male partner was briefed to be dominant and critical (assertive phase). Also unknown to the patient the role-partners were briefed to introduce periodic silences. The task was designed in this way to test for various skills.

First, how did the skilled patients perform over all? They spoke for about half the time (48 per cent), and so achieved an almost exact balance of conversation sharing. They also looked at the other for about half the time (52 per cent). They smiled occasionally (6 per cent), gestured occasionally (11 per cent) and shifted their postures periodically (average number: 19). In comparison, the unskilled patients on the whole did less of everything. They spoke for less than a third of the time (31 per cent) and looked less (41 per cent). Most smiled less (4 per cent) but a proportion smiled a great deal (35 per cent) and for long periods. They gestured considerably less of the time (4 per cent) and on the whole made fewer postural shifts, with 40 per cent not moving at all.

Looking at performance differences within phases, we find the skilled group more able to speak upon request, and more sensitive to feedback, for instance by speaking less when others appeared disinterested, and initiating speech more when others fell silent. They also spoke much more than the unskilled group during the assertive phase (61 compared to 38 per cent). In their speech the unskilled group responded to overt situation cues, such as the instruction when to speak and listen, but were much less sensitive to the covert non-verbal cues of the other person, varying their amount of speech less than the skilled group.

The skilled group were more attentive listeners, as shown by amount of looking. They looked about 75 per cent of the time while listening, which is about average for most subjects studied (Argyle, 1975). The unskilled group looked for only 50 per cent while listening.

The skilled group responded more to the others in other ways. They smiled more during the listening phase, and gestured more during the assertive phase.

We note that Gillingham *et al.* (1977) also report that patients with 'interpersonal problems' spoke significantly less than patients without such difficulties, and also looked less of the time, though the latter finding is not reported as statistically significant. However, these figures were obtained in a non-comparable (interview) situation. Eisler *et al.* (1973) found that un-assertive patients spoke less than assertive controls, and also spoke more softly, and with less spontaneity.

Relative Importance of Social Signals

Are some elements of social behaviour more important than others in contributing to over-all impressions of social competence? To answer this, the scores on all elements were separately correlated with global ratings of social skill made by three judges (two clinicians and one lay person), and multiple regression analysis carried out to find which combination of elements best predicted judgements of skill. The direct correlations showed that the amount spoken was by far the most important element in contributing to an impression of skill—the less subjects spoke, the less skilled they appeared, and vice versa. This corroborated a finding by Marzillier and Lambert (1976) in a similar study on a separate group of patients. Amount of looking during the listener phase was also important, with gesture during the assertive phase next most important. Multiple regression analysis showed a low amount of speech and looking combining to give a high multiple correlation with impressions of poor skill (0.81). Adding low frequency of gesture and a low amount of smiling increased the correlation slightly.

Marzillier and Lambert found that the total amount spoken (by patient and stooge), together with smiles and laughter, gestures, positional movements, hesitations, and self disclosure produced, in combination and in that order, the best prediction of impressions of conversational skill. They also found that the total amount spoken, direction of gaze, fiddling movements, hesitations, subject's speech and subject's questions produced, in combination, and in that order, the best prediction of level of social anxiety. As these authors point out, the high correlation of amount spoken with impressions of skill and anxiety is not unexpected. Anxious patients may be expected to speak less, and inadequate patients often complain of not knowing what to say. From this and further analyses, we conclude that where speech is lacking or minimal, patients will be judged unskilled almost irrespective of other aspects of behaviour. However, when amount of speech is roughly average or 'normal', judges will be influenced by other, non-verbal deficits more, and in particular the amount they look and smile.

Interpretation

Different Kinds of Failure

Social skills can be grouped into several categories according to the function they serve in communication, such as in expressing feelings and attitudes, in generating conversation, in influencing the behaviour of others. There are also different components involved in the production of skilled behaviour such as goal setting and motivation, perception, decision-making, skill repertoire and feedback. Failure in skills such as described above can be usefully analysed in terms of these categories and components.

1. Interpersonal Attitudes
Research has consistently found that body language is a much more import-ant communicator of interpersonal attitudes like dominance and liking than verbal language (Mehrabian, 1972; Argyle, 1975). We have seen that unskilled patients often fail to use non-verbal signals and are perceived as inexpressive

and cold. They may also send unintentional negative signals, communicating hostility, sarcasm, etc.

2. Conversation

This involves a complex and carefully-timed integration of verbal and non-verbal signals. Verbal utterances are supported by non-verbal ones to (a) elaborate and punctuate verbal messages (for example gestures, postures, intonations), (b) provide feedback (for example by fine changes in facial expression), and (c) control the synchronising of utterances, for example by gaze shifts. Gaze serves several functions, acting simultaneously as a source of feedback, a synchronising signal, and as a signal commenting on utterances and conveying interpersonal attitudes. A number of patients were quite unable to sustain a conversation, through failure in the use of these non-verbal signals. There were also a range of verbal deficits as we have seen.

3. Rewardingness

Social psychologists have often emphasised the importance of rewards and punishments in social behaviour. We believe that these play an important part in the accommodation of interactors to each other. A sends small rewards (head nods, smiles, praise) whenever B does what A wants (and punishments when he does not); this modifies the behaviour of B; at the same time B is modifying the behaviour of A. Furthermore the stronger the rewards A receives from B, the more strongly attracted A is to B. It is essential for interactors to reward the behaviour of others in this way. Our patients were found to be significantly lacking in rewardingness.

4. Empathy

Effective social interaction also depends on the ability to perceive the world from another person's point of view—to 'take the role of the other' (Sarbin and Allen, 1969). Patients are often said to be 'egocentric', and the unskilled patients in the Elms study were found to talk about themselves too much and to take little interest in the other.

5. Situation Rules and Social Routines

Socially skilled behaviour has to be appropriate to the situation and this implies an understanding of situation rules and the common social routines of a given sub-culture (Goffman, 1972). Unskilled patients had greater difficulty in a wide variety of situations, and complained of not knowing what to do in such situations.

6. Self-presentation

The presenting of a self-image to others is an essential part of social behaviour, but it has to be done in appropriate ways (Goffman, 1956). Some patients typically presented themselves poorly, for instance by being too modest, by dwelling on the negative things about themselves, and by inattention to appropriate dress and appearance. A few over-presented, for example by boastfulness. One patient dressed in clothes and spoke in a voice of a woman 40 years older.

7. Beliefs and Attitudes

All behaviour is affected by the individual's beliefs and attitudes, and there are a number of theories about this, such as Kelly's Personal Construct Theory (1955), Bandura's Social Learning Theory (1977a), Bem's Self-perception Theory (1972), and Rotter's Locus of Control Theory (1966) (p. 216). Bandura (1977b) for example, says that individuals develop certain expectations of self-efficacy which determine whether they will initiate and sustain coping behaviour. Poor performance is one of several causes of low levels of efficacy expectations. Certain negative attitudes will affect these expectations, such as faulty appraisal of performance and expectation of aversive consequences, because of unrealistic criteria, misperception regarding performance and negative self-evaluation (Curran, 1977).

8. Components of Skilled Behaviour

Skilled performance requires the setting of goals and motivation to achieve them, accurate perception of the environment, decision-making, possession of a repertoire of skills and ability to monitor and modify performance in the light of feedback. This model (Argyle and Kendon, 1967) suggests a number of ways in which social performance might fail. There could be problems with feedback, for example from aversion of gaze or misperception of cues; poor motivation and lack of goal-setting; indecision and insufficient skills. Finally the performance may be disrupted by anxiety or other symptoms.

The above categories of social behaviour and the social signals they subsume tend to fall into two sub-groups of skills. There are *facilitation* skills which seem to have the purpose of maintaining social interaction and encouraging (reinforcing) the behaviour and interest of the other. There are *controlling* skills which have the purpose of controlling and directing the interaction. Patients lacking in the first group would tend to be seen as cold and unrewarding, those in the second group as submissive. In the Elms study coldness was associated with one set of elements (for example silences, failure to hand over the conversation, dull expression and still posture) and unassertiveness was associated with a different set of elements (for example lack of initiative in conversation, lack of spontaneous speech, brief speech and soft volume). Mehrabian (1972) found that elements of behaviour fell into similar sub-groups.

Aetiology of Social Inadequacy

How does the above way of looking at social behaviour link up with mental disorder? There are two possible links between failure in social skills and other aspects of mental disorder: (a) social skill failure may be primary, due to faulty socialisation or lack of experience, resulting in a limited skill repertoire, failure to assimilate social rules and misperception of social cues. This could lead to social isolation, and hence frustrations and deprivations which then lead to other symptoms. (b) Failure may be secondary to some other problem, such as social anxiety or other symptoms, and to problematic attitudes such as low expectations of self-efficacy, which may lead to disruption or inhibition of social performance. The two problems may present in some ways as superficially similar, but different in aetiology. The idea of two kinds of social failure was tested in a recent study (Trower *et al.*, 1978*b*) in which support was found for the primary form of social failure but the existence of a secondary form was not established. However we will concentrate now on primary social failure and its causes

We can approach the question of aetiology by examining how social behaviour is acquired. Social skills are normally learned through the natural process of socialisation, by means of imitation, reinforcement, instruction and so on, and through exposure to skilled models such as parents, siblings, relatives, peers and others. Primary social failure may arise, as stated earlier, through poor socialisation. Unfortunately research on exactly how this process takes place is comparatively scant. A review is given in Trower *et al.* (1978*a*), and only a summary of evidence will be given and some speculations made here.

Our studies reviewed above showed that social inadequacy was a long-standing problem, often dating back to childhood and in most cases at least to adolescence.

Unskilled patients were judged by the clinic psychiatrist to have had social difficulties long before their presenting 'illness'. From the standpoint of skills acquisition the earliest environment and the first models available to the child are the parents. Most research on parent—child relationships has emphasised the development of emotional bonds rather than skills acquisition. However, Sherman and Farina (1974) have shown that inadequate male college students were more likely than adequate students to have socially inadequate mothers, which the authors interpreted as supporting the idea of acquiring skills through imitation of the parents, although a genetic explanation is possible. Maccoby and Jacklin (1975) conclude after a review of the literature on sex-typed behaviour that direct reinforcement and imitation are clearly involved, but that the cognitive ability to deduce rules from observation is an essential component. We take the view that sex-typed behaviour is only one of many groups of skills acquired in this way.

Research on the effect of siblings and peers on skills acquisition is also limited. Later born children have been found to be more socially outgoing and stronger on measures of sympathy than first-born and only children, and later born boys and girls to be less submissive to authority (Sampson, 1965). The processes involved are not clear, but presumably are related to the effects of having siblings from the earliest years of life, and the effect this has on family dynamics. Research in this area has been somewhat contradictory and inconclusive.

As regards peers outside the family, it has been shown that children use social techniques such as imitation to gain admission to groups (Phillips *et al.*, 1951). Peer groups have norms of their own, and provide models for imitation and opportunities for learning to influence others. We speculate that it is essential that the child and adolescent have experience with and exposure to others in their own age group, as well as parents, in order to acquire relevant skills.

Another factor in skills acquisition is the *type* of experience—whether or not the growing child and adolescent learns that he can influence his environment. Lewis and Goldberg (1959) have explored how the infant may acquire this experience if the mother follows a certain pattern of contingent reinforcement. Rotter (1966) put forward the now well-known 'locus of control' scale which classifies people into internal controllers who feel in control of the environment and external controllers who feel controlled by it. We have already commented on the importance of control as a dimension of social skills, and the unskilled patients in the Elms study were characterised by their inability to control and manage the situation. Experience of and subsequent belief in external control could also be relevant to certain aspects of depression. Seligman (1974) has put forward the theory (and a body of supporting research) that reactive depression is a form of learned helplessness, where, because of past failures, the individual believes he cannot influence and control his environment (external controller) and thus feels helpless. Ability to influence others involves social skills, and failure to acquire these may lead to depression. We found a weak but none the less important link between depression and social inadequacy in the male outpatients. Libet and Lewinsohn (1973) showed that a group of depressed students were less socially skilful than a group of non-depressed students.

Treatment

Social Skills Training

Primary social inadequacy is marked by lack of skills and most established treatments such as drugs, psychotherapy and the anxiety-reduction techniques in behaviour therapy cannot be expected to be totally effective treatments in themselves. However, the past 10 years or so has seen the parallel growth of behaviour acquisition techniques (for example Bandura, 1977a) and research into the elements and processes of social interaction referred to earlier. Out of these have developed such methods as social skills and assertive training, for which therapist manuals are now available (Liberman *et al.*, 1975; Goldstein *et al.*, 1976; Trower *et al.*, 1977), and an improved technology of assessment (Eisler, 1976; Bellack and Hersen, 1976).

The training method adopted and developed by ourselves is briefly as follows: (a) A problem situation or skills theme is taken and analysed into component steps and described (instruction). (b) A coping strategy is performed by one or more role-partners (modelling). (c) The patient imitates and rehearses the new skill (behaviour rehearsal). (d) The patient modifies his performance in the light of video/audio playback and his own and others' observations (feedback). In practice, training begins with a role-play simulation of a problem situation and the patient's faulty performance. The faulty sequence is then broken down into components, each of which is analysed and explained, helping the patient to bring each of them more under cognitive control. The components are modelled in easily mastered steps and then practised. After successful performance, increasing realism and variety are introduced, with new role-partners or transferred to a real-life venue and the training sequence repeated. Finally the patient carries out the same or similar task unaided as a homework assignment. Thus patients are taken from safer and simpler tasks to more difficult, realistic and complex ones. The procedure for the more unskilled patients is augmented by training in basic, general skills in such areas as perception and performance of non-verbal signals, conversation production and management and common social routines such as greetings, partings, apologies and requests.

A similar approach to acquiring competence is participant modelling (Bandura, 1975) where a number of response induction aids are used, such as graduated sub-tasks (as above), joint performance with the therapist or other aide (such as a volunteer) who facilitates required actions, graduated length of exposure and variation in severity of the threatening situations.

There has been modest experimental support for the efficacy of social skills and related training techniques with patients, but a review of this is beyond the scope of the present discussion. Critical reviews are published for assertiveness training (Rich and Schroeder, 1976), for heterosexual skills training (Curran, 1977) and for social skills and assertiveness training (Marzillier, 1978).

References

Argyle, M. (1975). *Bodily Communication*. Methuen, London
Argyle, M. (1976). *Gaze and Mutual Gaze*. Cambridge University Press, Cambridge
Argyle, M. (1978). *The Psychology of Interpersonal Behaviour*. Penguin, Harmondsworth
Argyle, M. and Kendon, A. (1967). The experimental analysis of social performance. In *Advances in Experimental Social Psychology*, Vol. 3 (Ed. L. Berkowitz), Academic Press, New York
Bandura, A. (1975). Generalizing change through participant modeling with self-directed mastery. *Behav. Res. Ther.*, 13, 141–152
Bandura, A. (1977a) *Social Learning Theory*. Prentice-Hall, Englewood Cliffs, New Jersey
Bandura, A. (1977b). Self-efficacy: toward a unifying theory of behavioral change. *Psychol. Rev.*, **84**(2), 191–215

Bellack, A. S. and Hersen, M. (1976). Use of self-report inventories in behavioral assessment. In *Behavioral Assessment: New Directions in Clinical Psychology* (Ed. J. D. Cone and R. P. Hawkins), Brunner/Mazel, New York

Bem, D. J. (1972). Self-perception theory. In *Advances in Experimental Social Psychology*, Vol. 6 (Ed. L. Berkowitz), Academic Press, New York

Bryant, B., Trower, P., Yardley, K., Urbieta, H. and Letemendia, F. J. J. (1976). A survey of social inadequacy among psychiatric outpatients. *Psychol. Med.* **6**, 101–12

Curran, J. P. (1977). Skills training as an approach to the treatment of heterosexual-social anxiety: a review. *Psychol. Bull.*, **84**, 140–57

Eisler, R. M. (1976). The behavioral assessment of social skills. In *Behavioral Assessment: A Practical Handbook* (Ed. M. Hersen and A. S. Bellack), Pergamon Press, New York

Eisler, R. M., Miller, P. M. and Hersen, M. (1973). Components of assertive behavior. *J. Clin. Psychol.*, **29**, 295–9

Gillingham, P. R., Griffiths, R. D. P. and Care, D. (1977). Direct assessment of social behaviour from videotape recordings. *Br. J. soc. clin. Psychol.*, **16**, 181–7

Goffman, E. (1956). *The Presentation of Self in Everyday Life*, Edinburgh University Press

Goffman, E. (1972). *Relations in Public: Micro-studies of the Public Order*. Penguin, Harmondsworth

Goldstein, A. P., Sprafkin, R. P. and Gershaw, N. J. (1976). *Skill Training for Community Living*, Pergamon Press, Oxford and New York

Kelly, G. A. (1955). *The Psychology of Personal Constructs*. Norton, New York

Lewis, M. and Goldberg, S. (1959). Perceptual-cognitive development in infancy: a generalised expectancy model as a function of the mother-infant interaction, *Merrill-Palmer Q.*, **15**, 81–100

Liberman, R. P., King, L. W., DeRisi, W. and McCann, M. (1975). *Personal Effectiveness: Guiding People to Assert Themselves and Improve their Social Skills*. Research Press, Chicago, Ill.

Libet, J. M. and Lewinsohn, P. M. (1973). Concepts of social skill with special reference to the behaviour of depressed persons. *J. consult. clin. Psychol.*, **40**, 304–12

Maccoby, E. E. and Jacklin, C. N. (1975). *The Psychology of Sex Differences*. University Press, Stanford

Marzillier, J. S. and Lambert, C. (1976). The components of conversational skills: talking to a stranger. Unpublished report, Birmingham University

Marzillier, J. S. (1978). Outcome studies of skills training. In *Social Skills and Mental Health* (Ed. P. Trower, B. Bryant and M. Argyle), Methuen, London

Mehrabian, A. (1972). *Nonverbal Communication*. Aldine-Atherton, Chicago

Phillips, E. L., Shenker, S. and Revitz, P. (1951). The assimilation of the new child into the group. *Psychiatry*, **14**, 319–325

Rich, A. R. and Schroeder, H. E. (1976). Research issues in assertiveness training. *Psychol. Bull.*, **83**(6), 1081–1096

Rotter, J. (1966). Generalized expectancies for internal vs. external control of reinforcement. *Psychol. Monogr. Gen. Appl.*, whole number 609

Sampson, E. E. (1965). The study of ordinal position: antecedents and outcome. *Prog. exp. pers. Res.*, **2**, 175–228

Sarbin, T. R. and Allen, V. L. (1969). Role theory. In *Handbook of Social Psychology*, Vol. 1 (Ed. G. Lindzey and E. Aronson), Addison Wesley Reading, Mass. pp. 488–567

Seligman, M. E. P. (1974). Depression and learned helplessness. In *The Psychology of Depression: Contemporary Theory and Research* (Ed. R. J. Friedman and M. Katz), Winston-Wiley, Washington

Sherman, H. and Farina, A. (1974). Social adequacy of parents and children. *J. abnorm. Psychol.*, **83**, 327–30

Trower, P. E. (1976). Analysis of situation effects on elements of social behaviour in patients. Paper given at British Psychological Society conference, York, March

Trower, P. E., Bryant, B. M. and Argyle, M. (Eds) (1978a). *Social Skills and Mental Health*. Methuen, London

Trower, P. E., Yardley, K., Bryant, B. M. and Shaw, P. (1978b). The treatment of social failure: a comparison of anxiety-reduction and skills-acquisition procedures on two social problems. *Behav. Mod.*, **2**, 41–60

17 The Behavioural Treatment of Obsessional Neurosis

M. S. Lipsedge

Response Prevention and Prolonged Exposure in the Treatment of Compulsive Rituals

It is generally agreed that obsessional neurosis has a poor prognosis. In one large series of 82 patients who were followed up for a period of 13–20 years, significant improvement in symptoms was observed in only 21 cases (Kringlen, 1965). Systematic desensitisation, which in the 1960s was giving such satisfactory results in specific phobic states, was on the whole ineffective in the treatment of both obsessional rituals and ruminations (see for example Furst and Cooper, 1970). This gloomy outlook has considerably improved since 1966, when Meyer developed a novel approach to the behaviour therapy of compulsive rituals. His method was influenced by reports in the animal experimental literature of response prevention (Lomont, 1965) and was partly derived from the patients' own explanation for the urge to carry out ritual checking, cleaning or washing. Some patients say that they feel compelled to perform rituals in order to avert eventual disaster to themselves or their families. Meyer (1966) predicted that the compulsive behaviour would stop if one could modify the patient's own expectation of the disastrous effects of failing to wash or to check. 'Cognitive restructuring' would occur if the patient could be persuaded to remain in intimate contact with 'contaminated' or 'dangerous' objects or situations. Two patients with severe chronic handwashing rituals were encouraged to handle contaminating objects while excessive washing was prevented by continuous supervision from nurses. This treatment led to a marked reduction in handwashing and the improvement had been maintained one year later. Since then Meyer *et al.* (1974) have followed up the progress of fifteen similar patients whose symptoms had lasted on average $15\frac{1}{2}$ years before behaviour therapy. These patients were all prevented from carrying out their rituals by nurses who diverted them into alternative activities. Curtailment of rituals continued while the patients were required to handle 'noxious' objects or remain in those situations which tended to trigger off handwashing or checking. At the end of this treatment (dubbed 'apotrepic therapy' from a Greek neologism meaning to turn away or dissuade) two-thirds of the subjects had a reduction in ritual score of at least 75 per cent and reassessment after an interval of from 6 months to 6 years showed that six patients had maintained this level of improvement, while two others had managed to make a further reduction in their rituals. Although this study was uncontrolled and the ratings (visual analogue scales) were relatively crude, the results were very encouraging.

The apotrepic or response prevention technique has two major components—curtailment of rituals and confrontation with situations which evoke anxiety. A small-scale pilot study of 12 obsessional handwashers (Lipsedge, 1974) attempted to compare the short-term effect of supervised prevention of rituals with prolonged exposure to 'contamination' or 'danger'. A fairly typical patient in this series had the following 3-year clinical history: He was a 40-year-old telegraphist who had developed a morbid preoccupation with luminous dials after reading that luminous paint is radioactive. The fear that exposure to minute amounts of radioactivity could cause cancer had generalised from close contact with watches and clocks to television sets and to any person who wore a wrist watch. This had led him to destroy the clothes of any members of his family who might have had contact with a watch and the construction of a *cordon sanitaire* around any part of his house which might have become polluted. In addition he was spending many hours each day in washing his hands to remove any possible trace of radioactivity. He had requested treatment after his wife took an overdose. She had begun to feel desperate when he prevented the family from using rooms that he considered contaminated with radioactivity. The patient was persuaded to handle a large old fashioned alarm clock with luminous dials whose glass cover had been removed. He was allowed to wash for as long as he wanted but was repeatedly re-contaminated by handling the clock. After only a few hours of this procedure he showed a marked and lasting reduction in the frequency of handwashing.

In this pilot study, prevention of washing conferred no significant additional benefit and it appeared that continuous exposure to anxiety-provoking situations ('flooding') was the effective component of the apotrepic treatment package. This conclusion accorded with the outcome of systematic studies of specific phobic and agoraphobic patients (Marks *et al.*, 1971) treated with prolonged exposure. The role of response prevention may be simply to prolong the period of exposure to pollution or to a feeling of imminent danger so that habituation can occur.

A third potentially therapeutic element is the sight of confident handling by the therapist of materials which the patient perceives as dangerous or polluted. The therapist's behaviour can be construed as a form of modelling which re-educates the patient by a process of learning by imitation (Bandura *et al.*, 1969). The relative contributions of modelling and exposure (flooding) have been elucidated in a series of controlled studies in 20 in-patients with chronic obsessional neurosis (Rachman *et al.*, 1971; Hodgson *et al.*, 1972; Rachman *et al.*, 1973; and Marks *et al.*, 1975). All the patients had been carrying out compulsive rituals for at least 1 year before the trial. Treatment consisted of a mean of 23 sessions lasting 40–60 minutes over a period of 1–3 months. Significant reduction of rituals occurred after 3 weeks of exposure to objects or situations which triggered off rituals. At 2 years follow-up, 14 patients were much improved. Modelling appeared to help a few patients but conferred no advantage over exposure alone for the group as a whole. Patients were encouraged to maintain any contamination and to refrain from rituals between treatment sessions, but very little supervision was provided. This self-imposed and limited response prevention contrasts markedly with the apotrepic procedure in which it was thought that close surveillance by nursing staff to curtail rituals was the critical therapeutic ingredient (Meyer *et al.*, 1974). Mills had also concluded that supervised prevention of rituals following exposure was a necessary condition for the eventual elimination of rituals (Mills *et al.*, 1971; Mills *et al.*, 1973). More recently, however, Meyer himself has reported successful domiciliary treatment with only minimal supervision of a patient with severe obsessional neurosis (Meyer *et al.*, 1974). The need for inter-session surveillance is an issue of practical significance because of the vast amount of specialised nursing time required for a programme of continuous supervision of each obsessional patient.

Catts and McConaghy (1975) have also reported on a combination of flooding and modelling with a limited degree of supervision outside treatment sessions in a series of six in-patients. They emphasise the importance of continuing treatment in the obsessional patient's home. Marks and his colleagues (1975) considered domiciliary treatment with involvement of family members to be crucial in some cases and they suggest that group treatment of patients with their families might increase motivation. Domiciliary treatment can be carried out by nurses (Marks *et al.*, 1975), by medical students (Stern, 1975) or by relatives. Catts and McConghy (1975) describe the sensible straightforward advice given to the relatives of their obsessional patients who were discharged from hospital within 6 weeks even if they had residual symptoms. 'His family was instructed that pressure of the kind applied to the patient in hospital, that is to enter situations evoking anxiety and rituals while resisting the latter, should be continued in the home, though without undue observation of the patient. Whenever, in the course of his daily activities, he was seen to stop because of intrusive thoughts or rituals, the spouse or parent was instructed to say directly and forcibly to the patient "Keep going" or "Put it down". If he did not respond, the relative was to take his hand and lead him through the appropriate behaviour. This was to be done in an unemotional manner without any annoyance and reinforced with praise.'

Primary Obsessional Slowness

Rachman (1974) has described a group of patients whose pathological slowness in the carrying out of ordinary day to day routines is not secondary to checking or washing rituals. Such patients spend many hours each day in washing, shaving and dressing. Encouraging results were obtained in ten chronic patients by the vigorous application of a common-sense approach. The therapist achieved a persisting speeding up of these activities by performing the task himself at a normal rate at the same time as his patient ('modelling' and 'pacing'), exhorting the patient to act more quickly while reminding him of the passage of time ('prompting') and praising the successful completion of tasks within a certain time ('shaping'). The patients were also shown how to monitor their own performance. This form of behaviour therapy has perhaps an antecedent in Janet's 'Treatment by Excitation' (Janet, 1925, quoted in Stern, 1977), 'The guide will specify the action as precisely as possible, and will analyse it into its elements if it should be necessary to give the patient's mind an immediate and approximate aim; by continually repeating the order to perform the action; by words of encouragement at every sign of success however insignificant, for encouragement will make the patient realise these little successes and will stimulate him with the hope aroused by glimpes of greater successes in the future'.

Obsessional Ruminations: Thought-stopping and Paradoxical Intention

Behaviour therapy techniques recently used to treat obsessional ruminations include thought-stopping (Wolpe and Lazarus, 1966; Stern, 1970; Yamagami, 1971), paradoxical intention (Frankl, 1960; Solyom et al., 1972), flooding (McCarthy, 1972) and satiation (Rachman, 1976). A common ingredient in these diverse techniques is the emphasis on direct confrontation with distressing ideas or situations, as opposed to the more passive approach in systematic desensitisation where the patient waits until he is free from anxiety before attempting to face his phobic or obsession-evoking situation in real life.

In thought-stopping, the patient is instructed to deliberately dwell on his particular obsessional theme (for example that he has inadvertently stabbed a child or is about to utter a blasphemous statement). The therapist then interrupts the induced rumination by making a sudden loud noise and shouting 'stop'. The patient is taught to shout (and eventually to whisper) 'stop' each time he conjures up his obsessional idea or theme. Several sessions of practice have led to a significant reduction in the frequency of spontaneous obsessional ruminations (Stern, 1970; Yamagami, 1971). In a controlled trial of thought-stopping which used tape-recorded instructions (Stern et al., 1973), four patients reported as much diminution in frequency of distressing intrusive ideas after learning to induce and then stop neutral thoughts, as they did by deliberately thinking and then extinguishing obsessional thoughts. This method may work by providing training in self-regulation (Kanfer and Seidner, 1973) and the same mechanism may be operating in Frankl's (1960) technique of paradoxical intention. Six sessions of instruction in deliberately magnifying and exaggerating obsessional ideas produced a marked decrease in the occurrence of obtrusive unwanted thoughts in five out of ten patients treated by paradoxical intention (Solyom, et al., 1972). Hackman and

McLean (1975) found that thought-stopping was almost as effective as flooding in practice, in patients with both rituals and ruminations.

Satiation or Habituation Training

Rachman (1976) has recently described a satiation method in which patients were asked to obtain their obsessional idea and hold it in consciousness for as long as 15 minutes per trial. He has found that with successive trials patients have increasing difficulty in conjuring up or retaining the obsessional thought or image. This technique differs from paradoxical intention in that no attempt is made to amplify the obsession. Prolonged exposure to obsessional thoughts appears to deprive the ruminations of their unpleasant quality, and habituation can occur more readily. Rachman also proposes that obsessional ruminators should be advised to refrain from inwardly 'putting right' the effects of their ruminations. (This is presumably the internal equivalent of what Freud (1959) described as the 'undoing' ('ungeschehenmachen') aspect of obsessional rituals.) 'Putting right' or neutralising activities include counter-images, numbers,words or incantations and Rachman predicts that if neutralising behaviour is the ruminative equivalent of compulsive rituals, then patients should respond to a combination of instructions to deliberately expose themselves to the provoking trigger (that is ruminative thought) and then refrain from internal or external neutralising rituals. This novel amalgam of satiation (or 'habituation training') and self-imposed response prevention has already produced promising results.

The Measurement of Obsessional Symptoms

There are a number of problems associated with the measurement of obsessional symptoms. Comprehensive questionnaires are unwieldy because of the enormous range of symptoms, while tailor-made individual measures are unsuitable for comparison between patients. Obsessional patients may hesitate for hours before committing their ratings to paper, and subjects in behaviour therapy trials have been known to destroy their ratings for fear of making an irrevocable error (Stern et al., 1973). Such patients report that they are afraid to give an inaccurate and misleading account and prefer not to commit themselves. The Leyton Obsessional Inventory (Cooper, 1970) has been used in clinical trials of clomipramine (Allen and Rack, 1975) and in studies of exposure treatment in obsessionals (Rachman et al., 1973). In the latter study the inventory correlated poorly with behavioural tests, partly because it was originally devised to separate houseproud housewives from normal housewives and obsessional neurotics in a study of family relationships and was not designed to measure response to treatment.

Technical apparatus may assist accurate measurement of frequency and duration of rituals and avoidance. Mills *et al.* (1973) employed a cumulative recorder which was automatically activated whenever their subjects (ritual handwashers) approached a wash basin. The 'safe' (that is non-polluted) distance which subjects attempt to keep between themselves and contaminants can be assessed by allowing the patient to control the approach of a trolley laden with dirty or dangerous objects by means of a hand-held compressed air apparatus (Lipsedge, 1974). Philpott (1975) has devised a flexible battery of both clinicians' and self-rating scales which reliably assess the amount of time spent on rituals and ruminations and the degree of discomfort experienced. Provision is also made on these scales for recording the avoidance or bizarre performance of everyday activities.

Developments in Descriptive Psychopathology and the Implications for Behaviour Therapy

Obsessional neurosis is a relatively rare condition. Kringlen (1965) found an incidence of 2.5 per cent in a psychiatric in-patient population. With the development and refinement of the treatment techniques described in this chapter, behaviour therapists have had access to unusually large numbers of patients and have been able to re-examine aspects of the phenomenology of this condition. For example Stern and Cobb (1977, in press) noted four main types of compulsive ritual in a sample of 45 patients: cleaning, avoiding, repeating and checking. Replies to questions about the phenomena generally used as criteria for the diagnosis of an obsessional state showed that recognition of senselessness was commoner than the experience of internal resistance. Over three-quarters of these patients recognised that their rituals were senseless, while only just over half the subjects stated that they attempted to resist the urge to carry out their compulsive repetitive acts. Resistance was commoner in patients with predominantly repeating rituals. About one-third of the patients only performed their rituals at home; this supports the view that domiciliary treatment can be more effective than hospital treatment especially if members of the family can be enlisted as co-therapists.

Rachman and his colleagues (Hodgson and Rachman, 1972; Roper *et al.*, 1973; Roper and Rachman, 1976) have carried out experiments to test the anxiety-reduction hypothesis according to which compulsive rituals persist because they lessen anxiety and discomfort. Ten patients with cleaning rituals were required to touch a contaminated object. This led to a marked increase in subjective discomfort which rapidly dissipated on completing a satisfactory wash. A similar experiment was carried out in twelve patients with repetitive checking who experienced an increase in anxiety after performing a 'provoking act'; the discomfort was relieved in the majority of subjects by completion of the checking ritual. (These observations contrast with those of Walker and Beech (1969) who have observed a number of obsessional patients whose rituals actually cause a deterioration in mood.) Rachman and his colleagues found that the increase in anxiety was more pronounced when the patient was alone. The presence of another person appeared to diminish the discomfort associated with checking rituals more than with washing rituals. This may be because the checkers tend to transfer on to the other person some of the responsibility for the effects of not carrying out the ritual and this leads to the therapeutic implication that obsessional checkers, even more than ritual washers, need to carry out a variety of self-directed and self-monitored tasks in their own environment. A 50-year-old caretaker in a city office block was a typical obsessional checker. He was spending 3–4 hours each night checking and re-checking locks and light switches on a night round that should have taken 20 minutes. He was treated with a few sessions of behaviour therapy by a medical student who hurried him round the building at a brisk pace, deliberately withholding reassuring comments when the patient asked him if everything was safe. The student-therapist spent progressively less time with the patient and encouraged him to complete the task within a specified time. At first he monitored the patient's progress by telephone calls and then withdrew his supervision as the patient's self-confidence increased. The caretaker was soon able to complete his night round in a reasonable period of time without undue anxiety or checking.

References

Allen, J. and Rack, P. H. (1975). Changes in obsessive/compulsive patients as measured by the Leyton Inventory before and after treatment with clomipramine. *Scot. med. J.*, **20**, 41–44

Bandura, A., Blanchard, E. B. and Ritter, B. (1969). The relative efficacy of desensitisation and modelling approaches for inducing behavioural, affective and attitudinal changes. *J. Pers. soc. Psychol.*, **13**, 173–199

Catts, S. and McConaghy, N. (1975). Ritual prevention in the treatment of obsessive-compulsive neurosis. *Aust. N. Z. J. Psychiat.*, **9**, 37–41

Cooper, J. (1970). The Leyton Obsessional Inventory. *Psychol. Med.*, **1**, 48–64

Frankl, V. E. (1960) Paradoxical intention: a logotherapeutic technique. *Am. J. Psychother.*, **14**, 520–535

Freud, S. (1959). *Inhibitions, Symptoms and Anxiety* (1926). Standard ed., Vol. 20, Hogarth Press, London

Furst, J. B. and Cooper, A. (1970). Failure of systematic desensitisation in 2 cases of obsessive-compulsive neurosis marked by fears of insecticide. *Behav. Res. Ther.*, **8**, 203–206

Hackman, A. and McLean, C. (1975). A comparison of flooding and thought stopping in the treatment of obsessional neurosis. *Behav. Res. Ther.*, **17**(4), 263–269

Hodgson, R. and Rachman, S. (1972). The effects of contamination and of washing in obsessional patients. *Behav. Res. Ther.*, **10**, 111–117

Hodgson, R., Rachman, S. and Marks, I. M. (1972). The treatment of obsessive-compulsive neurosis: follow up and further finding. *Behav. Res. Ther.*, **10**, 181–189

Janet, P. (1925). *Psychological Healing.* (Translation) Eden & Cedar Paul, London. George Allen & Unwin, London, p. 978

Kanfer, F. M. and Seidner, M. L. (1973) Self-control; factors enhancing tolerance of noxious stimulation. *J. Pers. soc. Psychol.*, **25**, 381–389

Kringlen, E. (1965). Obsessional neurotics. A long-term follow-up. *Br. J. Psychiat.*, **111**, 709–722

Lipsedge, M. S. (1974). Therapeutic Approaches to Compulsive Rituals. Unpublished M.Phil. dissertation, University of London

Lomont, J. F. (1965). Reciprocal inhibition or extinction? *Behav. Res. Ther.*, **3**, 209–219

Marks, I. M., Boulougouris, J. and Marset, P. (1971). Flooding versus desensitisation in phobic disorders. *Br. J. Psychiat.*, **119**, 353–375(a)

Marks, I. M., Hallam, R. S., Philpott, R. and Connolly, J. C. (1975). Nurse therapists in behavioural psychotherapy. *Br. med. J.*, **iii**, 133–148

Marks, I. M., Hodgson, R. and Rachman, S. (1975). Treatment of chronic obsessive-compulsive neurosis by in vivo exposure. *Br. J. Psychiat.*, **127**, 349–364

McCarthy, B. W. (1972). Short-term implosive therapy: case study. *Psychol. Rep.*, **30**, 589–590

Meyer, V. (1966). Modification of expectancies in cases with obsessional rituals. *Behav. Res. Ther.*, **4**, 273–280

Meyer, V., Levy, R. and Schnurer, A. (1974). The behavioural treatment of obsessive-compulsive disorders. In *Obsessional States* (Ed. H. R. Beech), Methuen, London

Meyer, V., Robertson, J. and Tallow, A. (1975). Home treatment of an obsessive-compulsive disorder by response prevention. *J. Behav. Ther. exp. Psychiat.*, **6**, 37–38

Mills, H. L., Barlow, D. H. and Baugh, J. (1971). An experimental analysis of response prevention in the treatment of obsessive-compulsive behaviour. Paper read at the Association for the Advancement of Behaviour Therapy Meeting, Washington, D.C.

Mills, H. L., Agras, W. S., Barlow, D. W. and Mills, J. R. (1973). Compulsive rituals treated by response prevention. *Archs gen. Psychiat.*, **28**, 524–529

Philpott, R. (1975). Recent advances in the behavioural measurement of obsessional illness. Difficulties common to these and other measures. *Scot. med. J.*, **20**, Suppl. 1, 35–42

Rachman, S. (1976). The modification of obsessions: a new formulation. *Behav. Res. Ther.*, **14**, 437–443

Rachman, S. (1974). Primary obsessional slowness. *Behav. Res. Ther.*, **12**, 9–18

Rachman, S., Marks, I. M. and Hodgson, R. (1971). The treatment of obsessive-compulsive neurotics by modelling and flooding in vivo. *Behav. Res. Ther.*, **9**,   –

Rachman, S., Marks, I. M. and Hodgson, R. (1973). The treatment of obsessive-compulsive neurotics by modelling and flooding in vivo. *Behav. Res. Ther.*, **11**, 463–471

Roper, G. and Rachman, S. (1976). Obsessional-compulsive checking: experimental replication and development. *Behav. Res. Ther.*, **14**, 25–32

Roper, G., Rachman, S. and Hodgson, R. (1973) An experiment on obsessional checking. *Behav. Res. Ther.*, **11**, 271–277

Solyom, L., Garze-Perez, J., Ledwidge, D. L. and Solyom, C. (1972). Paradoxical intention in the treatment of obsessive thoughts; a pilot study. *Compreh. Psychiat.*, **13**, 291–297

Stern, R. S. (1970). Treatment of a case of obsessional neurosis using thought-stopping technique. *Br. J. Psychiat.*, **117**, 539

Stern, R. S. (1975). The medical student as behavioural psychotherapist. *Br. med. J.*, **iii**, 78–81

Stern, R. S. (1977) Problems of obsessional illness in behavioural treatment. Open lecture April 5th, Institute of Psychiatry

Stern, R. S. and Cobb, J. P. (1977). Phenomenology of obsessive-compulsive neurosis. *Br. J. Psychiat.*, (in press)

Stern, R. S., Lipsedge, M. S. and Marks, I. M. (1973). Thought-stopping of neutral and obsessive thoughts; a controlled trial. *Behav. Res. Ther.*, **11**, 659–662

Walker, V. J. and Beech, H. R. (1969). Mood state and the ritualistic behaviour of obsessional patients. *Br. J. Psychiat.*, **115**, 1261–1268

Wolpe, J. and Lazarus, A. A. (1966). *Behaviour Therapy and Techniques*. Pergamon Press, Oxford

Yamagami, T. (1971). The treatment of an obsession by thought-stopping. *J. Behav. Ther. exp. Psychiat.*, **2**, 233–239

18 Treatment of Deviant Sexual Behaviour

John Bancroft

Deviance is primarily a social concept. Behaviour is deviant when it is socially unacceptable, stigmatised and in many instances legally proscribed. This aspect of sexual deviance is relevant to the question of treatment. First, social values change and this leads to changes in attitudes to treatment. I have noticed a definite fall in the number of patients seeking treatment for homosexual feelings in the past ten years; this probably reflects changing attitudes to homosexuality and greater acceptance of homosexual lifestyles. The social nature of the concept of deviance means that we are not dealing with illness and it is unusual for deviant sexual behaviour to be usefully regarded as a manifestation of illness.

Intervention or treatment is therefore of two main types—when its concern is the interest of the individual, that is counselling and psychotherapy, and when it is the interests of society, that is social control. There is a tendency to confuse these two forms of intervention and I hope to make clear as we proceed the distinction between them and the importance of maintaining it.

The main difference lies in the nature of the patient/therapist relationship. In the first case, counselling, this relationship is of an 'adult—adult' kind. The therapist offers help, advice and information but the responsibility for change lies with the patient. In the second, social control, responsibility lies with the 'agent' of society, the objectives are not those necessarily sought by the patient. This is not medical treatment even when drugs or psychosurgery, requiring medical expertise, are involved.

I shall be dealing mainly with the first type of intervention, counselling or psychotherapy. Whether the deviant sexual behaviour be in the category of homosexuality, fetishism, trans-sexualism, exhibitionism, or paedophilia the principles underlying counselling and the range of objectives are basically the same. Except where the objectives are very limited, and largely those of reassurance, effective help for people in these categories is time consuming and needs a considerable range of therapeutic resources. It should not be undertaken lightly. There are four principal types of objectives which should be considered in each case.

(1) The establishment of rewarding sexual relationships (either hetero-sexual or homosexual).

(2) The improvement of sexual function within a sexual relationship (whether it be hetero- or homo-sexual).

(3) Increase in self-control over sexual behaviour.

(4) Adjustment to a deviant role, from the non-sexual point of view.

Frequently more than one of these objectives is relevant in a particular case.

Counselling or psychotherapy for these problems can be very roughly divided into directive and non-directive forms. I will not be dealing with the latter as first, I am not qualified to do so, and secondly I am of the opinion that these are much less important and relevant than the directive, particularly behavioural kinds of counselling. Before discussing the therapeutic methods in more detail, I will first outline the fundamental principles of treatment which are in fact of general relevance to counselling for behaviour change.

(1) *Check the patient's motivation.* Attempt to clarify to what extent the patient is seeking treatment because of pressures either from society at large or from family, the courts or the Church. Where such pressures exist, it is important to confront the patient with them. Significant depression of mood should be looked for. Not infrequently, a deviant pattern of behaviour, for example homosexuality, will be rejected in a depressed state, and when the depression lifts will be re-accepted. Sometimes, as part of the grief following the break-up of a homosexual relationship, homosexuality *per se* will be blamed and rejected. Obviously such reactions are not the grounds for treatment aimed at altering sexual preferences. Non-sexual motives for sexual behaviour should be looked for, particularly in the case of certain types of sexual offence such as exhibitionism. When this seems likely, the sexual behaviour should be seen as an indicator of other problems and help should be aimed at those in the first instance.

(2) Agree on the objectives of treatment and arrive at an explicit contract which spells out not only the goals but also the extent and nature of the therapist's involvement and the patient's responsibilities.

(3) Emphasise the educational nature of the treatment. The patient is being helped to learn new ways of behaving rather than being 'cured' of an illness.

(4) Use the following basic principles of behavioural psychotherapy:

(a) At each treatment session target behaviours are defined and the patient is asked to carry them out before the next session. These usually represent small steps towards the final treatment goal.

(b) At the next session, the patient is asked in detail about his efforts to carry out those behaviours and any problems or negative feelings that resulted.

(c) In this way, key attitudes or resistances to change are identified.

(d) These attitudes are then modified if possible.

(e) A next set of target behaviours is agreed on when appropriate.

This sequence is followed in each treatment session and throughout the course of treatment, moving from one target behaviour to another as each is carried out satisfactorily. If behavioural progress is blocked for too long, then either the objectives of treatment are renegotiated or treatment is stopped.

The essence of this approach is that the patient is always given something to do between treatment sessions and that his attempts to carry out these tasks and the difficulties that he has in doing so provide the main subject matter for the treatment sessions themselves. The therapist's method of dealing with these problems is usually the main source of variance between therapists and of overlap between psychotherapeutic approaches. (For detailed discussion of these counselling techniques, see Bancroft (1975 and 1977).)

With this set of principles in mind, we can now consider some of the more detailed behavioural approaches.

Establishment of Rewarding Sexual Relationships

The problems in this category usually are of four types:

(1) A general lack of sexual interest or responsiveness. The reasons for the considerable variation in levels of sexual arousability between individuals are far from clear and are likely to be multifactorial. It is however therapeutically useful to consider low levels of sexual arousability to be due, at least in part, to psychological inhibition and to aim treatment at reducing this inhibition. In many instances, the principal focus of counselling should be on encouraging the individual to accept his or her own sexual feelings and give advice on the use of self-touching and masturbation, similar to the Masters and Johnson sensate focus but applied on an individual rather than couple basis. In the course of pursuing these behavioural goals, attitudes about guilt, moral values and fear of losing control are often expressed and need to be dealt with.

(2) A lack of responsiveness to particular types of person. The commonest example is of someone who can respond to partners of the same sex but not of the opposite sex. Whereas early attempts to help with this problem aimed at suppressing the initial pattern of responsiveness in the hope of encouraging a new form, for example by use of aversive techniques, it is now generally agreed that the emphasis should be on encouraging a new approach rather than suppressing the old (Bancroft, 1974).

The most direct approach is in the modification or 'shaping' of sexual fantasies. If the subject normally uses a particular type of fantasy during masturbation involving the initial sexual preferences, then he is encouraged to masturbate while gradually and systematically modifying the content of the fantasy in the desired direction. That means that on the first occasion, he may just alter one relatively small part of the fantasy content, providing that is compatible with continuing sexual responses and orgasm, on the next occasion he adjusts the fantasy a little further. Details of this technique as used with a masochist are given in Bancroft (1971). Although some writers have advocated the so-called masturbatory conditioning procedure, whereby the subject is advised to switch from the deviant fantasy to a normal or desired fantasy immediately preceding orgasm, I have not found this approach helpful, most patients finding the switch far too difficult to carry out.

A variety of ingenious and usually technically sophisticated methods for generalising sexual responsiveness from one set of stimuli to another have been described in the literature. In most cases their general usefulness has not been adequately assessed. (For detailed description see Bancroft (1974).)

(3) Anxiety or uncertainty about sexual relationships. Anxiety, which may be associated with either the social or sexual part of the relating process, may be sufficient to inhibit the initiation or seeking-out of such a relationship. Such anxiety is often fostered by ignorance, lack of or insensitivity to feedback from other people or physical or emotional handicaps which make interpersonal adjustment more difficult. In any case, a vicious spiral of anxiety or lack of self-confidence and social incompetence may become established and either keep the individual away from potential sexual relationships altogether or encourage him to enter into relationships of a kind which make no demand on him (as in some of the forms of deviant sexual behaviour). Although such anxiety and uncertainty is considered normal in the adolescent individual, social and sexual competence is expected of him as he gets older and the failure to adjust tends to aggravate the problem for this reason. The anxiety involved may not only inhibit the appropriate sexual approach behaviour, it can also inhibit sexual interest and responsiveness itself whilst in others it may lead to an anxious preoccupation with sex.

The therapeutic approach to such anxiety is to agree on limited behavioural goals of the socio-sexual kind while reporting back to the therapist on details of each such encounter. The therapist's task is to give as much information and interpretation of what happens as is appropriate as well as suggesting alternative forms of behaviour. Reduction of guilt and other forms of reassurance are often helpful.

Social skills training in mixed sex groups using videotape feedback (Argyle et al., 1974) can be helpful in such cases but is difficult to provide with limited resources.

(4) Problems in *maintaining* a relationship with a sexual partner other than those involved in specifically sexual dysfunction, for example inappropriate 'dating' behaviour, general communication difficulties, problems in coping with anger, role conflicts. Counselling can be provided in certain fundamental aspects of relationships, in particular defective communication and dealing with feelings as well as the emphasis on positive rather than negative methods of reinforcing behaviour in one's partner (for fuller discussion see Bancroft (1975)).

Improving Sexual Function within the Relationship

Whatever the form of deviant sexual relationship that brings the patient to the therapist, if there is sexual dysfunction existing in an on-going and otherwise desirable relationship, then the method of helping that dysfunction is the same as that used for sexual dysfunction in general. This also applies whether the relationship is of a homosexual or heterosexual kind. Such counselling has been adequately described elsewhere and will not be dealt with here (see Masters and Johnson, 1970; Kaplan, 1974; Bancroft, 1975 and 1977; LoPiccolo, 1977).

Self-control of Unwanted Sexual Behaviour

It is reasonable to assume that undesirable behaviour is frequently maintained by the lack of more desirable behavioural alternatives. It is on that basis and to some extent on the results of research that emphasis has shifted much more to building up rewarding behaviours rather than reducing unrewarding or undesirable ones. Nevertheless there remain some patients who either because of the negligible potential for positive change or because of the risk that their current behaviour entails, leave the therapist with little to offer except help in controlling their unwanted sexuality. Self-control is something that is necessary and desirable in any social situation and when sexual offences are concerned, it is as often the lack of control as it is the nature of the behaviour that needs modification. Fantasies, however bizarre, are not necessarily harmful and may be enriching to the person's experience. When he ceases to control the transition from fantasy to reality, however, that individual is in a potentially vulnerable or dangerous situation.

Types of behaviour that most commonly present themselves in this respect are exhibitionism, paedophilia and rape (although in the case of rape it is still infrequent for this problem to be presented outside penal institutions or special hospitals). In these cases, there is something unusual about the content of the behaviour as well as its control. Nevertheless, the enhancement of self-control is still the most direct and immediate means of keeping out of trouble.

The first step is a careful analysis of the sequence of events leading up to the unwanted acts. When this proves to be relatively predictable then the therapist has reasonable scope for intervention. When it is not, the behaviour seemingly arising out of the blue or precipitated by a variety of non-specific stressful events, the therapist's task is much more difficult. A predictable sequence may offer a number of stages when alternative or incompatible behaviour can be introduced. These are then clearly defined and rehearsed repeatedly either in fantasy or reality. In this way the patient knows full well that when the crucial point of the sequence is reached, he has a well-rehearsed alternative behaviour pattern to carry out. If, for example, a businessman finds that opportunities for carrying out his unwanted sexual behaviour occur on certain types of business trip, then he is in a position to organise these trips in advance, at a time when the urge for the behaviour is unimportant, and in such a way that these opportunities are removed.

The ability to comply with such self-regulatory rules obviously requires a strong wish to succeed in increasing self-control. It is also necessary to accept that such compliance may be made more difficult by the strength of the urge to carry out the deviant act. It is often helpful, therefore, to combine this type of self-regulating rule setting with some procedure that reduces the strength of the behavioural drive. It is here that either aversive techniques or covert sensitisation may be useful.It is not clear from the available evidence how these techniques work when they are helpful, but at the present time it is appropriate to regard them as a means of facilitating self-control by providing well-rehearsed aversive fantasy situations which can be used to avert or weaken the urge to act. It remains a possibility that aversive procedures in some way actually reduce the attractiveness of the behaviour or alter the strength of sexual drive associated with it. However, it is better to emphasise the self-control aspect of management rather than reliance on the 'curative' action of such techniques. In some cases where these methods are insufficient, then the use of libido reducing drugs can be considered. Although oestrogens have been used in the past for this purpose their side-effects and the disadvantages make them inappropriate when there are preferable alternatives, i.e. cyproterone acetate, an anti-androgen or benperidol, a butyrophenone (Bancroft, et al., 1974; Tennent et al, 1974). The proper clinical place for these drugs is yet to be clarified and at the present time they should be used with caution and only in those cases where there is an obvious clinical need to reduce sexual arousability per se. Of particular importance in using such drugs is the need to distinguish between their proper use in a therapeutic relationship, when the patient takes advantage of their effects to facilitate his own self-control and their use as a method of social control imposed upon the person, as indicated earlier. It is also important to counteract the effects that the use of drugs has in encouraging the patient to see himself in a passive role dependent on the therapist for the solution to his problems.

Adaptation to a Deviant Role

Although several of the objectives and methods outlined above are appropriately applied to improving homosexual relationships, there are problems which stem more directly from the deviant nature of the behaviour and which can benefit from appropriate counselling. This help is of two rather contrasting types; for the homosexual and for the trans-sexual.

For the Homosexual

The following objectives are frequently relevant:

(a) The reduction of guilt by helping to distinguish between deviant interest and behaviour which is morally acceptable and that which is irresponsible or antisocial, a distinction that is all too often blurred.

(b) Counselling in methods of coping with the effects of stigmatisation, for example how to cope with hostility, alienation, etc.

(c) Introduction to minority groups.

For the Trans-sexual

The problem here is not so much one of coping with stigmatisation but learning how to 'pass' effectively in society without being noticed as being abnormal. The typical trans-sexual does not want to be regarded as deviant, but as a normal member of the anatomically opposite sex. Counselling involves confronting the trans-sexual with the reality of how people react to him as well as suggesting methods of changing his behaviour to make it more effective in the desired role. Once again social skills training with video or audio feedback can be useful in this respect. Most experts in this field advocate a reasonably prolonged period of attempting to work and live in the desired sex role before any irreversible treatment such as sex re-assignment surgery. The use of hormones has an intermediate role, being used for a period of time before surgery is considered and as a means of enhancing the effectiveness of the behavioural re-assignment (Money and Walker, 1977).

References

Arygle, M., Trower, P. and Bryant, B. (1974). Explorations in the treatment of personality disorder and neurosis by social skills training., *Br. J. med. Psychol.*, **47**, 63–72

Bancroft, J. (1971). The application of psychophysiological measures to the assessment and modification of sexual behaviour. *Behav. Res. Ther.*, **9**, 119–130

Bancroft, J. (1974). *Deviant Sexual Behaviour: Modification and Assessment*. Clarendon Press, Oxford

Bancroft, J. (1975). The behavioural approach to marital problems. *Br. J. med. Psychol.*, **48**, 147–152

Bancroft, J. (1977). The behavioural approach to treatment. In *Handbook of Sexology* (Ed. J. Money and H. Musaph), Excerpta Medica, Amsterdam

Bancroft, J., Tennent, G., Loucas, K. and Cass, J. (1974). The control of deviant sexual behaviour by drugs: behavioural changes following oestrogens and anti-androgens. *Br. J. Psychiat.*, **125**, 310–315

Kaplan, H. S. (1974). *The New Sex Therapy*. Brunner/Mazel, New York

LoPiccolo, J. (1977). Direct treatment of sexual dysfunction in the couple. In *Handbook of Sexology* (Ed. J. Money and H. Musaph), Excerpta Medica, Amsterdam

Masters, W. H. and Johnson, V. E. (1970), *Human Sexual Inadequacy*. Churchill, London

Money, J. and Walker, P. A. (1977). Counselling the transsexual. In *Handbook of Sexology* (Ed. J. Money and H. Musaph), Excerpta Medica, Amsterdam

Tennent, G., Bancroft, J. and Cass, J. (1974). The control of deviant sexual behaviour by drugs: a double-blind controlled study of benperidol chlorpromazine and placebo. *Archs sex Behav.*, **3**, 261–271

SECTION 4
SPECIFIC ISSUES

19 The Psychophysiology of Schizophrenia

P. H. Venables

Psychophysiology

Psychophysiology is probably best defined by contrasting it with physiological psychology. This latter sub-discipline is concerned with the alteration of physiological status and examination of the resultant changes in behaviour. Consequently, because of the need for surgical intervention this area of work is normally undertaken with animals as subjects or exceptionally on patients with accidental injury.

In contrast, psychophysiological techniques employ largely non-invasive measures of physiological status and examine them in relation to deliberately manipulated psychological states or states which have become changed as a result of some naturally occurring process or disease condition.

It is not surprising, therefore, that one of the areas in which psychophysiological techniques have had large usage has been in psychiatry or abnormal psychology.

It has been convenient to loosely divide the areas of psychophysiology into those largely using measures of 'central' activity—namely, EEG and its derivatives such as event-related potentials—and measures of 'peripheral' activity—mainly of autonomic function. These latter include cardiovascular activity in the form of measures of heart rate, vasomotor tone or blood pressure, electrodermal activity measured as skin conductance or skin potential, or activity of the pupil measured photographically or by televisual means. Not all peripheral measures are concerned with autonomic function and other important measures are EMG and eye movement measured by electro-oculographic techniques.

The 'central—peripheral' division is not a good reflection of the state of knowledge of brain function. While EEG measures probably reflect cortical processes in general, peripheral measures, used correctly, do more than reflect peripheral activity and may be useful measures of sub-cortical function.

The Use of Psychophysiological Techniques in Psychiatry

It is important before presenting the results of psychophysiological investigations in this area to examine the aims and intentions of the work.

In the past it is probable that investigations have used psychophysiological techniques to answer such questions as 'Is this group of patients more aroused than normal?' In a sense what has been sought is an additional description to add to the psychiatric description, in the same way as one might ask for a blood sample to be taken and analysed and the results added to the general body of descriptive data on the patient.

The anomaly, however, is that it is at the present time extremely rare for a psychophysiological description of a patient ever to be used in a diagnostic or prognostic sense where functional disorders are concerned. Of course, clinical EEG techniques are used where the main aim is to eliminate the presence of focal or diffuse organic pathology but it would be fairly rare for a routine EEG measurement to be taken from a patient otherwise diagnosed as almost certainly schizophrenic, and even more rare for a measure of his electrodermal activity to be considered to be of diagnostic value.

To some extent, therefore, psychophysiological techniques are more realistically considered as research tools. If this is so, then it is essential that the physiological mechanisms underlying the measurements be understood and the measures be used as more than mere descriptors. Because of this the interaction of psychophysiology and physiological psychology becomes important, and the investigation, using *suitable* animal models, of the mechanisms controlling peripherally measured variables is a *sine qua non* for the interpretation of psychophysiological data. This latter type of data is unfortunately fairly rare and appropriate new work may only be stimulated by the process of the psychophysiologist raising in his work points of interest which the physiologist may think worthwhile to investigate.

Another area where some mutually beneficial interaction has taken place but where more is needed is that of psychopharmacology. In the psychophysiological investigation of many psychiatric conditions the fact that the patients are medicated has a major influence on the measurements taken and the need for data in this area is a paramount necessity.

Earlier it was stated that psychophysiological techniques were rarely used for diagnostic purposes. This is true at least in part because of lack of adequate normative data and base rates of incidence of abnormal responses. Psychophysiological techniques have developed markedly over the past ten or twenty years and controversies over systems of measurement have diminished. There is thus a possibility that over the next decade data will be produced which will enable some norms to be established against which abnormalities of function may be recognised.

Areas of Work on the Psychophysiology of Schizophrenia

It is obvious that the major area of investigation has been with adult schizophrenics, and this largely with hospitalised patients. Almost all research papers have given lip service to the need for careful sub-diagnosis of the patients to be investigated. The development over the past ten or so years of standardised diagnostic tools such as the PSE (Wing *et al.*, 1974) and the CAPPS (Endicott and Spitzer, 1972) have made possible the selection of schizophrenic samples that can be replicated in other studies. To date, however, there have been few attempts to use these sorts of techniques to select samples for psychophysiological investigations. Another major source of difficulty is that the majority of hospitalised patients are under some form of medication.

Attempts to control this factor are fraught with ethical and methodological difficulties. Chronic schizophrenic patients not currently on medication are often those for whom neuroleptic drugs appear to have been ineffective and consequently they probably form an unusual sample. Newly admitted patients commonly reach the psychiatrist having been medicated by the G.P., and the collection of an unmedicated sample entails considerable patience. Taking patients off drugs probably demands that they are maintained in an untreated state for at least a month to allow for total elimination of medication. Such a tactic clearly involves ethical problems.

Because of this, and also for other reasons, there has been a major growth of studies of children in the pre-morbid state who are at 'high-risk' for schizophrenia. The common tactic of these studies is to look at children of a schizophrenic parent thereby increasing (from 0.85 per cent to around 16 per cent) the chance that members of the sample may break down and thus yield useful data. The economics of the study are thus improved. While the escape from the problems of the medicated patient is one of the reasons for this type of study, it is not the only one. Mednick and McNeil (1968), for instance, drew attention to the fact that the state of the patient by the time he reaches hospital is the product of his original disease process plus the anxiety, misery and loneliness that the developing disease has engendered, plus the reactions of society to the increasing unusualness of behaviour of the 'patient-to-be'.

An area of considerable neglect in experimental studies of schizophrenia is that of the female patient. This applies not only to psychophysiological work but other areas of investigation. In part this is because of the laudable recognition of the interfering variables of the menstrual cycle and the difficulty of controlling for it and the lack of knowledge of its effect on the measurements to be undertaken. On the other hand, it is to be suspected that the acknowledged greater difficulty of doing experimental work with female patients may underlie some of the avoidance of this sex.

Data Available in Psychophysiological Work on Schizophrenia

Among peripheral measures the distribution of data is markedly skew. The amount of work on electrodermal activity is large. Among cardiovascular measures, work on heart rate is fairly extensive, but other measures in this area have received hardly any attention.

Two other areas which have had rather specific investigation are those of

pupillography and eye movement. The literature on the EEG in schizophrenia covers a long period of time but tends to be somewhat inconclusive
in its impact. Some recent developments using event-related potential
techniques, however, offer promise.

Electrodermal Activity

There are two forms of electrodermal activity: 'exosomatic', in which the
conductivity of the skin is measured in response to an external source of
potential, and 'endosomatic', in which the potential generated at the skin
surface of palmar and plantar areas is measured. The former gives rise to
measurement of tonic activity skin conductance level (SCL) and phasic
activity skin conductance response (SCR) having the components amplitude,
latency, rise time and half-recovery time. Tonic endosomatic activity is
measurable as skin potential level (SPL) and phasic activity as skin potential
response (SPR). The latter measure is difficult to quantify and is generally used
as a counted variable. Details of measurement techniques and the peripheral
and central mechanisms underlying them are presented in Venables and
Christie (1973).

Effect of Medication

In summary it can be said that studies show that neuroleptic medication has
the effect of lowering skin conductance level (SCL) and reducing the number
of spontaneous skin conductance fluctuations, both of which may be thought
of as measures of tonic activity (or 'arousal'). On the other hand, phasic
responses to simple stimuli appear not to be affected by medication although
responses to more meaningful stimuli (for example anxiety eliciting slides)
may be.

A good example of a study examining the effect of phenothiazines on
electrodermal activity in schizophrenics is that of Spohn et al. (1971). Fifteen
members of a group of twenty-nine schizophrenic patients on phenothiazines
were taken off and remained off drugs for three months. When off drugs, the
SCL of these patients increased in relation to their 'on drug' status. This
finding is supported by work of Bernstein (1967) and Gruzelier and
Hammond (1977a).

When the effect of medication on phasic activity (SCL) was investigated, it
was found that numbers of responses increased when patients were taken off
drugs. When, however, the effect of SCL was removed by partial correlation
techniques from SCR, then the effect of medication on SCR frequency was not
significant. No effect of drugs on SCR amplitude was found. Later in this
chapter, responsivity versus non-responsivity in the electrodermal activity of
schizophrenics will be discussed. Gruzelier and Hammond (1977a) investigated the effect of chlorpromazine on this dichotomy in a 4 weeks on/4

weeks off/4 weeks on drug paradigm. No clear effect of chlorpromazine upon responsivity was found. These same authors provide data to suggest that chlorpromazine reduces response rise time and recovery time but not latency.

No data appear to be available on the effect of medication on skin potential activity.

Skin Conductance: Phasic Activity

A degree of inconsistency is apparent in the data although investigations to establish the grounds for the inconsistencies themselves appear to throw up areas of possible importance. Reviews of the area from somewhat opposing viewpoints are given by Zahn (1976) and Venables (1977).

In 1972 Gruzelier and Venables reported that there appeared to be a dichotomous distribution of electrodermal responsivity in schizophrenics. Approximately 50 per cent of subjects showed no responses to simple tone stimuli while the other 50 per cent tended to be hyper-responders showing maximal orientation responses and diminished habituation. The 50 per cent rate for non-responsivity should be compared with a rate of about 7 per cent in adult normal subjects. Venables (1977) examined the data then available from a variety of sources and reached the conclusion that the high level of non-responsivity among schizophrenics was a real phenomenon. Zahn's (1976) data, however, suggest that non-responding among his schizophrenic patients amounted only to about 15 per cent. Zahn's patients were drug free and those of Gruzelier and Venables were on various levels of neuroleptic medication. However, Zahn himself suggested that the results were unlikely to be due to drug effects and the data reviewed in the previous section also suggest that this is unlikely. Venables (1977) examined the possible factors leading to the differences between the two sources of data and reached the conclusion that it was a feasible suggestion that the source of the difference probably lay in the saliency of the types of stimuli used.

Patterson and Venables (1978), while confirming in general the finding of a high level of electrodermal non-responsivity among schizophrenic patients, showed that in addition a further group of patients could be distinguished who, while initially giving normal amplitude SCRs, showed very fast habituation and exhibited one, or at the most two, responses only. This type of minimal responsivity tends to be shown in the work reported by Bernstein (1964, 1967, 1970).

In summary, there appear to be four types of responsivity which can be distinguished in a schizophrenic population: (a) non-responsivity, (b) fast habituation, (c) normal habituation, and (d) non-habituation. The relatively simplistic findings of Gruzelier and Venables (1972), suggesting that schizophrenics were confined to classes (a) and (d) and normals to class (c), appear to require modification by the inclusion of class (b), and in some few instances class (c) among the schizophrenics, while as stated earlier some 7 per cent of normals appear in class (a).

Speculation concerning the role of malfunctioning of the limbic system in producing these patterns of responsivity are presented in Venables (1973, 1975); in short, it is suggested this non-responsivity is a concomitant of dysfunction of the amygdala while non-habituation reflects malfunction of the hippocampus. Behavioural data may be assembled by which the differences in performance associated with differences in electrodermal responding give theoretical support to malfunction of underlying limbic mechanisms.

So far the temporal components of the SCR have not been discussed. One of the findings which has come to the fore over recent years is the importance of the recovery limb of the SCR as a feature of adult schizophrenia and a predictor of breakdown among children at risk for schizophrenia. In 1968 Mednick and Schulsinger reported a faster rate of electrodermal recovery in data collected six years previously among those offspring of schizophrenic mothers who had succumbed to psychiatric illness than among those who remained well or among low-risk controls. This finding stimulated workers using adult schizophrenics as their subjects to examine the SCR recovery of data from their patients. For instance, Ax and Bamford (1970), Venables and Gruzelier (1972) and Zahn et al. (1975) showed that the recovery of the SCR was faster in schizophrenics than normals. The only major set of disparate findings is that of Maricq and Edelberg (1975) who reported that schizophrenics show longer recovery times than normal. Close examination of the types of patients included in Maricq and Edelberg's study, however, suggests that the differences between them and the other findings may not be so marked as at first appeared.

Patterson and Venables (1978), as stated above, showed that a sub-group of schizophrenic patients have a pattern of fast habituation of response. These patients also show an abnormally long time of SCR recovery. The extent to which this type of patient is present in a sample of schizophrenics will markedly alter the mean recovery time shown by that group.

The earlier reports of the high-risk study of Mednick and Schulsinger (1968) have been recently extended (Mednick et al., 1977). This study reports findings on the relation between birth data, psychophysiological data collected in 1962 when the subjects had a mean age of 15 years, and a full psychiatric assessment in 1972 at mean age 25 years. It was shown that for *male* subjects a set of perinatal variables predicted electrodermal status, and electrodermal status predicted schizophrenic breakdown. The electrodermal measure used was the product of number of responses given and recovery rate (that is numbers of micromhos recovered per second). The measure of psychiatric status was taken in a standard psychiatric interview (Schulsinger, 1976) and is built up for CAPPS and PSE variables. There are essentially four parts to the measure: hallucinations and delusions, hebephrenic features, thought disorder and autistic features. For *female* subjects, the perinatal data significantly predict electrodermal status, as with the male subjects, but the electrodermal data do not predict psychiatric breakdown.

One possibility is that further time has to elapse before sufficient female subjects break down and produce a significant association between electrodermal and psychiatric status. The results with the males are, however, encouraging and indicate the usefulness of the electrodermal measures outlined.

Skin Conductance: Tonic Activity

It is not possible to make general statements about the 'arousal level' of schizophrenics as reflected in tonic levels of skin conductance. Depue and Fowles (1973) in their review show little consistency of results using SCR as a variable and advocate the use of habituation rate of the orientating response and frequency of spontaneous responses as measures which 'appear to reflect arousal and yield results indicating that chronic schizophrenics are over-aroused'.

In the previous section, however, it was shown that it was feasible to divide patients into four groups on the basis of responsivity and habituation rate. Gruzelier and Venables (1972) and Patterson and Venables (1978) provide data to show that phasic non-responders have a lower SCL than schizophrenic and normal responders, and that fast-habituating subjects have an SCL which is intermediate in value between that of responders and non-responders. The mean skin conductance level shown by a group of schizophrenics thus is dependent on the composition of that group. Another finding of theoretical interest but one that makes interpretation of any single set of data difficult is the 'paradoxical' diminution of SCL in some schizophrenic patients with increase in behavioural arousal. This work has been reviewed by Jordan (1974) and is shown in data presented by Gruzelier et al. (1972). In this study the SCL of non-paranoid patients fell as activity on a bicycle ergometer increased beyond moderate levels. This was not shown by paranoid patients whose SCL increased in a monotonic fashion with increase in behavioural arousal.

Laterality of Skin Conductance Activity

Data published by Gruzelier (1973) and Gruzelier and Venables (1974) show that, while in general there appears to be no difference in SC responsivity of the two hands to simple tones in normal subjects, there is a tendency for the responsivity of the right hand to be higher than that of the left in those schizophrenic subjects that give electrodermal responses. The available neuro-anatomical data on pathways for hand to brain are scanty but Luria and Homskaya (1963) and Sourek (1965) provide data which suggest that the pathway is ipsilateral. Thus defective responding on the left hand might be considered to indicate defective functioning of the left hemisphere and thus be in line with the work of Flor-Henry (for example 1974). Recently, Gruzelier and Hammond (1977b) have provided data which suggest that one of the effects of chlorpromazine medication is to reduce the lateral imbalance found in unmedicated schizophrenics. They further suggest that this reduction of asymmetry may underlie the therapeutic efficiency of the drug.

Skin Potential

The amount of work with schizophrenics using skin potential as a dependent variable is small compared with that using skin conductance. Because the mechanisms and principles of propagation of the two electrodermal measures are not equivalent (Venables and Christie, 1973), it is worthwhile taking both measures when this is possible. In practice, however, it appears to be rare to do so.

Gruzelier et al. (1972) showed that the 'paradoxical' effect in skin conductance reported above was not shown in SPL, which thus appears to behave in a different fashion. Venables and Wing (1962) showed that SPL was directly related to rated withdrawal (Venables, 1957) in non-paranoid but not in paranoid patients and this finding was replicated by Spain (1966) but not by Crider et al. (1965).

Because phasic skin potential activity commonly has a biphasic waveform, quantification is difficult. However, Edelberg (1970) has shown that the speed of recovery of the SCR is paralleled by the type of SPR which the subject produces. Fast recovery SCRs tend to be accompanied by biphasic SPRs and slow recovery SCRs tend to be shown alongside uniphasic negative going SPRs.

With this in mind, Janes and Stern (1976) examined the SPRs of three groups of children; two 'high-risk' groups having schizophrenics or manic depressives as parents and one group having normal parents. The biphasic responders were rated as being more disturbed than the uniphasic responders; the response form was not, however, related to risk status, but as the children were only $8\frac{1}{2}$ years old, and only a small number of each risk group would be expected to become sick, the chances of finding statistically significant differences between the groups are small.

Cardiovascular Activity

Data in this area are not as extensive as those using electrodermal measurement and most of what there is, is confined to measures of heart rate.

The Effect of Medication

The general finding of studies on the effect of phenothiazines on heart rate is that they raise tonic level of activity.

The work of Spohn *et al.* (1971) which was quoted earlier in connection with electrodermal data also provides material which supports the finding of rise in heart rate under neuroleptic medication. The on/off/on paradigm of Gruzelier and Hammond (1977*a*) also provides support for this position, as does the work of Goldstein *et al.* (1966) and Goldstein and Acker (1967).

The phasic response of the heart may be conveniently considered in three parts: an initial deceleration lasting up to 2 s post-stimulus, an acceleratory phase up to 5 s post-stimulus, and a secondary deceleratory phase up to 8 s post-stimulus. While this description is somewhat arbitrary, it serves as a possible framework for description.

The effect of phenothiazine medication appears to be to reduce the acceleratory ('defensive') response to anxiety provoking material (Goldstein *et al.*, 1966). However, Spohn *et al.* (1971) report that the deceleratory orientation response to simple stimuli appears to be unaffected by medication.

Tonic Levels of Heart Rate (HR)

The fairly universal finding is that HR levels in schizophrenics are higher than normal. Spohn *et al.* (1971) for instance reported that even when phenothiazine medication was withdrawn HR of schizophrenic patients was elevated in relation to normals. These findings support those reviewed by Lang and Buss (1965) and a study by Zahn *et al.* (1968). The universality of the finding appears to be substantiated by the data of Fenz and Velner (1970) who show equally elevated HRs in process and reactive schizophrenics. Perhaps more surprising is the finding of higher than normal HRs in both SCR responder and non-responder groups in the data reported by Gruzelier and Venables (1975)—both groups on the occasion being under medication.

Data from the Mednick and Schulsinger high-risk study reported by Herman (1972) suggest that tonic levels of HR are not significantly different in high and low risk groups during rest. However, differences do show up during a fairly stressful conditioning period and the HR of high risk subjects is significantly higher than that of low risk subjects.

Phasic Heart Rate Responses

It has been widely recognised since the work of Kraepelin (1919) that impairment of attention is a major symptom of schizophrenia and more recent work, for example of Venables (1964) and McGhie (1969), has reviewed data to support this point of view. For this reason it is rather surprising that the amount of work done with schizophrenics using phasic HR response as a dependent variable is slight when the work, for instance, of Lacey (1967) and Obrist *et al.* (1970) indicates the role of HR changes in attentional processes.

In general it may be said that HR deceleration as part of the orientation response occurs in situations where the subject appears to be 'open' to the environment while HR acceleration is part of a 'defensive' response system in which the attentional strategy is one of 'closure' to the environment.

Zahn et al. (1968) report that schizophrenics show HR acceleration to 72 dB tones. This level of intensity would be expected to produce an HR decelerative orientating response in normals. In support Dykman et al. (1968) report HR acceleration to 60 dB tones in a group of schizophrenics. Gruzelier (1973), using the SC responder −non-responder dichotomy outlined above, reported that SC responders showed an accelerating response to 75 dB tones after initial two beat post-stimulus deceleration. In contrast, SC non-responders after the initial deceleratory component show a fractional return to baseline and no acceleratory phase.

An otherwise unpublished study in a Ph.D. thesis by De Vault (1955) reported HR deceleration to pictorial stimuli denoting themes of hostility, dependency and sex, and to a verbal warning preceding a loud sound. These would be the sorts of response to be expected with normal subjects. However, in another unpublished Ph.D. thesis Lobstein (1974) reported deceleration to loud tones of 100 dB, which would have been expected to produce acceleration in normal subjects.

The data available do not therefore enable useful conclusions to be drawn by which the functioning of the cardiac system of schizophrenics might be related to the extensive body of similar data on normal subjects.

Pupillography

The data from the cardiac system, as has just been shown, do not provide definitive material; however, the use of the other dually innervated system which is readily measurable, the pupil, has produced some satisfactory results. It must, however, be borne in mind that in interpreting the results from a dually innervated system it is not always possible to say that a change in one direction—dilation or contraction—is due to increase in one type of innervation or decrease in another.

Two types of measurement of pupillary activity have been carried out with schizophrenics. These are the pupillary response to light pulses used by Hakerem and Sutton (1964) and Lidsky et al. (1971); and the light−dark reflex used by Rubin (1960, 1961, 1962), Rubin and Barry (1972a,b,c), Patterson (1976a,b) and Venables and Patterson (1977).

In the light pulse procedure the subject is dark adapted and presented with a series of light pulses. In the Rubin procedure the subject is light adapted, then given a period of darkness and a subsquent period of light. The pupil in darkness is photographed using infra-red illumination. No substantive data appear to be available on the effect of antipsychotic medication on pupillary activity.

Light Pulse Studies

In a study by Hakerem and Sutton (1964) chronic and acute schizophrenic patients, unmedicated at the time of testing, were presented with one-second pulses of light after a period of dark adaptation. The initial diameter after adaptation was smaller in acute patients than in chronic patients or normals. Both groups of patients showed a shorter time of contraction than normals although the extent of this contraction did not differentiate the groups. In a subsequent study, Lidsky *et al*. (1971) used a similar method to examine pupillary differences between acute schizophrenic patients and normals.

The results replicated the earlier study in finding a smaller pupil diameter after adaptation in patients as compared to normals. In this study, however, the patients showed a smaller extent of contraction than normals, and the speed of contraction was greater in normals. The authors favour an interpretation of their data in terms of reduced parasympathetic activity in the patient sample.

Light—Dark Reflex Studies

References to some of the large number of studies by Rubin and his colleagues have been given above, where the stimulation paradigm is also described. In support of the Hakerem *et al*. studies schizophrenics showed a less dilated pupil than normal after dark adaptation . Rubin's work distinguishes two classes of patients who show larger or smaller levels of dilation although these are always smaller than normal; two groups can also be distinguished in terms of speed and extent of constriction . The conclusions reached from these studies suggest that there are probably seven distinguishable ways in which the pupillary response of schizophrenics may differ from that of normals.

Patterson (1976*a* and *b*), Venables and Patterson (1977) have carried out work which in essence follows the Rubin paradigm. This work shows that a chronic medicated group of patients taken as a whole differed from normals in showing a lesser extent of constriction. The extent of dilation was also smaller in patients than in normals, in accord with previous studies but the difference did not reach significance.

If the pupillometric results are related to electrodermal parameters, then the skin conductance non-responders show smaller dilation and constriction than normal while the SC responding patients show a larger than normal constriction at 500 ms post-light onset.

Using the parameter of SC recovery time, the patients with fast SC recovery showed the longest time to maximal pupil constriction, while those with the slowest SC recovery showed the shortest time, although this latter group also showed smaller dilation and constriction than the fast recovery groups.

Interpretation of these results is possible in terms of a cholinergic depletion hypothesis to account for the slow constriction time of the fast SC recovery subjects. This is in accord with the suggestion that the hippocampus inactivity which is a factor in fast SC recovery is akin to cholinergic depletion; a point of view formulated by Douglas (1972).

Smooth Pursuit Eye Movements

The data reviewed to this point have been concerned with autonomic variables. However, other electrical signals may readily be recorded; for instance, with electrodes placed in the outer canthi of each eye and the potentials thus produced amplified by a d.c. recording system, eye movements may readily be recorded.

Eye movements are normally of two kinds: smooth tracking of slow-moving targets and saccades, being fast movements to alter eye position to new targets. Using a pendulum as a target the smooth pursuit eye movement which is the feature of normal behaviour produces a sinusoidal type of recording. Faulty eye tracking of psychotic patients was first investigated by Diefendorf and Dodge in 1908 but their findings were virtually forgotten until re-investigated by Holzman and Shagass and their colleagues (Holzman *et al.*, 1973; Holzman *et al.*, 1974; Holzman *et al.*, 1976; Shagass *et al.*, 1974; Shagass *et al.*, 1976).

These authors showed that the eye tracking of schizophrenic patients is not smooth but shows irregularities and has a 'cogwheel' appearance. Instead of smooth pursuit, tracking tends to stop, and there are 'velocity arrests' which show up clearly on a differentiated record. Records are scored either by a rating procedure which shows high inter-rater reliability or by counts of velocity arrests which give high correlations to the subjective ratings.

Holzman's work shows a clear-cut differentiation in eye tracking performance between schizophrenics and normals, but Shagass's work, while supporting Holzman's, also finds disturbances in tracking performance in other psychotic patients. Among schizophrenics it is those having a diagnosis based on the presence of thought disorder that show major tracking dysfunction.

Perhaps the most interesting finding of Holzman's is that poor eye tracking is found in a large percentage of the otherwise normal relatives of schizophrenics. A study by Holzman in conjunction with the Norwegian genetist Kringlen (Holzman *et al.*, 1977) shows that in a twin sample the concordance rate for monozygotic twins is 0.77 and for dizygotic twins 0.40. Studies by both Shagass and Holzman show that when steps are taken to maximise attention to the target pendulum the eye tracking of schizophrenics improves, but even under these circumstances tracking remains inferior to normal. The poor eye tracking appears to be uninfluenced by tranquillising medication. Few steps have been taken to relate eye tracking to other psychophysiological variables; however, an unpublished study by Owen (personal communication) suggests that poor eye-tracking is not found among schizophrenics who are SC non-responders but is confined to SC responders. As this latter type of response is that which in the study of Mednick *et al.* (1977) predicts schizophrenic breakdown of a florid kind with thought disorder as a major feature, the value of pursuing this association in further research seems evident.

Cortical Activity

The literature in this field is very extensive and at this point it is not possible to do anything other than indicate some of the more promising areas.

Perhaps the most directly interpretable work on the EEG is that of Goldstein and his colleagues (Goldstein *et al.*, 1963; Goldstein *et al.*, 1965) using Drohocki (1948) type integration. This work, integrating the whole of the EEG spectrum, shows a smaller 'mean energy content' (MEC) and coefficient of variation (CV) of that content in schizophrenics in comparison with normals. These measures, which may be roughly interpreted as indices of 'arousal', provide cortical equivalents to the findings reviewed earlier suggesting (in part) higher electrodermal and cardiac levels of 'arousal' in patients than in normals.

The association between MEC and CV and 'arousal' may be drawn from the study by Murphree *et al.* (1962) which shows a 20 per cent decrease in MEC and a 35 per cent decrease in CV in normal subjects under dextro-amphetamine medication.

The use of small laboratory computers, however, makes the relatively crude integration of the whole frequency band by the Drohocki method obsolete and the use of the Fast Fourier Transform makes possible the investigation of the power in particular frequency bands within the EEG spectrum.

In a series of studies, Itil *et al.* (1972), Itil *et al.* (1974), Itil *et al.* (1976), using visual evaluation of EEG records and computer analysis of the same material, showed that in adult schizophrenics, children at risk for schizophrenia and psychotic children, there is evidence of more slow and fast activity and less activity in the alpha band than in normal subjects. Itil and his colleagues suggest on the basis of these findings that 'the findings are characteristic of the psychophysiology of schizophrenia'.

The availability of small laboratory computers, either of a 'hand-wired' or programmable variety, is of course the basis for the considerable amount of work being pursued on event-related potentials (ERPs) in schizophrenic patients.

One of the most productive workers in this field, Shagass, has reviewed his work very completely in 1976 and it would be redundant to attempt to cover it here. However, it is worthwhile drawing attention to two conclusions which he notes at the end of his review. These are the possibility of distinguishing electrophysiologically different sub-types of schizophrenia and the suggestion that what the ERP data particularly indicate is 'impaired attentive and perceptual functioning in chronic schizophrenia' resulting from a 'filtering defect'. Shagass's data thus support views that have been developed from other psychophysiological and behavioural investigations.

Another area of particular promise in the ERP investigation of schiz-ophrenia is that of Buchsbaum and his colleagues, for example Landau *et al.* (1975), Buchsbaum (1975).

This work is concerned with the application of the concept of 'augmentation-reduction' to the field of investigation of schizophrenia. The concept is that there are individual differences in the extent to which a person tends to 'amplify' or 'turn down the gain' on the input to his nervous system and that these differences may be exemplified by examination of components of the event-related cortical potential.

In those who may be labelled as *reducers*, the amplitude of the P100–N140 component decreases as the intensity of stimuli increases. On the other hand, in those labelled as *augmenters*, the same ERP component increases in parallel with increases in stimulus intensity.

Work on schizophrenic patients shows that the majority of them tend to give a reducing type of response. Landau *et al.* (1975), for instance, provide data to show that schizophrenic patients (diagnosed by careful research-orientated procedures) could be distinguished from normals using ERP variables with 71 per cent accuracy. While still requiring further work, the promise shown by this technique indicates the value of progress in this area.

The work reviewed in this chapter suggests that development can valuably take place in the direction of producing greater understanding of some of the mechanisms involved in the processes underlying overt schizophrenia. A further step in parallel with this understanding is the possibility of developing means of improved diagnosis and sub-diagnosis and in addition techniques for the monitoring of the effectiveness of therapeutic processes.

References

Ax, A. F. and Bamford, J. L. (1970). The GSR recovery limb in chronic schizophrenia. *Psychophysiology*, **7**, 145–147

Bernstein, A. S. (1964). The galvanic skin response orienting reflex among chronic schizophrenics. *Psychon. Sci.*, **1**, 391–392

Bernstein, A. S. (1967). Electrodermal base level, tonic arousal and adaptation in chronic schizophrenics. *J. aborm. Psychol.*, **72**, 221–232

Bernstein, A. S. (1970). Phasic electrodermal orienting response in chronic schizophrenics. *J. abnorm. Psychol.*, **75**, 146–156

Buchsbaum, M. (1975). Average evoked response, augmenting/reducing in schizophrenia and affective disorders. In *Biology of the Major Psychoses* (Ed. D. X. Freedman), Raven Press, New York

Crider, A. D., Greenspoon, L. and Maher, B. A. (1965). Autonomic and psychomotor correlates of pre-morbid adjustment in schizophrenia. *Psychosom. Med.*, **27**, 201–206

Depue, R. A. and Fowles, D. C. (1973). Electrodermal activity as an index of arousal in schizophrenics. *Psychol. Bull.*, **79**, 233–238

De Vault, S. H. (1955). Physiological responsiveness in reactive and process schizophrenia. Unpublished doctoral dissertation. Michigan State University

Diefendorf, A. R. and Dodge, R. (1908). An experimental study of the ocular reactions of the insane from photographic records. *Brain*, **31**, 451–489

Douglas, R. J. (1972). Pavlovian conditioning and the brain. In *Inhibition and Learning* (Ed. R. A. Boakes and M. S. Halliday), Academic Press, New York, Chapter 20

Drohocki, Z. (1948). L'integrateur de l'électro-production cérébrale par l'encephalographie quantitative. *Rev. Neurol.* (*Paris*), **80**, 619–624

Dykman, R. A., Reese, W. G., Galbrecht, C. R., Ackerman, P. T. and Sunderman, R. S. (1968). Autonomic responses in psychiatric patients. *Ann. N. Y. Acad. Sci.*, **147**, 237–303

Edelberg, R. (1970). The information content of the recovery limb of the electrodermal response. *Psychophysiology*, **6**, 527–539

Endicott, J. and Spitzer, R. (1972). Current and past psychopathology scales (CAPPS). *Archs gen. Psychiat.*, **27**, 678–687

Fenz, W. D. and Velner, J. (1970). Physiological concomitants of behavioural indexes in schizophrenia. *J. abnorm. Psychol.*, **76**, 27–35

Flor-Henry, P. (1974). Psychosis, neurosis and epilepsy. *Br. J. Psychiat.*, **124**, 144–150

Goldstein, L., Murphree, H. B., Sugerman, A. A., Pfeiffer, C. C. and Jenney, E. H. (1963). Quantitative electroencephalographic analysis of naturally occurring (schizophrenic) and drug induced psychotic states in human males. *Clin. Pharmac. Ther.*, **4**, 10–21

Goldstein, L., Sugerman, A. A., Stolberg, H., Murphree, H. B. and Pfeiffer, C. C. (1965). Electro-cerebral activity in schizophrenics and non-psychotic subjects. Quantitative EEG amplitude analysis. *EEG clin. Neurophysiol.*, **19**, 350–361

Goldstein, M. J. and Acker, C. W. (1967). Psychophysiological reaction to films by chronic schizophrenics II: individual differences in resting level and reactivity. *J. abnorm. Psychol.*, **72**, 23–29

Goldstein, M. J., Acker, C. W., Crockett, J. T. and Riddle, J. J. (1966). Psychophysiological reactions to films by chronic schizophrenics I: Effects of drug status. *J. abnorm. Psychol.*, **71**, 335–344

Gruzelier, J. H. (1973). The investigation of possible limbic dysfunction in schizophrenia by psychophysiological methods. Unpublished doctoral dissertation. University of London

Gruzelier, J. H. and Hammond, N. V. (1977a). The effect of chlorpromazine upon psychophysiological endocrine and information processing measures in schizophrenia. *J. psychosom. Res.*, in press

Gruzelier, J. H. and Hammond, N. V. (1977b). The effect of chlorpromazine upon bilateral asymmetries in bioelectrical skin reactivity of schizophrenics. *Stud. Psychol.*, **19**, 40–51

Gruzelier, J. H., Lykken, D. T. and Venables, P. H. (1972). Schizophrenia and arousal revisited. Two flash thresholds and electrodermal activity in activated and non-activated conditions. *Archs gen. Psychiat.*, **26**, 427–432

Gruzelier, J. H. and Venables, P. H. (1972). Skin conductance orienting activity in a heterogeneous sample of schizophrenics. *J. nerv. ment. Dis.*, **155**, 277–287

Gruzelier, J. H. and Venables, P. H. (1975). Bimodality and lateral asymmetry of skin conductance orienting activity in schizophrenics: Replication and evidence of lateral asymmetry in patients with depression and disorders of personality. *Biol. Psychiat.*, **8**, 55–73

Hakerem, G. and Sutton, S. (1964). Pupillary reactions to light in schizophrenic patients and normals. *Ann. N.Y. Acad. Sci.*, **105**, 820–831

Herman, T. M. (1972). Heart rate functioning in children with schizophrenic mothers. Unpublished doctoral dissertation. New School for Social Research, New York

Holzman P. S., Kringlen E., Levy D. L., Proctor L. R., Haberman S. J. and Yasillo N. J. (1977). Abnormal pursuit eye movements in schizophrenia. *Archs gen. Psychiat.*, **34**, 802–805

Holzman, P. S., Levy, D. L. and Proctor, L. R. (1976). Smooth pursuit eye-movements, attention and schizophrenia. *Archs gen. Psychiat.*, **33**, 1415–1420

Holzman, P. S., Proctor, L. R. and Hughes, D. W. (1973). Eye-tracking patterns in schizophrenia. *Science*, **181**, 179–181

Holzman, P. S., Proctor, L. R., Levy, D. L., Yasillo, N. J., Meltzer, H. Y. and Hurt,

S. W. (1974). Eye tracking dysfunctions in schizophrenic patients and their relatives. *Archs gen. Psychiat.*, **31**, 143–151

Itil, T. M., Hsu, M. S., Saletu, B. and Mednick, S. (1974). Computer EEG and auditory evoked potential investigations in children at high risk for schizophrenia. *Am. J. Psychiat.*, **131**, 892–900

Itil, T. M., Saletu, B. and Davis, S. (1972). EEG findings in chronic schizophrenics based on digital computer period analysis and analog power spectra. *Biol, Psychiat.*, **5**, 1–13

Itil, T. M., Simeon, J. and Coffin, C. (1976). Qualitative and quantitative EEG in psychotic children. *Dis. Nerv. Syst.*, **37**, 247–252

Janes, C. L. and Stern, J. A. (1976). Electrodermal response configuration as a function of rated psychopathology in children. *J. nerv. ment. Dis.*, **162**, 184–194

Jordan, L. S. (1974). Electrodermal activity in schizophrenics: further considerations. *Psychol. Bull.*, **81**, 85–91

Kraepelin, E. (1919). *Psychiatrie*. Barth, Leipzig

Lacey, J. I. (1967). Somatic response patterning and stress: some revision of activation theory. In *Psychological Stress* (Ed. M. H. Appley and R. Trumbull) Appleton-Century-Crofts, New York

Landau, S. G., Buchsbaum, M. S., Carpenter, W., Strauss, J. and Sacks, M. (1975). Schizophrenia and stimulus intensity control. *Archs gen. Psychiat.*, **32**, 1239–1245

Lang, P. J. and Buss, A. (1965). Psychological deficit in schizophrenia II. Interference and activation. *J. abnorm. Psychol.*, **70**, 77–106

Lidsky, A., Hakerem, S. and Sutton, S. (1971). Pupillary reactions to single light pulses in psychiatric patients and normals. *J. nerv. ment. Dis.*, **153**, 286–291

Lobstein, T. J. (1974). Heart rate and skin conductance activity in schizophrenia. Unpublished doctoral dissertation. University of London

Luria, A. R. and Homskaya, E. D. (1963). Disturbance of the regulating activity of the frontal lobes of the brain. In *The Human Brain and Psychic Processes*, Moscow, Academy of Psychological Sciences of the RSFSR, pp. 450–453

Maricq, H. R. and Edelberg, R. (1975). Electrodermal recovery rate in a schizophrenic population. *Psychophysiology*, **12**, 630–641

McGhie, A. (1969). *Pathology of Attention*. Penguin, Harmondsworth

Mednick, S. A. and McNeil, T. F. (1968). Current methodology in research on the etiology of schizophrenia. Serious difficulties which suggest the use of the high-risk group method. *Psychol. Bull.*, **70**, 681–693

Mednick, S. A. and Schulsinger, F. (1968). Some pre-morbid characteristics related to breakdown in children with schizophrenic mothers. In *The Transmission of Schizophrenia* (Ed. D. Rosenthal and S. S. Kety), Pergamon Press, New York, pp. 267–291

Mednick, S. A., Schulsinger, F., Teasdale, T. W., Schulsinger, H., Venables, P. H. and Rock, D. R. (1977). Schizophrenia in high-risk children. Sex differences and predisposing factors. Paper presented to Kittay Scientific Foundation 5th International Symposium, New York

Murphree, H. B., Jenney, E. H. and Pfeiffer, C. C. (1962). Quantitative electroencephalographic analysis of the effects of lysergic acid diethylamide (LSD-25) and D-amphetamine in man. *Fedn. Proc.*, **21**, 337

Obrist, P. A., Webb, R. A., Sutterer, J. R. and Howard, J. L. (1970). Cardiac deceleration and reaction time: an evaluation of two hypotheses. *Psychophysiology*, **6**, 695–706

Patterson, T. (1976a). Skin conductance responding/nonresponding and pupillometrics in chronic schizophrenia: a confirmation of Gruzelier and Venables. *J. nerv. ment. Dis.*, **163**, 200–209

Patterson, T. (1976b). Skin conductance recovery and pupillometrics in chronic schizophrenia. *Psychophysiology*, **13**, 189–195

Patterson, T. and Venables, P. H. (1978). Detailed examination of the skin potential and bilateral skin conductance records of schizophrenic and normal subjects: the identification of the fast habituation group of schizophrenics. *Psychophysiology* (in press)

Rubin, L. S. (1960). Pupillary reactivity as a measure of autonomic balance in the study of psychotic behaviour: a rational approach to chemotherapy. *Trans. N.Y. Acad. Sci.*, **22**, 509–518

Rubin, L. S. (1961). Patterns of pupillary dilation and constriction in psychotic adults and autistic children. *J. nerv. ment. Dis.*, **133**, 130–142

Rubin, L. S. (1962). Autonomic function in psychoses. *Archs gen. Psychiat.*, **7**, 1–14

Rubin, L. S. and Barry, T. J. (1972a). The reactivity of the iris muscle as an index of autonomic dysfunction in schizophrenia. *J. nerv. ment. Dis.*, **155**, 265–276

Rubin, L. S. and Barry, T. J. (1972b). The effect of the cold pressor test on pupillary reactivity of schizophrenics in remission. *Biol. Psychiat.*, **5**, 181–197

Rubin, L. S. and Barry, T. J. (1972c). The effects of conjuctival instillation of eserine and homatropine on pupillary reactivity in schizophrenics. *Biol. Psychiat.*, **5**, 257–269

Schulsinger, H. (1976). A ten-year follow up of children of schizophrenic mothers: clinical assessment. *Acta psychiat. scand.*, **53**, 371–386

Shagass, C. (1976). An electrophysiological view of schizophrenia. *Biol. Psychiat.*, **11**, 1–30

Shagass, C., Amadeo, M. and Overton, D. A. (1974). Eye-tracking performance in psychiatric patients. *Biol. Psychiat.*, **9**, 245–260

Shagass, C., Roemer, R. A. and Amadeo, M. (1976). Eye-tracking performance and engagement of attention. *Archs gen. Psychiat.*, **33**, 121–125

Sourek, K. (1965). *The Nervous Control of Skin Potential in Man*. Nakladalelstri Ceskoslovenske Akadamie Ved, Praha

Spain, B. (1966). Eyelid conditioning and arousal in schizophrenic and normal subjects. *J. abnorm. Psychol.*, **71**, 260–266

Spohn, H. E., Thetford, P. E. and Cancro, R. (1971). The effects of phenothiazine medication on skin conductance and heart rate in schizophrenic patients. *J. nerv. ment. Dis.*, **152**, 129–139

Venables, P. H. (1957). A short scale of rating 'activity-withdrawal' in schizophrenics. *J. ment. Sci.*, **103**, 197–199

Venables, P. H. (1964). Input dysfunction in schizophrenia. In *Advances in Experimental Personality Research 1* (Ed. B. Maher), Academic Press, New York

Venables, P. H. (1973). Input regulation in psychopathology. In *Psychopathology* (Ed. M. Hammer, K. Salzinger and S. Sutton), Wiley, New York, Chap. 14

Venables, P. H. (1975). A psychophysiological approach to research in schizophrenia. In *Clinical Applications of Psychophysiology* (Ed. D. C. Fowles), Columbia University Press, New York

Venables, P. H. (1977). The electrodermal psychophysiology of schizophrenics and children at risk for schizophrenia: controversies and developments. *Schizophren. Bull.*, **3**, 28–48

Venables, P. H. and Christie, M. J. (1973). Mechanisms, instrumentation, recording techniques and quantification of responses. In *Electrodermal Activity in Psychological Research* (Ed. W. F. Prokasy and D. C. Raskin), Academic Press, New York, Chap. 1

Venables, P. H. and Patterson, T. (1977). Speech perception and decision processes in relation to skin conductance and pupillographic measures in schizophrenia. In *Schizophrenia* (Ed. L. Wynne, R. Cromwell and S. Matthysse), Wiley, New York, Chap. 16

Venables, P. H. and Wing, J. K. (1962). Level of arousal and the subclassification of schizophrenia. *Archs gen. Psychiat.*, **7**, 114–119

Wing, J. K., Cooper, J. E. and Sartorius, N. (1974). *The Measurement and Classification of Psychiatric Symptoms*. Cambridge University Press, London

Zahn, T. P. (1976). On the bimodality of the distribution of electrodermal orienting responses in schizophrenic patients. *J. nerv. ment. Dis.*, **162,** 195–199

Zahn, T. P., Carpenter, W. T. and McGlashan, T. H. (1975). Autonomic variables related to short term outcome in acute schizophrenic patients. Paper presented to Society of Psychophysiological Research, Toronto

Zahn, T. P., Rosenthal, D. and Lawlor, W. G. (1968). Electrodermal and heart rate orienting reactions in chronic schizophrenia. *J. psychiat. Res.*, **6,** 117–134

20 The Influence of Family and Social Factors on the Course of Schizophrenia

C. E. Vaughn and J. P. Leff

Introduction

Although the aetiology of schizophrenia continues to puzzle clinicians and researchers alike, enough is now known about the precipitants of relapse in a patient with an established schizophrenic illness to suggest that he is highly responsive to his social environment. Of particular interest is a series of studies carried out by George Brown and his colleagues concerning the influence of family life on the course of a schizophrenic illness. In the most recent study (Brown *et al.*, 1972) a standardised method was used to assess the *quality* of the emotional relationship between a schizophrenic patient and the relative with whom he lives. The authors found that they could predict relapse of schizophrenia during a nine months period following discharge by using an index of the expressed emotion (EE) shown by the relative during an interview shortly after the patient was admitted to hospital. This index of expressed emotion had three components, the most important of which was the number of critical comments made by the relative when talking about the patient and his illness. Additional measures of EE were hostility, which rarely occurred in the absence of high criticism, and marked emotional over-involvement.*

The index was used to categorise patients as coming from high EE or low EE homes. During the nine months after discharge from hospital, 58 per cent of the patients from high EE homes relapsed, compared with only 16 per cent of the low EE group, a highly significant finding ($P < 0.001$). This association was independent of the patient's previous behaviour disturbance and work impairment.

Results did suggest that patients living with relatives who expressed high emotion at the time of key admission were less likely to relapse if they either received regular phenothiazine medication (this trend did not reach significance) or managed to avoid close contact with the family. But the index of the relative's expressed emotion remained the best single predictor of symptomatic relapse.

* Criticism and hostility were based on either negative emotion (judged by tone of voice) or a 'clear statement of resentment, disapproval, dislike or rejection'. Marked emotional over-involvement tended to be found in parents rather than in other relatives and is best characterised by excessive anxiety, overconcern, or overprotectiveness toward the patient. It is rated on the basis either of feelings expressed in the interview or of behaviour reported outside it.

The unequivocal nature of these results, and their practical and theoretical implications, made a replication of the study highly desirable. The present authors, although sharing the same research tradition as Brown and his colleagues, were determined to approach this work in a critical frame of mind. We were interested in whether the results concerning the factors influencing the outcome could be replicated with another sample of schizophrenic patients.

In most respects the present study is identical to the earlier study in its design and execution. A similar prospective nine months follow-up design is used, featuring independent assessments of past behaviour, present emotional response of relatives and any subsequent relapse. As before, the hypothesis to be tested is 'that a high degree of expressed emotion is an index of the characteristics in the relatives which are likely to cause a florid relapse of symptoms, independently of other factors such as length of history, type of symptoms or severity of previous behaviour disturbance'. And again, two basic assumptions are made: first, that the index of the relative's expressed emotion is a reasonable indicator of family relationships, which can be relied upon even though his everyday behaviour toward the patient is not being observed directly; second, that the attitude shown by the relative toward the patient during the interview is representative of an enduring relationship over time. Findings in the 1972 study by Brown *et al.* appeared to justify these assumptions.

Design

Patients included in the study were collected sequentially at point of relapse, on admission to one of three hospitals in South East London (Bethlem, Maudsley, St Francis). The case records were screened of all patients aged 17–64 whose native language was English and who were living with relatives at the time of admission. Any persons with suspected organic illnesses were excluded. The psychiatrist (J.L.) interviewed all patients whose records suggested a diagnosis of schizophrenia, using the 9th edition of the Present State Examination to make clinical ratings (Wing *et al.*, 1974). If the diagnosis was confirmed the patient was included in the study and his relatives were approached by the psychologist (C.V.).

Using these criteria, 43 schizophrenic patients were initially selected. Of this original number, five schizophrenic patients had to be excluded because their relatives refused to participate.* One more patient was eliminated from the study during the nine months follow-up period because he left home shortly after discharge from hospital. The remaining 37 schizophrenic patients

---

* These were all cases in which the patient had a long psychiatric history and the relatives, generally very critical of the patient, were unwilling to retell the whole story yet another time. A typical response was 'It's an agony to me and a waste of your time'. All the excluded schizophrenic patients were living with parents.

comprised the final follow-up group, and represent 86 per cent of the original sample. The patients were distributed by sex and living group as shown in table 20.1

Table 20.1
Distribution of patients by sex and living group

Type of household	Male	Female	Total
Parental	11	6	17
Marital	4	9	13
Other (patient living with adult child or other relative)	0	7	7
Total N	15	22	37

The mean age of the schizophrenic patients was 33.1 years.

The first patient was seen in October 1971, and the last follow-up interview took place in January 1975.

The current mental state (PSE) interviews were carried out by the psychiatrist shortly after the patient's admission to hospital, and again at readmission or nine months follow-up. An abbreviated version of the main family interview (Brown and Rutter, 1966; Rutter and Brown, 1966) was administered on a home visit by the psychologist within days of the psychiatrist's assessment. As in the original study, the husband or wife of a married patient was always seen. In cases where an unmarried patient lived with both parents, mother and father were interviewed on separate occasions. Of the 13 pairs of relatives, both were seen in 10 cases; in the remaining 3 pairs only one relative was seen.

In the study to be replicated the interview with the relative alone at the time of the key admission produced the significant finding. This therefore was considered to be the definitive interview. Family interviews were not repeated at the time of follow-up or readmission, nor given to the patient alone. For similar reasons the 'joint' interview was dropped. Certain measures, however, were reapplied by the psychiatrist at the time of follow-up, if changes were thought to have occurred during this period. For example, the patient was questioned about the family time budget if there had been changes in the amount of face to face contact between him and his relatives.

All but two of the 37 patients who qualified for the follow-up study were personally revisited by the psychiatrist. The two exceptions, both of whom had left the South East London area, were reassessed through hospital case notes and personal correspondence. In addition to repeating the Present State Examination, the psychiatrist took a careful history of drug treatment during the months since discharge, checking with out-patient records wherever possible. Criteria for judging whether a discharged patient had taken phenothiazines regularly were strictly adhered to. If drugs were discontinued or taken irregularly for more than one month of the nine months follow-up period, a person was considered to be off regular medication.

Techniques of Measurement

The techniques of behavioural, psychiatric and family measurement were identical to those used in the earlier study, with one important difference: the abbreviated length of the main family interview schedule. The rationale for the abbreviated interview is given by Vaughn and Leff (1976). The psychologist spent several months learning to use the interview schedule. High inter-rater reliability with the original interviewers was established by rating tapes from the 1972 study. The psychiatrist also learned the technique for the rating of criticism; inter-rater reliability between psychologist and psychiatrist over 15 interviews was 0.86 (product moment correlation).

1. Ratings of Emotional Response

Ratings were made on all the scales employed in the 1972 study, including the three which form the components of the overall index of relatives' expressed emotion (EE): number of critical comments made about the patient, hostility, and emotional over-involvement. Detailed descriptions, with examples, of these and other measures (for example demonstrated warmth, dissatisfaction on four-point scales describing areas of family life) may be found in references already cited.

2. Relapse

The criteria used to assess relapse of schizophrenia were the same as those employed in the 1972 study. Brown *et al.* distinguished between two types of relapse: Type I involved a change from 'normal' or 'non-schizophrenic' state to a state of 'schizophrenia' as defined by the CATEGO clinical classification procedure, classes S or P (Wing, *et al.*, 1974). Type II involved a 'marked exacerbation' of persistent schizophrenic symptoms. At the time of reassessment the psychiatrist was unaware of the original level of relatives' expressed emotion.

Results

The mean numbers of critical comments made by relatives of schizophrenics in the two series do not differ significantly ($z = 0.173$) despite the much abbreviated length of the family interview in our study. The mean number of critical remarks made by the 46 relatives in the present study was 8.22 (s.d. $= 11.11$). The mean number of comments for all 126 relatives interviewed in the 1972 study was calculated and found to be 7.86 (s.d. = 14.40). When one considers that these two series of patients and relatives were assessed by different research teams a decade apart in time, this seems an impressive result.

In the present sample, the mean number of critical remarks does not differ significantly for the two main living groups (Parental $\bar{x}$ = 7.04, s.d. = 7.63; Marital $\bar{x}$ = 11.92, s.d. = 17.14; t = 1.07, 36 d.f., NS).

1. Overall Index of Relatives' Expressed Emotion (EE)

As before, the individual scales were first related to relapse. In the 1972 study a threshold of 7 critical comments was used to divide the families into two expressed emotion subgroups roughly equal in size. Using this same cut-off point, and including relatives who showed marked emotional over-involvement (that is scores of 4 or 5 on a five-point scale) in the high EE subgroup, we obtained the relapse figures shown in table 20.2 (a). This

Table 20.2
Relationship of relatives' expressed emotion to relapse in the 9 months after discharge

(a) Using a criticism threshold of 7 critical comments

EE of relatives	No relapse	Relapse	Per cent relapse
High 7+ critical comments and/or marked EOI	9	9	50
Low 1–6 critical comments; no marked EOI	17	2	12 $\chi^2, P < 0.02$

(b) Using a criticism threshold of 6 critical comments

EE of relatives	No relapse	Relapse	Per cent relapse
High 6+ critical comments and/or marked EOI	11	10	48
Low 1–5 critical comments; no marked EOI	15	1	6

Fisher's exact test

$P = 0.007$

threshold gives a split close to the median. However, a closer inspection of results revealed that a cut-off point of 6 critical remarks gave a better separation in terms of relapse rates (table 20.2 (b)). In view of the arbitrary nature of the original cut-off point, we felt justified in making an adjustment in the level of criticism required for allocation to the high EE subgroup. All results presented below are based on this new criticism threshold.*

2. Relationship between Index of Expressed Emotion and Relapse

The relapse figures for 37 schizophrenic patients from high EE and low EE homes are shown in table 20.2 (b). A total of 11 schizophrenic patients (28 per cent) relapsed during the follow-up period. Of these all but one had a Type I relapse. They had been well for some time after their key discharge, but had definite schizophrenic symptoms at readmission or nine months follow-up. Six patients (16 per cent of the total sample) were readmitted to hospital. As in the 1972 study, there is a significant association between high EE and relapse (Fisher's exact $P = 0.007$).

It is evident, however, that relatives' EE is not the sole determinant of relapse, for more than half of the patients from high EE homes managed to remain well during the follow-up period. Other factors—social, clinical, environmental—must be operating to influence outcome. A series of analyses was carried out to see whether the relationship between EE and relapse was linked with any other factors. Only the most important of these will be mentioned here.

3. Other Factors Related to Relapse

(a) Clinical and Demographic Factors
A comparison was made between those schizophrenic patients who relapsed and those who remained well in terms of the clinical PSE syndromes present at key admission. Only one item was related to outcome at the 5 per cent level of significance: Grandiose Delusions were more common in those patients who relapsed.

Within the high EE subgroup a comparison was also made between those who relapsed and those who remained well. In this analysis two items, Grandiose Delusions and Residual Schizophrenia, were found more commonly in those who relapsed. As 38 comparisons were being made, these could well be chance findings.

No other clinical variable measured, nor any feature of psychiatric history assessed, added anything to the value of the EE index for predicting relapse. This is in accord with findings in the 1972 study.

Of the many demographic factors considered, only two were related to

---

* In no case was hostility found in the absence of high criticism, so it was not used in the compilation of the high EE group.

outcome: sex and marital status. The relapse rate for schizophrenic men is double that for women, and the rate for the unmarried is significantly greater than for the married (exact $P = 0.033$):

Married: men, 25 per cent; women, 0 per cent; total 8 per cent.

Unmarried: men, 54 per cent; women, 31 per cent; total 42 per cent.

Very similar marital status and sex differences were revealed in the 1972 study. These differences do not affect the main association between expressed emotion and relapse.

(b) Previous Work Impairment and Behaviour Disturbance

Using the criteria of Brown *et al.* for work impairment, 43 per cent of the present sample of schizophrenic patients were rated as impaired, two-thirds of these being found in high EE homes. The relapse rate in the impaired group was 37 per cent, and in the non-impaired group 24 per cent (NS). As in the 1972 study, it was found that work impairment was only associated with relapse because of its association with level of EE. No work-impaired patients in a low EE home relapsed; 55 per cent of those in a high EE home did so.

Many measures of the patient's behaviour before admission were made from the relative's account. Their relationship both to the relative's EE and to relapse was examined in a variety of ways. When we employed the same criteria used by Brown *et al.*, to rate severe behaviour disturbance as either present or absent, we obtained almost identical results. We too found that a majority of the schizophrenic patients (present study, 62 per cent; cf. 1972 study, 75 per cent) fall into one of two categories: either they are rated 'disturbed' in behaviour during the three months preceding admission and live with relatives showing a high degree of expressed emotion, or they are rated as 'not disturbed' and living with relatives with a low degree of expressed emotion. But in cases where patients are incongruent for the two factors the degree of EE is related to relapse (exact $P = 0.027$) and the degree of disturbance in the months before admission is not important.

The analysis of Brown *et al.* did not take into account the duration and persistence of symptoms or the possibility that certain behaviours might be differentially important both for the relative's response and for outcome. However, when the data were examined in a variety of ways, similar results were produced, indicating that the relationship between EE and relapse was independent of the patient's behaviour disturbance during the 3 months before admission.

(c) Factors after Discharge

Two other factors found to be important in the 1972 study were examined: maintenance therapy with phenothiazines and amount of face to face contact. As in the 1972 study, neither of these factors had significance for the low EE group, but each did relate to outcome for those in high EE homes (tables 20.3 and 20.4). In fact the result for maintenance therapy is statistically significant

TABLE 20.3
Relationship of relatives' EE, drug-taking after discharge and relapse

Relatives' EE	No drugs			Drugs			Significance (χ^2)
	No relapse	Relapse	Per cent relapse	No relapse	Relapse	Per cent relapse	Fisher's exact test
High	2	7	78	9	3	25	$P = 0.024$
Low	6	1	14	9	0	0	NS
Total	8	8	50	18	3	14	$P = 0.023$

Table 20.4
Relationship of relatives' EE, time spent in face to face contact per week after discharge and relapse

Relatives' EE	Time in face to face contact with relatives		
	Less than 35 hours		
	No relapse	Relapse	Per cent relapse
High	5	2	29
Low	6	1	14

χ^2 NS

Relatives' EE	Time in face to face contact with relatives		
	More than 35 hours		
	No relapse	Relapse	Per cent relapse
High	6	8	57
Low	9	0	0

Fisher's exact test $P = 0.006$.

($P < 0.05$). A similar trend failed to reach statistical significance in the 1972 study.*

---

* Fifty-seven per cent of the 37 schizophrenic patients satisfied our criteria for regular maintenance therapy. Equal proportions of low EE and high EE patients failed to take one of the phenothiazines regularly.

4. Relative Contribution of Various Factors to Relapse

Having identified a number of factors individually related to relapse, we determined their relative contribution by a correlation matrix. This matrix (table 20.5) shows that relatives' EE is more closely related to relapse than any other factor considered, including lack of preventive drug treatment. When behaviour disturbance (based on total symptoms score) is partialled out, the significance levels are unchanged. In fact, the correlation between EE and relapse is actually raised ($r = 0.52$; $P < 0.01$). This is conclusive evidence that for schizophrenic patients the relationship between EE and relapse holds independently of behaviour disturbance.

Table 20.5
Correlation matrix of factors

	1. Relapse	2. Behaviour disturbance	3. Critical comments	4. Drug treatment	5. Face to face contact	6. Expressed emotion
1.	1.00	−0.20	0.11	−0.39*	0.14	0.45†
2.			0.34*	0.32	−0.01	0.24
3.				0.24	0.13	0.58‡
4.					−0.01	0.01
5.						0.11

* $P < 0.05$.   † $P < 0.01$.   ‡ $P < 0.001$.

5. Additive Effects of Factors Related to Relapse

These separate analyses aroused interest in the ways in which the effects of the different variables on relapse—maintenance therapy, face to face contact, relatives' EE—might be additive. This particular analysis had not been done by Brown and his colleagues, but because the two studies were so similar in design and methodology it was possible to return to the original data, reanalyse them, and pool the resulting figures with our own, as shown in figure 20.1.

It is evident from the relapse rates that patients in high EE homes who spend much time with their relatives and are not protected by maintenance therapy (subgroup 6) have a very poor outcome. The relapse rates drop considerably if one of the two protective factors is operating (subgroups 4 and 5). The prognosis is best of all, however, for patients living in high EE homes but protected both by reduced contact and by maintenance therapy. For this group of patients (subgroup 3), the relapse rate drops to 15 per cent, a rate significantly lower than that of patients for whom neither protective mechanism is operating ($P < 0.001$), and as low as that of patients from low EE homes (subgroups 1 and 2).

The relapse rates in the six subgroups in figure 20.1 provide valuable information about the preventive role of maintenance therapy. It is clear from

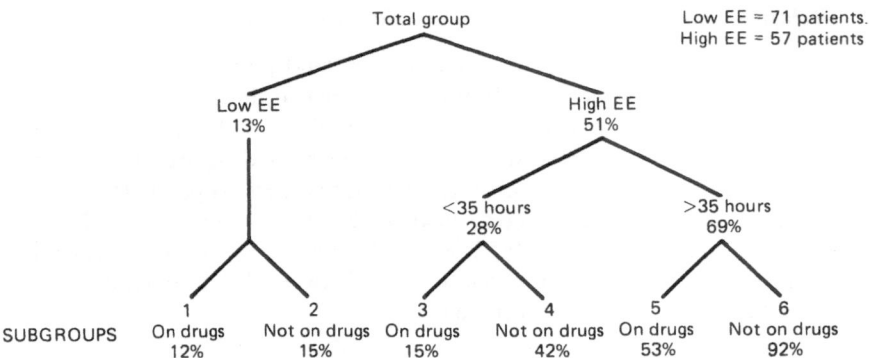

Figure 20.1   Nine month relapse rates of total group of 128 schizophrenic patients

the relapse rates in subgroups 1 and 2 that drugs make no difference for patients living in low EE homes. They are effective, however, in reducing the relapse rate in patients from high EE homes, especially in patients who spend less than 35 hours per week with their relatives.

Discussion

The main results of Brown *et al.* (1972) concerning the family and social factors influencing the course of schizophrenia have been almost exactly replicated. It has been possible to predict relapse patterns even more precisely than in the earlier study, by considering the additive effects of various biological and social factors shown to be individually important for outcome. A high degree of emotion expressed by the relative at the time of key admission remains the best single predictor of symptomatic relapse during the 9 months following discharge. But results suggest that the combination of maintenance therapy and reduction of face to face contact with a highly involved or critical relative will prevent relapse in nearly every instance.

Sex and Living Group Differences

Brown *et al.* believed the differences in relapse rates between the unmarried and married schizophrenics to be a consequence of the fact that if either or both parents live with the patient alone more emotion is expressed. But this was not the case in our study; parents were just as likely to show high EE if there were other persons in the household. Nor can the results be explained by differences in the amount of emotion expressed by parents and spouses; these were not significant.

Both the 1972 figures and our own show unmarried men to be at greatest risk of relapse, and married women to be least vulnerable. Evidence from both studies indicates that unmarried men from high EE homes are significantly less likely than their female counterparts to be protected by both drugs *and* reduced face to face contact (exact $P = 0.006$); only 5 per cent of these men had both protective mechanisms operating, compared with 50 per cent of the unmarried women.

One can only speculate about the reasons for the low relapse rate among married schizophrenic women; they may include such factors as premorbid personality and differing role expectations. This is not the place to expand on this finding at length. The importance of these results lies in the identification of a group which would be at high risk of relapse in any prevention programme.

Factors after Discharge

Compared with our series of schizophrenic patients, a higher proportion of patients in the 1972 study relapsed while on drugs. These differing relapse rates may be due to the more stringent criteria for 'regular' drug-taking in the present study. Then too, 10 years have passed since the original study was carried out. It may be that more discrimination is shown now in the way drugs are prescribed and given, the recipients now more often being those in greatest need.

Low face to face contact can result from the patient being away from the home, for example working or at a Day Centre, or can be produced by his staying in the home but withdrawing socially. A distinction must be made between two terms. 'Social withdrawal' refers to a decrease in *verbal* communication: a refusal to initiate conversation, failure to answer when directly addressed, seeming to be in another world. Face to face contact is a measure of actual physical proximity. Thus it is possible for a person to have high face to face contact with his relatives and still rate highly on social withdrawal.

Brown and others have suggested that social withdrawal can be a means of coping with a stressful situation, a protective mechanism which lessens chances of relapse of schizophrenia. Investigation of this possibility revealed a significant association between low face to face contact and social withdrawal in patients from high EE homes (exact $P = 0.023$). Within the high EE group, two-thirds of those who were socially withdrawn or avoided family members in the months preceding key admission were well at follow-up, while 58 per cent of those who did *not* show signs of withdrawal later relapsed. This suggests a general coping style, and provides further support for the notion that the person suffering from schizophrenia does exercise some control over the course of his illness.

Practical Applications

Throughout this paper, the importance of relatives' EE for outcome, first recognised by Brown and his colleagues, has been re-emphasised. Yet it is clear that the negative effects of relatives' high EE can be modified by the two protective mechanisms, drugs and lowered face to face contact (figure 20.1). One of the many difficulties in attempts to treat persons for schizophrenia has been a lack of knowledge of what the goals of intervention should be. Our data suggest that if one could actually intervene so as to ensure that patients from high EE homes, identified as being at high risk, were maintained on drugs and saw their relatives as little as possible, the likelihood is that the relapse rate could be lowered toward that of patients from low EE homes.

The summary of factors relating to relapse makes it immediately apparent who would be the highest risk subjects in any prevention programme. In order to be minimally protected against relapse, an unmarried male living in a high EE home should both be taking drugs regularly *and* seeing his family as little as possible. For unmarried women and married men, the presence of just one extra protective factor might be sufficient, while married women might conceivably remain well even if off drugs and in high contact with relatives.

The first step in any intervention programme would be the identification of families in which schizophrenic patients are at a high risk of relapse. Although the Brown–Rutter family interview has until now only been used as a research tool, it is possible that a streamlined version, such as the one developed by Vaughn and Leff (1976), could be adapted for use as a practical clinical instrument; but the importance of a standardised instrument, administered by a properly trained interviewer, cannot be too strongly emphasised.

Clearly it would also be an advantage to be able to identify patients at high risk in terms of some psycho-physiological measures of stress. 'Arousal' levels have been shown to be surprisingly high in chronic schizophrenics (Venables, 1960). It might be possible to pick up abnormalities of psycho-physiological response in patients and in this way identify those most sensitive to their social environment.

Once high risk patients have been identified, there are a number of possibilities for active intervention. Maintenance therapy is perhaps the single most important protective factor for patients in high EE homes. But with the patients at greatest risk, for example unmarried males, relapse will not be prevented with drugs alone. It is necessary to find ways of reducing face to face contact between the patient and his high EE relative. Various strategies for social intervention of this kind are set out in figure 20.2. The obvious solution for persons in parental households, removal to a hostel or other sheltered accommodation, is not always practicable. An alternative strategy would be to get the patient out to work or to a Day Centre, which would give the patient a measure of independence and cut down on the hours patient and family spend together. If the patient is an unemployable male living with his wife, it could be advantageous to get his wife to take a job.

Ultimately, however, these 'administrative' solutions are unlikely to be effective without the co-operation of the patient and his relatives. The subgroups in figure 20.1 are not randomly allocated, but self-selected. There

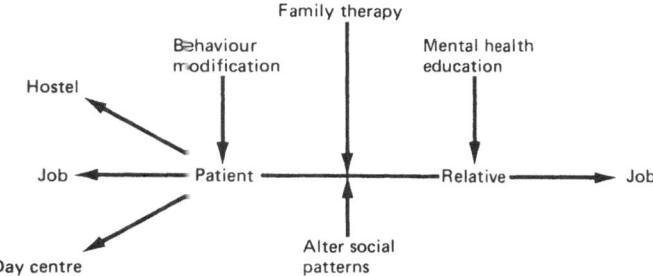

Figure 20.2   Strategies of social intervention

may be features of a relationship which bind family members together despite considerable tension and strain. In such cases, family members are likely to resist outsiders' attempts to prise them apart, however tactful the efforts may be; this is especially true of families in which the relative is emotionally over-involved. Unless these potential difficulties are recognised and dealt with early on in an intervention programme it may be doomed to failure.

This brings us to yet another kind of intervention; efforts to change the attitudes of over-involved or highly critical relatives.

For example, in considering how to deal with a highly critical relative, it would be useful to examine systematically the relative's complaints—to carry out, in effect, a content analysis of his responses. Are his remarks directed at long-standing personality traits of the patient, or are they primarily about illness-related behaviours?

In fact the bulk of criticism is directed, not at the florid symptoms such as delusions and hallucinations, but at the negative features of schizophrenia, such as apathy, lack of communication, and lack of emotional expression. These features were not recognised by the relatives as being part of an illness, but were seen rather as undesirable attributes of the person. Consequently the patients were described as lazy, awkward, stubborn, or difficult. It seems likely that if the relative can be induced to see these negative symptoms as part and parcel of schizophrenia and hence not under the patient's control, a reduction in criticism might follow. This is a strong argument for including a mental health education programme among possible strategies.

Family therapy could also be employed with the relatives, possibly including the patient as well, in an attempt to alter emotional reactions, but currently we have no idea as to the effectiveness of this form of treatment.

Fifteen years have passed since Brown and his colleagues first began to explore the complex relationships between the schizophrenic and his social environment. Present knowledge about the factors influencing outcome is such that we can at least begin to plan effective programmes for the prevention of relapse of schizophrenia. Possibly the new techniques in behaviour therapy may provide tools for intervening in a rational way. However daunting the prospect, there may never be a better time.

References

Brown, G. W., Birley, J. L. T. and Wing, J. K. (1972). Influence of family life on the course of schizophrenic disorders: a replication. *Br. J. Psychiat.*, **121**, 241–58

Brown, G. W. and Rutter, M. (1966). The measurement of family activities and relationships: a methodological study. *Hum. Relat.*, **19**, 241–63

Rutter, M. and Brown, G. W. (1966). The reliability and validity of measures of family life and relationships in families containing a psychiatric patient. *Soc. Psychiat.*, **1**, 38–53

Vaughn, C. E. and Leff, J. P. (1976). The measurement of expressed emotion in the families of psychiatric patients. *Br. J. Social Clin. Psychol.*, **15**, 157–165

Venables, P. H. (1960). The effect of auditory and visual stimulation on the potential response of schizophrenics. *Brain*, **83**, 77–92

Wing, J. K., Cooper, J. E. and Sartorius, N. (1974). *The Description and Classification of Psychiatric Symptoms: An Introduction Manual for the PSE and Catego System.* Cambridge University Press, London

21 Psychopharmacology of Manic-depressive Illness

Trevor Silverstone

The neurochemical and psychopharmacological hypotheses which have thus far been most frequently put forward to explain the pathogenesis of manic-depressive disorders have emphasised the possible role which noradrenaline (NA) and 5-hydroxytryptamine (5-HT) may play (Schildkraut, 1973). It is only recently that another neurotransmitter, dopamine (DA), has been seriously considered as being implicated in this condition.

There are at least three dopaminergic pathways within the central nervous system: the *nigrostriatal*, running from the substantia nigra to the corpus striatum; the *mesolimbic* going from the mid-brain to the limbic system; the *infundibulo-hypophyseal* passing from the hypothalamus to the pituitary gland (see figure 21.1). The nigrostriatal dopamine pathway is thought to be

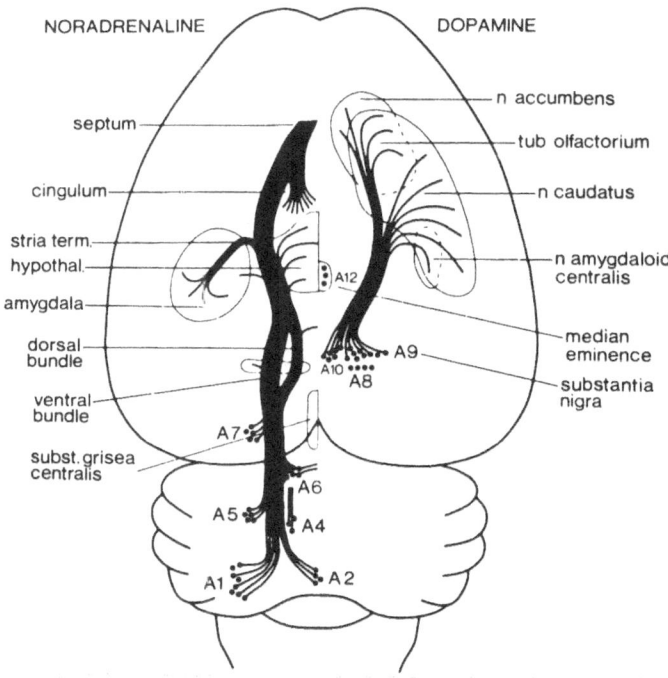

Figure 21.1   Horizontal projection of the ascending NA and DA pathway

mainly concerned with motor co-ordination, while the infundibulo-hypophyseal pathway is generally considered to be of particular relevance to neuroendocrine relationships, especially prolactin secretion. It is the mesolimbic dopamine pathway which is most likely to be involved in any mood regulating properties which dopamine may have, as the limbic system forms a major part of the so-called 'emotional circuit' originally described by Papez (1937).

There are a number of pharmacological compounds which, on the basis of animal experimentation are thought to influence DA pathways within the brain (see figure 21.2). Some of these drugs enhance dopaminergic activity (enhancers) while others diminish it (inhibitors). The enhancers are believed to act in one or more of the following ways: (1) by increasing the available amount of dopamine precursor—levodopa (Butcher and Engel, 1969); (2) by promoting the release of DA from presynaptic DA neurons—amphetamine (Am) (Carlsson, 1970); (3) by direct stimulation of postsynaptic DA receptors—piribedil (PBD) (Corrodi et al., 1972), bromocriptine (BMC) (Corrodi et al., 1973). The inhibitors probably act as follows: (1) by reducing the synthesis of DA through inhibition of the enzyme tyrosine hydroxylase—α-methyl-p-tyrosine (AMPT) (Spector et al., 1965); (2) by blocking postsynaptic DA receptors—neuroleptics such as pimozide (PMZ) and haloperidol (HP) (Anden et al., 1970); (3) by inhibiting receptor adenylate cyclase, and thereby reducing the transformation of adenosine triphosphate (ATP) to cyclic adenosine monophosphate (cyclic AMP)—lithium (Geisler and Klysner, 1977).

Provided always that we bear two points in mind: first, that the drugs we use are unlikely to be specific in their action on DA pathways, and second that activation or suppression of neurochemical activity in the DA system is going to affect other neurochemical pathways, I believe we can gain valuable information concerning the pathogenesis of mania and severe bipolar depression by observing in man the effect of drugs having a putative action on DA mechanisms in the brain. If the symptoms of mania and amphetamine-induced euphoria are due to increased DA activity, then they should be reduced by the inhibitor group of compounds. Conversely the depressive phase of manic depressive psychosis (bipolar depression) should be improved by the enhancer group. Furthermore, it could be expected that the DA enhancer drugs might themselves produce states resembling mania in those predisposed to the condition, while the inhibitor group might precipitate depressive symptoms.

Amphetamine-induced Euphoria and Arousal

Amphetamine (Am) has long been known to produce arousal and euphoria in normal subjects (Lasagna et al., 1955). In fact it was this property, together with its anorectic action, which originally made it so appealing as a slimming drug (Lesses and Myerson, 1938), and which later led to its becoming a popular drug of abuse. In addition amphetamine can lead to changes in objective measures of central arousal such as critical flicker fusion (Turner, 1971).

In animals amphetamine has been shown to promote release of newly synthesised DA and noradrenaline (NA) from presynaptic neurons (Carlsson, 1970) and to block their re-uptake, resulting in an increase of available neurotransmitter at the post synaptic receptors. It has been shown that the increase in locomotion produced by amphetamine in rats is due at least in part to release of DA in the nucleus accumbens (Kelly *et al.*, 1975). In man the subjective changes produced by amphetamine are attenuated by drugs of the DA inhibitor group.

1. α-Methyl-*p*-tyrosine (AMPT)

AMPT blocks the formation of DA and NA from tyrosine by inhibiting tyrosine hydroxylase (see figure 21.2). Behaviourally it has been found to reduce the central excitatory effects of amphetamine in experimental animals. In man AMPT administered in three successive doses of 1.5, 1.5 and 3 g at 12-hourly intervals, virtually abolished the euphoriant and stimulating effects of 160 mg amphetamine injected intravenously 2 hours after the last dose of AMPT (Jonsson *et al.*, 1969). Subsequent investigations revealed that the blocking effect of AMPT on amphetamine arousal and euphoria were less after one week's continuous medication with AMPT, although blocking the autonomic effects of Am persisted (Jonsson *et al.*, 1971). On the basis of these findings it was suggested that the euphoriant effects of Am were mediated by an AMPT-sensitive pool of catecholamines in the brain. It is of interest in this connection that the euphoriant effects of ethanol are also reduced by AMPT (Ahlenius *et al.*, 1973).

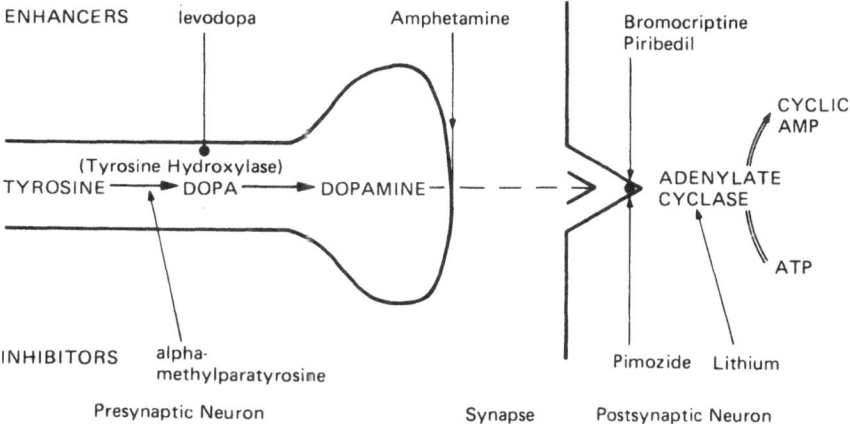

Figure 21.2

2. Neuroleptics

Carlsson and Lindqvist (1963) were the first to suggest that the neuroleptic drugs acted by blocking DA receptors. Subsequently Anden *et al.* (1970) demonstrated that of the neuroleptics PMZ was more specific in blocking monoamine receptors than most of the others which also blocked NA receptors to some extent. It is therefore significant in terms of dopaminergic mechanisms, that 5–20 mg PMZ was found to reduce amphetamine-induced euphoria in previously dependent subjects given 200 mg Am intravenously (Jonsson, 1972). In contrast, compounds which block noradrenergic receptors, either β receptors (propranolol) or α receptors (phenoxybenzamine), were without effect on amphetamine euphoria.

We have found that PMZ given as a 2 mg oral dose 2 hours before 10 mg *d*-amphetamine, also given orally, to eight female subjects, reduced their subjective experience of arousal which they had felt following Am alone; it is noteworthy that PMZ failed to attenuate the anorectic effect of Am. These results would suggest that Am-induced arousal and euphoria is DA-mediated, whereas the anorectic action of Am is not (Silverstone *et al.* in press).

3. Lithium

Among its many actions lithium (Li) prevents the enzymatic transformation of ATP to cyclic AMP by inhibiting adenylate cyclase (Geisler and Klysner, 1977). The post synaptic DA receptor is thought to be closely related to, if not identical with, adenylate cyclase (Iversen *et al.*, 1975) and DA may act by stimulating its receptor adenylate cyclase. Li should produce effects similar to blockade of the receptor itself. It is therefore of interest that Van Kammen and Murphy (1975) reported that Li, in depressed patients, attenuated the euphoriant effect produced by 30 mg *d*-Am. Similarly Flemenbaum (1974) described three subjects, taking Li for affective disorders, who noted that Am, which they had previously taken for its euphoriant and alerting effects, was no longer giving them the 'lift' they were used to.

In conclusion it would appear that the amphetamine-induced arousal and euphoria in man is blocked by drugs which are thought to act by inhibiting the dopaminergic system.

Mania

Mania is characterised by over-activity, elevation of mood, pressure of speech, flight of ideas, grandiose ideas, decreased sleep and distractability. The presence of mood elevation, plus any three other of the above symptoms persisting for a period longer than two weeks has been considered to be diagnostic of mania (Feighner *et al.*, 1972).

Unfortunately there are no good animal models of mania for, as Murphy and Redmond (1975) have pointed out '. . . the limited number of animal behaviours subject to outside scrutiny, and the 200 million years of evolutionary separation . .' greatly restricts the usefulness of behavioural experiments in animals in the study of human affects and moods.

Therefore, in order to determine the effect of drugs in mania we must have recourse to actual manic patients. By examining the effects in such patients of drugs with known neurochemical actions (the knowledge of which is based almost entirely on animal experiments) we might arrive at a position where we could extrapolate from the clinical changes observed, to the presumed neurochemical pathways involved, and thereby draw tentative conclusions about possible mechanisms underlying pathogenesis. Limiting ourselves for the purpose of this presentation, to drugs acting on dopaminergic pathways, we can approach the problem in two ways; first by reviewing the actions of drugs inhibiting DA pathways (see figure 21.2) on relieving the characteristic symptoms of mania in patients with the condition; secondly, by seeing whether any of the DA enhancer drugs precipitate mania in patients who are predisposed to develop the illness. (The fact that certain of the latter group of drugs, such as levodopa, have failed to precipitate mania, or even euphoria, in normal subjects, should not deter us, for the underlying neurochemical homeostatic mechanisms in the brains of potential patients may differ from those of normal subjects.)

1. α-Methyl-p-tyrosine (AMPT)

Brodie et al. (1971) reported that a dose of 2–4 g AMPT administered in a gradually increasing regimen, led to clinically significant amelioration of symptoms in five of seven manic patients treated. However, the fact that three patients remained better after the AMPT was withdrawn led Mendels and Frazer (1974) to question whether the clinical improvement noted in these three patients was, in fact, related to the AMPT which had been administered; indeed they stated '. . . there is relatively little evidence that AMPT has a direct effect on mood in either normal or psychiatrically disturbed persons'.

Undeterred by this view, Sack and Goodwin (1974) went on to investigate in a further eight manic patients, the effect of fusaric acid, a drug which inhibits the enzymatic transformation of DA to NA by dopamine-β-hydroxylase. While the patients with mild symptoms did improve a little on fusaric acid, those patients with severe manic symptoms became much more disturbed. In conjunction with the exacerbation of manic symptomatology there was a pronounced rise in the level of homovanillic acid (HVA), the metabolite of DA, and a fall in 3-methoxy-4-hydroxyphenylglycol (MHPG), the metabolite of NA, in the cerebrospinal fluid, suggesting that brain DA levels had risen and brain NA levels had fallen as a result of treatment with fusaric acid. On the basis of these findings Sack and Goodwin concluded that the amelioration of mania was related more to a reduction in DA, than to any change in NA.

However, in contrast to the report by Brodie *et al.* (1971), Shopsin *et al.* (1976) failed to detect any antimanic activity of AMPT.

2. Neuroleptics

The neuroleptics have long been used in the treatment of mania, and haloperidol in particular has been recommended (Pare, 1968). All members of this class of drugs show a DA receptor blocking activity (Anden *et al.*, 1970). In man they cause a rise in the level of HVA in the CSF (van Praag and Korf, 1976), and in the serum levels of prolactin, a hormone generally believed to be under central dopaminergic control (Rubin *et al.*, 1976).

Of the neuroleptics, PMZ is one of the most specific in terms of DA receptor blockade (Anden *et al.*, 1970). We have compared the effect of PMZ to fenfluramine (FF), a 5-HT re-uptake inhibitor (Garattini and Samanin, 1976) in five patients with unequivocal mania (Cookson and Silverstone, 1976). Using a modification of the manic state rating scale devised by Beigel *et al.* (1971) we found the PMZ produced significant improvement in all the patients within three days over the whole range of symptoms rated. While FF also produced some improvement, it was limited to a reduction in motor activity; manic ideation seemed to be less affected. We have subsequently treated a substantial number of manic patients with PMZ, the great majority of whom responded well. Our experience with PMZ is in keeping with the single case report of Gerner *et al.* (1976); in their patient daily doses of up to 14 mg PMZ led to rapid improvement of the manic state according to ratings made on a scale similar to the one we used.

The findings in these two clinical studies are consistent with the view that over-activity within DA pathways in the brain plays a part in the psychopathology of mania.

3. Lithium

Following the initial reports by Cade (1949) and Schou *et al.* (1954) there have been a great many publications attesting to the efficacy of Li in the treatment of mania, although the onset of its antimanic action would appear to be slower than that of the neuroleptics (see Johnson, 1975, for reviews). As I have already indicated, one of the many pharmacological actions of Li is the inhibition of adenylate cyclase, an enzyme closely associated with the DA receptors. It is not inconceivable, therefore, that the antimanic action of this drug is due to interference with DA transmission in the CNS.

All the clinical studies reviewed (apart from the unpublished report of Shopsin and Gershon) are consistent with the view that DA mechanisms are involved in mania. This, of course, does not preclude other neurochemical pathways being involved, especially a serotonergic one. The fact that fenfluramine, a drug which acts as a serotonergic agonist, can alleviate some of the symptoms of mania (Cookson and Silverstone, 1976) is consistent with the view that activity of serotonergic mechanisms may be reduced in this condition (Prange *et al.*, 1974). Further support for this view comes from a recent report that cyproheptadine, a serotonergic blocking drug, can precipitate mania (Pearce *et al.*, 1977).

Bipolar Depression

Bipolar depression is the name given to that form of depressive illness which occurs in the course of a recurrent cyclic affective disorder with both manic and depressive phases. Genetically, bipolar depression would appear to be distinguishable in terms of family history from other depressive states (Winokur *et al.*, 1969; Allen, 1976); furthermore, Shapiro *et al.* (1976) have recently reported that patients presenting with bipolar depression are much more likely than patients with unipolar depression to possess particular specific histocompatability antigens, particularly HLA-BW16. There are also certain clinical features which distinguish patients with bipolar depression from those with the unipolar form; for example the onset of the illness tends to occur at an earlier age among bipolar patients. Follow-up from the time of initial diagnosis of depression infrequently leads to a change in diagnostic category; the chance of patients who had been diagnosed as having unipolar depression, later having the diagnosis changed to bipolar depression is less than 5 per cent (Dunner *et al.*, 1976).

1. Levodopa

The catecholamine precursor levodopa is thought to increase preferentially the amount of DA in the brain (Butcher and Engel, 1969) and the levels of both HVA and MHPG increase in the CSF of patients being treated with levodopa (Bunney *et al.*, 1972). Administration of levodopa under double-blind conditions to seven patients with bipolar depression resulted in the appearance of brief hypomanic episodes in six. In contrast, only one of the eleven patients with unipolar depression showed a similar response (Murphy *et al.*, 1971). There would thus appear to be a specific susceptibility to develop manic symptoms among patients with bipolar depression who have, by definition, a past history of manic episodes. Other studies have confirmed the lack of response to levodopa in unipolar depression, but none, so far as I know, has specifically examined the response in bipolar patients.

2. Amphetamines

In the single case of manic depressive illness already referred to (Gerner *et al.*, 1976), 15 mg *d*-amphetamine given in a single intravenous infusion during a bipolar depressive episode precipitated a florid attack of mania within 36 hours. The manic symptoms remitted spontaneously after 3 days and the patient reverted to his previous depressed state. A second intravenous infusion of d-Am, this time at a dose of 20 mg, produced a similar sequence of changes in the patient's clinical state. Although Gerner et al. reported that such a response to Am in a patient with bipolar depression was atypical in their experience, Van Kammen and Murphy (1975) observed a hypomanic response in two out of three bipolar depressed patients given 30 mg d-Am orally on two consecutive days, whereas none of the six unipolar patients given Am responded in this way.

3. Dopamine Receptor Agonists

Piribedil (previously known as ET-495) is a DA receptor agonist which acts directly on the receptor itself (Corrodi et al., 1972). Arbuthnott and Murray (1975), in order to test their hypothesis that mania was due to supersensitivity of DA receptors, administered piribedil to seven manic patients. They reasoned that any such supersensitivity might be reversed by chronic treatment with a receptor agonist. Increasing doses of piribidel, starting at 20 mg daily and rising to 240 mg over 3—6 weeks, helped 'one or two patients' but the rest failed to respond and required alternative treatment. The authors concluded that the drug had little to offer in the treatment of mania. Approaching the use of DA agonists in a rather different way, that is using them as DA enhancers in bipolar depression with a view to activating a possibly unresponsive DA system, Gerner et al. (1976) gave piribedil to a patient suffering from bipolar depression. This patient became manic after twelve days of treatment with piribedil.

Bromocriptine (BMC) is another direct-acting DA receptor agonist (Corrodi et al., 1973; Johnson et al., 1976). We have given BMC to ten depressed patients; these included three with bipolar depression and seven with unipolar depression. None of the patients with unipolar depression responded to BMC in doses up to 20 mg given daily for over 2 weeks. The three bipolar patients treated with BMC had all become depressed when taking PMZ for a recent manic episode. Stopping PMZ for two or three days did not result in any improvement. BMC in gradually increasing doses starting at 2.5 mg daily in one patient, 2.5 mg b.d. in the second, and 2.5 mg t.i.d. in the third was associated with definite, if temporary, improvement in all three within two to three weeks. Thus three patients with a manic-depressive diathesis, when given the DA receptor block drug PMZ during a manic episode, subsequently became depressed, and when the PMZ was stopped and BMC substituted, they became less depressed. To what degree administration of the DA receptor agonist BMC was a significant factor in the improvement noted, and how much was due to stopping PMZ, is uncertain.

Conclusions

All the psychopharmacological findings in bipolar depression which I have

Table 21.1
Drugs inhibiting CNS dopaminergic activity

	AMPT	Neuroleptics	Lithium
Pharmacological action	Inhibits synthesis of DA	Block DA receptors	Inhibits adenylate cyclase in DA receptors
Effect on amphetamine-induced euphoria and arousal	Reduced	Reduced	Attenuated
Effects in mania	Improved	Improved	Improved

Table 21.2
Drugs enhancing CNS dopaminergic activity

	Levodopa	Amphetamine	Piribedil and bromocriptine
Pharmacological action	DA precursor—increases synthesis	Promotes release and blocks re-uptake of DA	Direct DA receptor agonist
Effect in bipolar depressive illness	Leads to brief hypomanic episodes	Can precipitate manic symptoms	Precipitates mania, improves bipolar depression

discussed, when considered together, would appear to point to DA mechanisms playing an important part in the onset and course of this illness.

If mania, and amphetamine euphoria, were due to increased DA activity, then drugs, which in animals have been found to inhibit activity in DA pathways in the CNS, should ameliorate the symptoms of these conditions in man; this was in fact found to be the case. Furthermore if DA inhibitors were to ameliorate mania, they should also precipitate depressive illness in patients who were constitutionally predisposed to develop the illness; this too was found to be true. Conversely if, as was found, drugs, which in animals enhance DA activity, improved the clinical state of patients suffering from bipolar depression, and at times precipitate manic symptoms in predisposed individuals, this would further support the role of DA in manic-depressive psychosis. These ideas would appear to be supported by almost all of the evidence presented—tables 21.1 and 21.2. It might, therefore, be concluded that any hypothesis which purported to explain the pathogenesis of manic-depressive illness in neurochemical terms, must find some place for dopaminergic mechanisms within its framework.

It should, however, be remembered that the DA pathways in the CNS do not act in isolation; they interact with other neurochemical systems to produce their effects. Changes in one pathway cause changes in others, and it is highly probable that the symptomatology of mania and of depression is related to a number of neurochemical mechanisms. These might well include serotonergic systems as suggested by Mendels and Frazer (1975), and cholinergic systems as implied by the finding that manipulation of acetylcholine levels of the brain, using the centrally acting anticholinesterase drug physostigmine, can ameliorate some of the symptoms of mania (Janowsky et al., 1973). However, such findings do not rule out a role for DA, they only imply that other pathways may also be involved, possibly acting in concert with DA pathways (Randrup et al., 1975).

References

Ahlenius, S., Carlsson, A., Engel, J., Svensson, T. and Persodersten, K. (1973). Antagonism by alpha-methyltyrosine of ethanol-induced stimulation and euphoria in man. *Clin. Pharmac. Ther.*, **14**, 586–591

Allen, M. G. (1976). Twin studies of affective illness. *Archs gen. Psychiat.*, **33**, 1476–1478

Anden, N. E., Butcher, S. G., Corrodi, H., Fuxe, K. and Ungerstedt, U. (1970). Receptor activity and turnover of dopamine and noradrenaline after neuroleptics. *Eur. J. Pharmac.*, **11**, 303–314

Arbuthnott, G. W. and Murray, L. G. (1975). Dopamine receptor agonists in psychiatric disease. In *Advances in Neurology* Vol. 9 (Ed. D. B. Calne, T. N. Chase and A. Barbeau), Raven Press, New York

Beigel, A., Murphy, D. L. and Bunney, W. E. (1971). The manic state rating scale. *Archs gen. Psychiat.*, **25**, 256–262

Brodie, H. K., Murphy, D. L., Goodwin, F. K. and Bunney, W. E. (1971).

Catecholamines and mania—the affect of alpha-methylparatyrosine on manic behaviour and catecholamine metabolism. *Clin. Pharmac. Ther.*, **12**, 218–224

Bunney, W. E., Gershon, E., Murphy, D. and Goodwin, F. K. (1972). Psychological and pharmacology studies of manic depressive illness. *J. Psychiat. Res.*, **9**, 207–226

Butcher, L. L. and Engel, J. (1969). Behavioural and biochemical effects of L-dopa after peripheral decarboxylase inhibition. *Brain Res.*, **15**, 233–239

Cade, J. F. (1949). Lithium salts in the treatment of psychotic excitement. *Med. J. Aust.*, **36**, 349–352

Carlsson, A. (1970). Amphetamine and brain catecholamines. In *Amphetamine and Related Compounds* (Ed. E. Costa and S. Garattini), Raven Press, New York

Carlsson, A. and Lindqvist, M. (1963). Effect of chlorpromazine or haloperidol on formation of 3-methoxytyramine and normetanephrine in mouse brain. *Acta Pharmac. Tox.*, **20**, 140–144

Cookson, J. and Silverstone, T. (1976). 5-Hydroxytryptamine and dopamine pathways in mania; a pilot study of fenfluramine and pimozide. *Br. J. clin. Pharmac.*, **3**, 942–943

Corrodi, H., Farnebo. L., Fuxe, K., Hamberger, B. and Ungerstedt, U. (1972). ET-495 and brain catecholamine mechanisms: evidence for stimulation of dopamine receptors. *Eur. J. Pharmac.*, **20**, 195–204

Corrodi, H., Fuxe, K., Hokfelt, T., Lidbrink, P. and Ungerstedt, U. (1973). Effects of ergot drugs on central neurones: evidence for stimulation of central dopamine neurones. *J. Pharm. Pharmac.*, **25**, 409–410

Dunner, D. L., Fleiss, J. L. and Fieve, R. B. (1976). The course of development of mania in patients with recurrent depression. *Am. J. Psychiat.*, **133**, 905–908

Feighner, J. P., Robins, E. and Guze, S. B. (1972). Diagnostic criteria for use in psychiatric research. *Archs gen. Psychiat.*, **26**, 57–63

Flemenbaum, A. (1974). Does lithium block the effects of amphetamine? A report of three cases. *Am. J. Psychiat.*, **131**, 820–821

Garattini, S. and Samanin, R. (1976). Anorectic drugs and brain neurotransmitters. In *Appetite and Food Intake* (Ed. T. Silverstone), Dahlem Konferenzen, Berlin

Geisler, A. and Klysner, R. (1977). Combined effect of lithium and flupenthixol on striatal adenylate cyclase. *Lancet*, **i**, 430–431

Gerner, R. H., Post, R. M. and Bunney, W. E. (1976). A dopaminergic mechanism in mania. *Am. J. Psychiat.*, **133**, 1177–1180

Iversen, L. L., Horn, A. and Miller, R. (1975). Actions of dopaminergic agonists on cyclic AMP production in rat brain homogenates. In *Advances in Neurology*, Vol. 9 (Ed. D. B. Calne. T. N. Chase, A. Barbeau), Raven Press, New York

Janowsky, D. S., El-Yousef, F. and Davis, J. M. (1973). Para-sympathetic suppression of manic symptoms by physostigmine. *Archs gen. Psychiat.*, **28**, 542–547

Johnson, A. M., Loew, D. M. and Vigouret, J. M. (1976). Stimulant properties of bromocriptine on central dopamine receptors in comparison to apomorphine (+)-amphetamine and L-dopa. *Br. J. Pharmac.*, **56**, 59–68

Johnson, F. N. (1975). *Lithium Research and Therapy*. Academic Press, London

Jonsson, L. E. (1972). Pharmacological blockade of amphetamine effects in amphetamine dependent subjects. *Eur. J. Clin. Pharmac.*, **4**, 206–211

Jonsson, L. E., Anggard, E. and Gunne, L. M. (1971). Blockade of intravenous amphetamine euphoria in man. *Clin. Pharmac. Ther.*, **12**, 889–896

Jonsson, L. E., Gunne, L. M. and Anggard, E. (1969). Effects of alpha-methyltyrosine in amphetamine dependent subjects. *Pharmac. Clin.*, **2**, 27–29

Kelly, P. H., Seviour, P. W. and Iversen, S. D. (1975). Amphetamine and apomorphine responses in the rat following 6 OHDA lesions of nucleus accumbens septi and corpus striatum. *Brain Res.*, **94**, 507–522

Lasagna, L., Von Felsinger, J. M. and Beecher, H. K. (1955). Drug induced mood changes in man. *J. Am. Med. Ass.*, **157**, 1006–1015

Lesses, M. F. and Myerson, A. (1938). Benzedrine sulphate as an aid to the treatment of obesity. *New Engl. J. Med.*, **218**, 119–124

Mendels, J. and Frazer, A. (1974). Brain biogenic amines and mood. *Archs gen. Psychiat.*, **30**, 447–451

Mendels, J. and Frazer, A. (1975). Reduced serotinergic activity in mania. *Br. J. Psychiat.*, **126**, 241–248

Murphy, D. L., Brodie, H. K. H., Goodwin, F. K. and Bunney, W. E. (1971). L-dopa: regular induction of hypomania in 'bipolar' manic depressive patients. *Nature*, **229**, 135–136

Murphy, D. L. and Redmond, D. E. (1975). The catecholamines: possible role in affect, mood and emotional behaviour in man and animals. In *Catecholamines and Behaviour* (Ed. A. Friedhoff), Plenum Press, New York

Papez, J. W. (1937). A proposed mechanism of emotion. *Archs Neurol. Psychiat.*, **38**, 725

Pare, C. M. B. (1968). The treatment of mania and hypomania. *Prescribers J.*, **8**, 113–116

Pearce, C. J., Isaacs, A. J. and Gomez, J. (1977). Treatment of Cushing's disease with cyproheptadine. *Lancet*, **i**, 1368–1369

Prange, A. J., Wilson I. C., Lynn, C. W., Alltop, L. B. and Stikeleather, R. A. (1974). L-tryptophan in mania. *Archs gen. Psychiat.*, **30**, 56–62

Randrup, A., Munkvad, I., Fog, R., Gerlach, J., Molander, L., Kjellborg, B. and Scheel-Kruger, J. (1975). Mania, depression and brain dopamine. *Curr. Dev. Psychopharmac.*, **2**, 207–247

Rubin, R. T., Poland, R. E., O'Connor, D., Govin, P. R. and Tower, B. B. (1976). Selective neuroendocrine effects of low dose haloperidol in normal adult men. *Psychopharmacology*, **47**, 135–140

Sack, R. L. and Goodwin, F. K. (1974). Inhibition of dopamine-β-hydroxylase in manic patients. *Archs gen. Psychiat.*, **31**, 649–654

Schildkraut, J. J. (1973). Neuropharmacology of the affective disorders. *A. Rev. Pharmac.*, **15**, 427–454

Schou, M., Juel-Nielson, N., Stromgren, E. and Voldby, H. (1954). The treatment of manic psychosis by the administration of lithium salts. *J. Neurol. Neurosurg. Psychiat.*, **17**, 250–260

Shapiro, R. W., Bock, E., Rafaelson, O., Ryder, L. P. and Svejgaard, A. (1976). Histocompatability antigens and manic depressive disorders. *Archs gen. Psychiat.*, **33**, 823–825

Shopsin, B., Gershon, S. and Selzer, G. (1976). Neuropsychopharmacology of mania. In *Drug Treatment of Mental Disorders* (Ed. L. Simpson), Raven Press, New York

Spector, S., Sjoerdsma, A. and Undenfriend, S. (1965). Blockade of endogenous norepinephorine synthesis by alpha-methyl-tyrosine, an inhibitor of tyrosine hydroxylase. *J. Pharmac. Exp. Ther.*, **147**, 86–95

Turner, P. (1971). Drugs and the special senses. *Seminars in Drug Treatment*, **4**, 335–352

Van Kammen, D. P. and Murphy, D. L. (1975). Attentuation of the euphoriant and activating effects of d- and l-amphetamine by lithium carbonate treatment. *Psychopharmacologia*, **44**, 215–224

Van Praag, H. M. and Korf, J. (1976). Importance of dopamine metabolism for clinical effects and side effects of neuroleptics. *Am. J. Psychiat.*, **133**, 1171–1177

Weiss, B. and Laties, V. G. (1962). Enhancement of human performance by caffeine and the amphetamines. *Pharmac. Rev.*, **14**, 1–36

Winokur, G., Clayton, P. J. and Reich, T. (1969). *Manic-depressive Illness*. C. V. Mosby, St. Louis

22 The Current State of Senile Dementia

Brice Pitt

The main concern of all who work with the elderly at the beginning of the last quarter of the twentieth century must be the prevalence of *dementia*.

Kay *et al.* (1964) showed that 10 per cent of those old people they surveyed in Newcastle upon Tyne were confused because of senile or atherosclerotic dementia, and that in half of these the condition was moderate or severe. Other prevalence studies give rates ranging from 4 per cent (Hobson and Pemberton, 1955) to 24 per cent (Williamson *et al.*, 1964). Bergmann (1977) points out that Newcastle studies have shown that the disease is 8 – 9 times as common in those over 75 as in those between 65 and 75. In the United Kingdom it is expected that by the end of the century the proportion of those in the population aged over 75 will have increased by one-third.

Only one-fifth of those confused old people in the Kay *et al.* study were in any kind of institutional care—general, geriatric or psychiatric hospital, or residential home for the elderly. Yet already most of these institutions feel over-burdened by the care of their demented elderly. In general hospitals beds are blocked by confused old people, admitted either because of their confusion or for some other reason, who, after appropriate medical or surgical treatment remain too confused to go home. Bergmann (1972) reports that 23 per cent of those over 65 admitted to an acute medical ward were confused, and only 59 per cent were mentally normal! In geriatric hospitals there is concern over restless, ambulant old people whose only serious disorder is dementia, ill-suited to an environment where most of the population are physically infirm. The proportion of patients over 65 in psychiatric hospitals has increased remarkably in the past 30 years, from less than a quarter to more than half, with a still higher figure for females. Perhaps half of these are chronic schizophrenics who have been in hospital for many years, but are becoming ever more infirm with ageing. The others, however, were admitted over the age of 65 with severe dementia. Their life expectancy is less than that of people of the same age without dementia (Roth, 1955), but improvements in the quality of care over the past 20 years may have increased it somewhat.

These very disabled and difficult patients who, with even the best care, inevitably deteriorate, daunt and oppress many of those doctors, nurses and other staff, who came into psychiatry expecting a more rewarding and less taxing clientele. The D.H.S.S. document 'Services for the Elderly Mentally Ill' (HM 72/71), having emphasised the importance of community support, predicted that the majority of the demented who require institutional care would be accommodated in residential homes for the elderly. However, the capacity of such homes to cope with a substantial number of confused residents may well have been over-estimated. These homes are frequently understaffed and also lacking in trained personnel. They are less able to deal with problems presented by muddled, irrational old people and the reactions of other residents than are hospital nurses. Those who become demented while resident in the Home are generally well tolerated, but the attitude to those confused at the time of referral to the Home is wary if not hostile; the confusion may be both exaggerated and exacerbated in consequence.

The main agency sustaining the demented elderly in the community is the family. Some families cope resourcefully and equably but others are sorely stressed. Sheldon, in 1947, found that almost 15 per cent of the old people in his survey were causing strain on those who looked after them, and in about half of these the strain was severe and almost intolerable. Grad and Sainsbury (1968) found that the burden of caring for 40 per cent of the elderly patients referred to psychiatric services was severe. Even when community care was good the burden remained heavy. The quality of community services available to the demented elderly at home and to their families varies considerably between districts and even within the same district. Especially since the Seebohm reorganisation, local authority generic social workers cannot be counted on to be informed or interested. The provision of day care, Home Helps, Meals-on-wheels, home bathing, luncheon clubs and incontinent laundry services varies, as does the awareness of old people and their families that such help may be available.

If a point is reached where through self-neglect, the loss of a key supporter (by bereavement or illness) or the family's understandable unwillingness to continue their care, admission to Home or Hospital is sought, it is rarely immediately forthcoming. There may be reluctance to take yet another demented old person into an over-burdened service, or a place may simply not be available. Intolerance of the situation in the community then rapidly intensifies, and anger, threats and desperation ensue. The cuts in public spending in the United Kingdom, forced by the state of the economy, affect the Health and Social Services for the elderly mentally infirm, even though the 'Priorities Document' (D.H.S.S., 1976) asks that the mentally ill and the elderly be given a bigger share of resources. The redistribution of finances evenly through the Regions is in fact impairing the provision in some previously 'privileged' areas where the facilities for the elderly and mentally ill were by no means as well endowed as the acute specialties.

This means that in many parts of the country (as no doubt in many other countries) the elderly demented are cared for under protest, or they and their families are simply not having their needs met in the community.

It is fortunate therefore that the M.R.C. have recently recognised the importance of research into dementia (Lishman, 1977), despite the evident difficulties, and have indicated ways in which this should be pursued. In the middle sections I shall discuss the present state of knowledge about dementia in the light of their suggestions, while the last section will deal with management, treatment and the best organisation of resources.

Diagnosis

For research and for treatment it is essential that the diagnosis of dementia should be correct, and that reversible causes of confusion should be recognised.

The *acute and sub-acute confusional states* (deliria) are readily identified if there is a reliable *history* of recent onset, but when there is no informant other than the patient, or when an acute episode of confusion occurs in the course of dementia, the diagnosis is less evident. The examination of the patient is then of the first importance. The Mental State Examination is of most value if the patient can be observed over the course of a day, when fluctuations in clouding of consciousness, predominently visual illusions and hallucinations, agitation and paranoia increasing towards nightfall, may be apparent. There may be physical signs of an underlying illness, such as pneumonia, stroke, heart failure, myocardial infarction, hypothermia or faecal impaction (and if the patient is seen at home the possibility of an iatrogenic cause may be suggested by the presence of various bottles of tablets). But often physical signs alone will not give the answer and radiological and laboratory investigations are required.

Respiratory and urinary tract infections, anaemia, uraemia, electrolyte disturbance, and disorders of liver function, are likely to be revealed by routine tests. Skull X-ray, blood sugar, blood gases, folate, B_{12} and other vitamin levels, serology and thyroid function tests are readily obtained. Beyond this an EEG and brain scan (which though somewhat costly do not hurt the patient) are indicated; say to help exclude a space-occupying lesion in the following: patients under 70; with confusion of unusually short duration for dementia though long for delirium; with an intermittent or atypical course; or with neurological signs. Air encephalography, ventriculography, or even lumbar puncture, all of which are potentially dangerous and can make the patient's mental condition slightly worse, are probably only indicated where there is the strong possiblity of a space-occupying lesion. Low pressure (communicating) hydrocephalus, which presents with ataxia, confusion and incontinence in patients usually with a past history of subarachnoid haemorrhage, or meningitis, may be remediable by a shunt operation. However, it is unlikely to be diagnosed without air encephalography, and it is highly questionable whether the (fair) chance that this diagnosis is overlooked in a number of older patients justifies the routine use of such an investigation. Incidentally, partial forms occur and shunt operations even without evidence of hydrocephalus have been performed in the United States with alleged benefit.

As Computerised Axial Tomography (E.M.I. Scan) becomes more generally available it may prove a valuable diagnostic instrument. Roberts and Caird

(1976) have shown good correlation between the maximum ventricular area on the E.M.I. Scan and measurements from pneumoencephalograms. In addition they have obtained statistically significant relations between the maximum ventricular area, scores on a memory and information test, and the Crichton Geriatric Behaviour Rating Scale in normal old people and groups with mild, moderate, and severe mental impairment. As more data become available it may be that disparity between intellectual impairment and ventricular size will also be of diagnostic importance, a large ventricle with slight impairment suggesting low pressure hydrocephalus, the reverse suggesting metabolic or psychogenic factors in impairment. However, so far observations on widening of cortical sulci have proved less valuable.

Functional Mental Illness as a cause of confusion or apparent confusion, especially *depressive pseudo-dementia*, can only be excluded by history, mental state examination or therapeutic trial. A past history of depression (and/or family history) and a story of depressive symptoms preceding confusion, the patient's bleak manner and a tendency to ignore questions rather than confabulate suggest the diagnosis, which will then be confirmed by an appropriate response to antidepressive therapy.

It is clear that dementia is not one disease. The distinction between the *parenchymatous* (senile) and *arteriopathic* forms, generally possible on clinical grounds, is largely confirmed at autopsy (Corsellis, 1962). In parenchymatous dementia there is usually an unremitting course, personality, intellect and memory being eroded to much the same extent throughout, and neurological signs are rare. The brain is generally shrunken with widened sulci, and histologically, senile plaques and neurofibrillary tangles are scattered throughout the cortex. Arteriopathic dementia runs a more intermittent course with greater disparity between impairment of memory and intellect and personality, greater fluctuations from day to day and during the day and various neurological signs as well as hypertension. The brain shows many areas of infarction.

The majority of old people die without showing signs of dementia, the relationship between which and the absent-mindedness of normal ageing or *Benign Senescent Forgetfulness* (Kral, 1962) is unclear. It is said that in the latter the old person remembers what she needs to remember for day to day living, though her general knowledge can be poor. However, follow up after a year suggests that by then a substantial proportion of the benignly forgetful have become demented. So 'BSF' may sometimes be the beginning of dementia. The distinction between *Alzheimer's pre-senile dementia* and the parenchymatous dementia of the senium is unclear. Pathologically the conditions appear identical, and some clinical differences may simply be due to their occurrence in different age groups, while the parietal lobe deficiencies, focal neurological signs and convulsions most often described in the pre-senile dementia also sometimes (though not typically) occur in the senile. However, genetic studies (see later) do not support the view that Alzheimer's disease and senile dementia are one and the same.

There is now considerable interest in *sub-cortical dementia*, in which the picture of dementia develops without changes in the cerebral cortex. Steele Richardson syndrome in which there is progressive Parkinsonism, rigidity of the trunk, abnormal eye movements and dementia, is a good example, but very rare. There is a failure of the reticular activating mechanism, and the possibility of a biochemical remedy. Dementia associated with some cases of Parkinson's disease may be sub-cortical. It is unlikely that senile dementia is a homogeneous disorder. As Bergmann (1977) states, it is tempting to speculate that as many antecedents will be discovered for the small shrunken brain as are now known to exist for the kidney disease once subsumed under the broad label of Bright's disease.

Those without parietal signs, or whose cortical abnormalities are less than would have been expected from their mental impairment during life, may have a form of sub-cortical dementia. Those who die soon, or late, may be distinct, as may those in whom the dementia appears eventually to arrest.

Clearly research will be handicapped if the final picture of dementia obscures the distinction between different disease processes which have reached the same result. Therefore early identification of subjects is essential.

To this end a community sample is required, as patients are unlikely to present until dementia is well established. As only 10 per cent of a random sample of elderly subjects are likely to develop the disorder, a large number is required to provide sufficient data for detailed longitudinal study. This might be obtained by studying subjects already in a community cohort study, such as the D.H.S.S. Nutrition Survey, or social surveys. Thus predisposing factors and precipitants might be identified, and patterns of evolution followed from the outset by clinical, psychological and laboratory investigations. In this way, it may be possible to ascertain the relevance of pre-morbid personality, such crises as bereavement, physical injury or illness, the significance of transitory confusion related to physical disorder, and the importance of living conditions including social stimulation and diet. It is not impossible that impairment of brain cell function, detected at a very early stage, may prove reversible.

Psychological Tests. The tests of cognition and rating scales now available are of limited diagnostic value, and are rather crude and unreliable measures of change. Frequently when the psychiatrist is unsure whether the patient shows organic impairment, so is the psychologist. However, the distinction between true and pseudo-dementia can be made by testing (Cowan *et al.*, 1975)—the WAIS (vocabulary only), Inglis Paired Associates Learning Test, Digit Copying Test, Bender Gestalt Test and Delayed Recall all having been found of value. Patients with established dementia are hard to test by such methods as the WAIS because their attention and co-operation are difficult to secure. Indeed, the whole test situation may be beyond their comprehension. Orientation tests, though of practical clinical value, are insensitive research instruments for recording change. Almost every new piece of research in the field throws up a new rating scale, indicating the dissatisfaction with those already available. Tests are needed which are reliable, valid, sensitive, acceptable to patients and repeatable without practice effects. It would be invaluable to have tests which would not only distinguish functional from organic impairment, but indicate the likely duration of any confusion since the history is in this respect so often faulty. The most relevant aspects of cognition may be speed and flexibility in processing information. These may be measured by relatively simple tests, such as pressing buttons in response to visual stimuli on automated testing apparatus. More needs to be known about the relationship between psychological defects and particular brain lesions, and also their site and speed of development. Studies of brain injury and animal experiments are helpful here.

Genetics

Genetic factors contribute to longevity, to adaptability in old age, and to some specific disturbances in the senium. While polygenes account for the first two, a single major mutant gene might bring about the last.

According to immunological theory, ageing is an autoimmune process devastating the cell population, and ending in the organism's self-destruction. Mutations interfere with the cell's capacity for self-recognition and an autoimmune response results.

The study of dementia is difficult because an accurate family history may not be obtained for a disease developing late in life, and autopsy material is rarely available to confirm the diagnosis. Despite this Larsson *et al.* (1963) found the morbidity risk for the parents and siblings of patients with senile dementia to be more than four times higher than that for the general population. Kallman (1956) found concordance rates for dementia of 43 per cent in MZ twins and 8 per cent in DZ. Only about 15 per cent of sufferers from Alzheimer's disease have a family history of the disorder, and Constantinidis *et al.* (1962) did not find an increased morbidity for this disorder in the families of patients with senile dementia. While Larsson suggests an incomplete dominance for the heredity of senile dementia, Kallmann and others argue for heterogeneity. It seems that an hereditary factor exists though it cannot be clearly recognised as yet.

Is there a continuous range of variation from normal old age through senile dementia to the pre-senile dementias? Is there a connection between any two of them? Or are they all different? Senile dementia is not the ultimate effect of physiological ageing. Sjogren (1956) found that mild dementia was not more common in the families of those with severe dementia. Family histories, geographical distribution and empirical morbidity rates do not support an identical aetiology for senile dementia and Alzheimer's disease (Zerbin-Ruedin, 1976). On the other hand the neuropathological differences between Alzheimer's disease and senile dementia seem, at present, only quantitative and topographical and between senile dementia and normal ageing again quantitative rather than qualitative.

Probably the best starting point for the quest for detailed family histories of the demented is from defined pathological material *post mortem*.

Pathology

Corsellis (1977) states that the evidence for depletion of *cortical neurons* is less certain than had been supposed. The multi-layering of cells in the cortex makes cell counts by eye over a large enough area and in a large enough number of cases excessively tedious and difficult. Image-analysing computers are able to size and count discrete objects in the microscopic field while allowing for the changes, such as shrinkage, in the volume of grey and white matter in the cortex. Such measures should determine whether any loss of neurons is global or in particular parts of the brain (for example loss of Purkinje cells with ageing has been demonstrated). Counts of *synapses*, small *blood vessels* and of *neuroglia* are also needed.

Corsellis has shown that, by and large, atherosclerotic and senile dementias are distinguishable *post mortem*. The changes—macroscopic such as flattening of gyri, widening of sulci, dilation of ventricles and shrinkage of the whole brain, and microscopic, particularly the presence of (Alzheimer's) neurofibrillary tangles, and senile plaques—correlate fairly well with the clinical condition before death (Corsellis, 1962). Blessed *et al.* (1968) found high plaque counts in the cortices of demented patients and a close correlation between the number of plaques and the morbid score on a clinical rating scale. Similar observations have been made on the incidence of granulovascular degeneration (Tomlinson and Kitchener, 1972) and of neurofibrillary tangles.

Electron microscopy has shown that the basis of the *neurofibrillary tangle* is a pair of helically wound filaments (PHF) replacing the normal straight neurotubules, and in which a new protein has been revealed. Although aluminium cream has induced a picture resembling neurofibrillary tangles under light microscopy, electron microscopy reveals that it is not the same. Terry and Wiesniwski (1970) have suggested that the tangle is a manifestation of altered tubular protein causing normal axoplasmic flow to be reduced and a form of 'dying back' to result. The axon and dendrites thus degenerate to form the senile plaque, in which amyloid deposition is a secondary phenomenon.

Senile plaques are thus aggregates of degenerating neuronal processes round an amyloid core. The processes are often still in contact with their parent cells, and their degeneration could represent an immune response to the new protein of the neurofibrillary tangle, or there could be a disturbance of axoplasmic transport. Plaques fill the space between capillaries, and it has been suggested that they could represent a response to some toxin derived from the blood.

Plaques can be induced experimentally in the cortex by undercutting the cortex and causing 'dying back'. They can also be induced in mice by the slowly replicating scrapie agent from sheep. This and the transmissibility of Jakob Creuzfeld disease by injecting diseased material into primates and the discovery of an infective factor in multiple sclerosis have suggested the possibility of, say, a slow virus as a cause of senile dementia.

The significance of *lipofuscin* accumulation in old age and dementia, the metabolites concerned and the cell groups afflicted, needs exploration. Likewise the role of *hypoxic ischaemia and small vessel pathology* in neuronal pathology needs to be clarified.

Biochemistry

Biochemical assays complement histological studies. Indices are available to monitor the loss of neuronal perikaryon, synaptic terminals and glial elements. Estimation of cell specific proteins is an alternative to cell counts, and of transmitter synthesising enzymes to counting synapses.

Specific brain proteins can be studied in the demented and non-demented, age matched controls, for example neuronin S-6 has been found to be markedly reduced in senile dementia.

Using material from brain biopsy as well as autopsy, the uptake and release of neurotransmitters, metabolites, the associated enzymes and glucose in different parts of the brain can be measured. A deficiency of γ-aminobutyric acid (GABA) in the basal ganglia of patients with Huntington's Chorea has been demonstrated, and this has led to studies of the more common dementias. An association between low homovanillic acid (HVA) concentration and a high degree of dementia suggests a possible disturbance of dopamine metabolism. However, three studies reported in one issue of the *British Journal of Psychiatry* (1977) (Davies; Perry and Perry; and Bowen and Davison) from three separate centres have shown that assays of choline acetylase and acetylcholinesterase *post mortem* from patients with Alzheimer's disease or senile dementia (of Alzheimer type) are markedly reduced relative to enzymes associated with other neurotransmitters when compared with controls, especially in the hippocampus and temporal and parietal cortex. This result suggests particular vulnerability of cholinergic neurons in these sites to whatever causes the dementia (and the possibility of pharmacological therapy by substitutes for acetylcholine or potentiation of cholinergic mechanisms).

The biochemistry and immunological state of *body fluids* may be informative, giving clues to pathogenesis and potential 'markers' of different forms of dementia. The turnover and fate of cortical neurotransmitters may be monitored at different stages by CSF levels. Enzymes, antigenic fragments of structured brain proteins, immunoglobulins, amines and metabolites may likewise be assayed in the CSF.

Cytology

Studies can be made of cell metabolism and longevity in tissue culture. It has been shown that the life span of fibroblasts is related to the age of the donor: is the same true of neuroglia and CNS capillaries? Is the loss of chromosomes in dementias a contributory factor, or a consequence? Might it be used as a marker? Studies of cell death may be informative, particularly the constituents of the CNS.

Other Studies

Studies also suggested by the M.R.C. include *electrophysiological*-evoked response, sleep patterns and other EEG derivatives. Peripheral nerve conduction is said to be reduced in senile dementia. Further understanding of the formation, flow and pressure of the *CSF* and of *cerebral blood flow* may prove relevant.

Research Strategies

Clinical Studies

The M.R.C. recommends that there should be:
a central referral agency for the intensive evaluation of dementia, taking cases from other hospitals and clinics over a wide area, and with extensive laboratory facilities;
specialised arrangements for clinical appraisal, periodic reviews and post mortem examinations;
small medical/psychological research teams to serve defined catchment areas, liaising with hospitals and residential homes;
cohort community studies based on G.P. lists or linked to other such studies in progress;
links between peripheral hospitals and centres of laboratory expertise;
closer liaison between biochemists and neuropathologists;
banks of brain tissue and sera from well-documented cases and control specimens from old people known not to be demented;
assessment of the effectiveness of the diverse health and social services for the elderly demented, with more precise measures and controls than heretofore (a lead has been given by techniques described by Kushlick (1972));
regular meetings between workers in the field.

Management and Treatment

There is no known treatment which will arrest, let alone reverse, the course of dementia, but it has been postulated, though not proven, that certain measures, such as the use of cerebral vascular dilators, and special training techniques (see below) may slow it down.

The value of *early diagnosis* (Harwin, 1975) has been contested. There are those who argue that since little can be done for those who are known to be demented, and even that little is performed poorly, if at all, there is no point in finding extra cases. On the other hand, if any new treatment, such as special diet or a stimulant or substitute for a failing neurotransmitter is ever to be effective it is highly likely that this will only be in very early cases, who will need, therefore, to have been identified. Further, scant resources could even now be better deployed if we had a fuller awareness of who is demented in the community and what problems of self-neglect, wandering, aggression, incontinence and dangerous forgetfulness there already are, or are likely to be. For example, the organisation of holiday relief admission, day care or a sitter-in, earlier rather than later, may enable a supporting relative to continue to look after a demented old person at home for much longer than if they battle alone and unrecognised until a crisis of anger and despair precipitates a demand for long-term institutional care.

The challenge of dementia is one that most doctors and indeed most other workers choose to avoid. This is as true of psychiatrists as of most other practitioners. These old people and their families are very likely to be neglected or left to over-burdened geriatric and social services unless psychiatric services are carefully organised to recognise and accept responsibility for (even if not always able to discharge that responsibility) the demented elderly in the community. The management of the difficult dement and the troubled ambivalent family requires psychiatric expertise; lacking this, other workers may do the job poorly, if at all.

The best organisation of resources usually follows the establishment of a *psychogeriatric team* within the district's department of psychiatry (Arie, 1971; Robinson, 1972; Pitt, 1974). This usually takes all psychiatric referrals of patients over 65, and not just the confused and demented. It is recommended (Royal College of Psychiatrists, 1975) that one in every four consultant psychiatrists providing a community service should specialise in the care of the elderly, with an appropriate proportion of medical, nursing, occupational therapy and secretarial staff, secondment of social workers and availability of psychologists and physiotherapists. The D.H.S.S. (HM 72/71) suggests that one bed per 2000 population over 65 be provided for functional illness, one for joint assessment and five or six for dementia. The adequacy of this latter provision has been questioned (Jolley, 1977) as it was simply based on an average of beds used for the demented in psychiatric hospitals throughout the country and took no account of difficult demented patients misplaced in, say, geriatric hospitals or residential homes. Most of these dementia beds are supposed ultimately to be found in community hospitals, but it may be questioned whether these will have enough day space, will attract suitably trained nurses, and if under the care of G.P.s will be sufficiently available to the psychogeriatric services. HM (72/71) also recommends two to three day hospital places per 1000 elderly population for the demented, and rather less than one place for the elderly with functional mental illness.

The psychogeriatric team should recognise its responsibility to advise and arrange services for and where necessary take over difficult problems of dementia. Having identified the scale of the problems the resources required can be ascertained. If, as is likely, existing resources are inadequate, pressure must be applied to have them improved, and until they are, what is already available should be given to those in the greatest need. Facing the problem in this way is to my mind far preferable to pretending that it is not there, or that it can be dealt with by others. A very important function of the psychogeriatric team is *liaison* with other services for the elderly, notably geriatric and social. One great advantage of the joint assessment unit, a ward in a general hospital to which both geriatrician and psychiatrist admit, meeting regularly to see the patients together and discuss referral, diagnosis, treatment and further arrangements, is that it brings the two specialties in close contact, and almost compels co-operation. Liaison with social services is more difficult as there are so many field social workers who may have something to do with the elderly, but no specialists. Secondment of workers to the psychogeriatric team, regular meetings with area social work team leaders and regular visits to residential Homes are ways of keeping in touch.

The main objective in the management of dementia is to *keep the patient at home* as far as possible. Most fare best in familiar surroundings, and deteriorate sometimes quite rapidly, especially in respect of personality preservation, in institutional care. The initial assessment is therefore best made in the patient's home. Here, the practical difficulties arising from her or his disability are readily identified, the special advantages or disadvantages of the situation noted (for example a day centre attached to a residential home just across the road, or a very helpful neighbour on the one hand, or very inadequate heating and a frequently vandalised lift on the other); and one can meet the key supporter, usually a spouse, a daughter or a son. If there is an obvious need for medical investigation, a subsequent assessment in an out-patient clinic or the joint assessment unit can be arranged, but this initial visit sets the scene for future care.

Treatment

In order to plan services realistically, it must be recognised that when all investigations have been concluded, the vast majority of those who appear to be demented at the initial assessment will prove to be so. Any hypothyroidism (Heneschke and Pain, 1977), vitamin B_{12} or folate deficiency, or positive serology will probably be coincidental, or at least its treatment will have little effect on the degree or the course of the dementia. It is very gratifying to find a treatable cause; it is also very rare. Treatment of any heart failure, chest infection, anaemia or malnutrition may well improve current functioning, but will not modify the underlying dementing process.

The place of *cerebral vascular dilators* is not very clear, but not very important either. Cyclandelate, naftidrofuryl, and dihydroergotoxine mesylate have all been reported (Judge, 1977) to have some effects in improving performance on cognitive tests and enhancing mood in double-blind crossover trials (though this has not been confirmed by Davies *et al.* (1977) in respect of cyclandelates), though not on daily living activities. Logically their place would seem to be confined to atherosclerotic dementia, though Sandoz, manufacturers of dihydroergotoxine mesylate, claim that it has some effects on senile dementia through reducing the osmotic pressure in astrocytes and thus improving capillary blood flow. However, the possible benefits of these drugs are so small, they are not without side-effects, and the problems of compliance by the confused patient are so great that their main value may be a placebo effect, giving the family (and sometimes the doctor!) the comfort that something is being done.

Sedatives and tranquillisers are two-edged weapons in the management of dementia. None, of course, actually relieves confusion, but they may control restless, difficult, disturbed or aggressive behaviour or troublesome nocturnal wandering. However, the side-effects—drowsiness, ataxia, Parkinsonism, dystonia, hypotension and dulling of the emotions, if not actual depression— increase the burden of physical care, contribute to falls and often turn a 'psychogeriatric' into a 'geriatric' problem. Probably the most useful tranquillisers are thioridazine and haloperidol, both of which are fairly effective; thioridazine is less likely than other tranquillisers to cause extrapyramidal side-effects, and haloperidol is less likely to induce drowsiness. Benzodiazepines have little place in the daytime, but nitrazepam is the most widely used hypnotic, though chloral and its derivatives and chlormethiazole (which has an interesting derivation from vitamin B_1) are very useful alternatives.

Psychologists, whose interest in therapy has been growing in most fields of psychiatry, have begun to turn their attention to the demented elderly, and Miller (1977) has reviewed some of the evidence for the value of active *psychological and social intervention* in behavioural problems. From the late 1960s onwards there has been a flow of reports, mainly of uncontrolled studies.

Brook *et al.* (1975) introduced an experimental group of patients to a room well equipped with stimulating materials, where therapists actively engaged them in various tasks (for example describing things, writing a diary) for 16 weeks. The control group went to the room for the same length of time, but the therapists were passive and left patients to their own devices. Ratings of social and intellectual functioning improved in both groups at first, but within two to four weeks the only gains were in the experimental group, while the control group fell back. The patients' active involvement was thus required to build upon the initial benefits. The less severely demented did best.

All studies involve an increase in social stimulation, and the commonest benefits are in social behaviour. These benefits disappear soon after the programme is over. This suggests that a programme shown to be beneficial should be continued indefinitely.

Folsom (1967) advocated *reality orientation* programmes, in which patients are continuously presented information about time, place and persons. The essence of reality orientation is to ensure that the patient relearns and continuously uses essential information about time, place and person, and the names and uses of commonly encountered objects. Formal daily classes are backed up by staff who keep stressing basic information. Whether the actual information is of value, or whether the forced interaction between staff and patients is of prime importance, is not yet clear.

Behaviour modification techniques which should be further explored include habit training, reward and exchange systems and special adaptations of the environment (for example blue lines leading to the men's lavatory). Interesting work is being done at Carlton Hayes Hospital, where an educationalist supervises the retraining of demented patients in daily living activities by simple stage by stage programmes derived from the field of mental subnormality (Lodge, 1974).

Community Care. At present 80 per cent of elderly dements are at home, thanks mainly to the support given by their families, and the main efforts of the professional services should be to help this support to continue. Requests for urgent admission far more often follow withdrawal of the services of the key supporter, because of personal illness, other commitments, holidays or despair, than any significant deterioration in the patient's clinical condition.

Practical help includes the provision of a home help or paid 'good neighbour', the supply of meals at home, day care at a day hospital or local authority day centre, holiday admission of the patient for a fortnight once or twice a year to hospital or a residential Home, the incontinent laundry service, the loan of a commode, district nursing, bathing attendants and 'sitters in'. An attendance allowance may compensate the supporter for not being able to go out to work. Baker and Byrne (1977) make extensive use of day hospitals for the demented and claim that in consequence less than 5 per cent of hospital admissions become long stay. Any reduction of these services (which in the present economic climate of the United Kingdom is all too probable) should be strongly resisted as a false economy, likely to cause hardship and to increase the demand for the more expensive and scarce institutional care.

Psychological support for the key supporter(s) includes a clear explanation of the nature of dementia and its likely course, of personality change, angry outbursts, accusations and obstinate irrationality arising from confusion; encouragement that the considerable patience, vigilance and effort demanded are worth while; reassurance that practical help will be available when needed; regular, reliable contact, and sympathetic listening. This is work for G.P.s, psychiatrists, community nurses, health visitors and, especially social workers. To recognise and deal with anxiety, depression, anger, guilt and over-protectiveness in the supporters requires skill, application and perseverance.

The effort is repaid by a reduction in crises of rejection, when frustration and a sense of futility end in angry desperation.

Institutional Care. If it is evident that a demented old person living alone is seriously at risk or already suffering from self neglect, despite the full use of community services, or if the key supporter is clearly carrying an insupportable burden and showing signs of serious strain, institutional care of one kind or another should be arranged speedily. The inability always to meet this recognised need because of insufficient accommodation is a sad reflection on the inadequacy of current Health and Welfare services and a serious morale problem for the psychogeriatric team forced to appear to condone what they actually deplore.

Most demented old people can be accommodated in residential Homes, Part III (Local Authority Old Peoples Homes), private and voluntary, though the problems for largely untrained staff and other residents of having a substantial proportion of the confused are often voiced. There is still controversy about the use of Elderly Mentally Infirm (EMI) Homes or wings. Most Social Services directors follow the line of Meacher's *Taken for a Ride* (1972) and advocate integrated rather than 'separatist' homes (the choice of these words well indicates their attitude) though in doing so one wonders how many are taking a realistic account of the day to day difficulties rather than a somewhat detached, idealistic view of how things ought to be. The Royal College of Psychiatrists (1976) supports the EMI Homes as best suited to the needs of the more demented elderly, having a higher staff – resident ratio and a higher proportion of staff with a nursing training (though the importance of the latter is questioned by the D.H.S.S.'s 1977 guidelines 'Residential Homes for the Elderly. Arrangements for Health Care') provided that the district has a psychogeriatric team who are in close liaison; otherwise there is a danger that the home's staff will feel too isolated with their many problems. As a good 30 per cent of residents in general are demented, EMI homes clearly cannot cope with them all, but only the more disabled.

Patients admitted to hospital are those who need assessment, those with a significant medical disorder requiring treatment, or heavy nursing, as well as their dementia—generally in geriatric wards—and those with serious behaviour disorder, who are best placed in psychiatric wards specialising in their care. The level of nurse staffing on these wards is frequently underestimated. The Group for the Psychiatry of Old Age (Royal College of Psychiatrists, 1978) recommends a ratio of 1 nurse to 1.2 patients on wards where the patients are heavily dependent.

This is unlikely to be attained immediately, but is a proper goal. Morale on these wards for dementia is enhanced by their being part of the resources of the psychogeriatric team, if occupational therapy and physiotherapy are available, and if the consultant psychiatrist and senior nursing officers are seen to take an interest.

In the institution, Home or hospital, recognition of the patient as still a person, enabling her to have personal clothing, glasses, hearing aid and dentures, a structured programme including regular exercise and occupation, unrestricted visiting, cheerful surroundings, accessible and comfortable lavatories, plenty of day space and a kind, calm, good-humoured staff help to sustain some quality of life during the final years.

At present such conditions, especially in hospitals, despite the efforts of the Health (formerly Hospital) Advisory Service are far from universal and too often little more is given than very basic care. However, the rapid growth of the Group (now Section) for the Psychiatry of Old Age (which after being founded in 1971 now has more than 700 members), the vigour of the British Geriatric Society, the development of some special interest groups among social workers and the energy and outspokenness of voluntary organisations, such as Age Concern and the National Corporation for the Care of Old People and Mind, at least indicate that the urgent needs of the demented elderly in the last quarter of the twentieth century will not be unvoiced.

References

Arie, T. (1971). Morale and the planning of psychogeriatric services. *Br. med. J.*, **3**, 166

Baker, A. and Byrne, G. (1977). Another style of psychogeriatric service. *Br. J. Psychiat.*, **130**, 123

Bergmann, K. (1972). Psychogeriatrics. *Medicine*, **9**, 643

Bergmann, K. (1977). Chronic brain failure; epidemiological aspects. *Age and Ageing*, **6**, Suppl., 4

Blessed, G., Tomlinson, B. E. and Roth, M. (1968). The association between quantitative measures of dementia and of senile change in the cerebral grey matter of elderly subjects. *Br. J. Psychiat.*, **114**, 797

Bowen, D. M. and Davison, A. M. (1977). Selective vulnerability of neurones in Alzheimer's disease. *Br. J. Psychiat.*, **131**, 319

Brook, P., Degun, G. and Mather, M. (1975). Reality orientation, a treatment for psychogeriatric patients: a controlled study. *Br. J. Psychiat.*, **127**, 42

Constantinidis, J., Garrone, G. and Ajuriaguerra, J. De (1962). L'hérédité des démences de l'age avancé. *Encéphale, Paris*, **51**, 301

Corsellis, J. A. M. (1962). *Mental Illness and the Ageing Brain*. Maudsley Monographs No. 9, London

Corsellis, J. A. M. (1977). Observations on the neuropathology of dementia. *Age and Ageing*, **6**, Suppl., 20

Cowan, D., Wright, M., Gourlay, A. J., Smith, A., Barron, G., De Gruchy, J., Copeland, J. R. M., Kelleher, M. J. and Kellett, J. M. (1975). A comparative psychological assessment of psychogeriatric and geriatric patients. *Br. J. Psychiat.*, **127**, 33

Davies, G., Hamilton, S., Hendrickson, E., Levy, R. and Post, F. (1977). The effect of cyclandelate in depressed and demented patients: a controlled study in psychogeriatric patients. *Age and Ageing*, **6**, 156

Davies, P. (1977). Cholinergic mechanisms in Alzheimer's disease. *Br. J. Psychiat.*, **131**, 318

D.H.S.S. (1972). Services for Mental Illness Related to Old Age (HM 72/71), H.M.S.O., London

D.H.S.S. (1976). Priorities For the Health and Personal Social Services. A Consultative Document. H.M.S.O., London

D.H.S.S. (1977). Residential Homes for the Elderly – Arrangements for Health Care. A Memorandum of Guidance. Welsh Office

Folsom, J. C. (1967). Intensive hospital therapy for psychogeriatric patients. *Curr. psychiat. Ther.*, **7**, 209

Grad, J. and Sainsbury, P. (1968). The effects that patients have on their families in a community care and a control psychiatric service. A two year follow up. *Br. J. Psychiat.*, **114**, 265

Harwin, B. (1975). Psychogeriatric Screening. In *Screening in General Practice* (Ed. C. R. Hart), Churchill Livingstone, Edinburgh and London

Heneschke, P. J. and Pain, R. W. (1977). Thyroid disease in a geriatric population. *Age and Ageing*, **6**, 151

Hobson, W. and Pemberton, J. (1955). *The Health of the Elderly at Home.* Churchill, London

Jolley, David (1977). Hospital in-patient provision for patients with dementia. *Br. med. J.*, **1**, 1335

Judge, T. C. (1977). Drug treatment of brain failure. *Age and Ageing*, **6**, Suppl., 70

Kallman, F. J. (1956). The genetics of ageing. In *Mental Disorders in Later Life* (Ed. O. J. Kaplan), Stanford University Press, Stanford

Kay, D. W. K., Beamish, P. and Roth, M. (1964). Old age mental disorders in Newcastle-upon-Tyne. I A study of prevalence. *Br. J. Psychiat.*, **110**, 146

Kral, V. A. (1962). Senescent forgetfulness; benign and malignant. *Can. med. Ass. J.*, **86**, 257

Kushlick, A. (1972). Research into Care for the Elderly. In *The Elderly Mind*. Br. Hosp. J./Hosp. Int. publication, London

Larsson, T., Sjogren, R. and Jacobson, G. (1963). Senile dementia. *Acta psychiat. scand.*, **39**, Suppl., 167

Lishman, W. (1977). Senile and presenile dementias. Report of an M.R.C. Sub Committee, M.R.C., London

Lodge, B. R. W. (1974). Personal communication

Meacher, M. (1972). *Taken for a Ride.* Longmans, London

Miller, E. (1977). The management of dementia: a review of some possibilities. *Br. J. soc. clin. Psychol.*, **16**, 77

Perry, E. K. and Perry, R. H. (1977). Cholinergic and G.A.B.A. systems in dementia and normal old age. *Br. J. Psychiat.*, **131**, 319

Pitt, B. (1974). *Psychogeriatrics.* Churchill Livingstone, Edinburgh and London

Roberts, M. A. and Caird, R. I. (1976). Computerised tomography and intellectual impairment in the elderly. *J. Neurol. Neurosurg. Psychiat.*, **39**, 986

Robinson, R. A. (1972). Organisation of Psychogeriatric Services. In *The Elderly Mind*. Br. Hosp. J. Hosp. Int. publication, London

Roth, M. (1955). The natural history of mental disorder arising in the senium. *J. ment. Sci.*, **101**, 281

Royal College of Psychiatrists (Group for the psychiatry of old age) (1975). Medical staffing for a population of 200,000. *Br. J. Psychiat.*, 'News and Notes', July

Royal College of Psychiatrists (Group for the psychiatry of old age) (1976). Memorandum on Residential Homes for the Elderly Mentally Infirm, *Br. J. Psychiat.* 'News and Notes', September

Royal College of Psychiatrists (Group for the psychiatry of old age) (1978). Memorandum on Nurse Staffing Needs for the Hospital Service for the Elderly Mentally Ill. *Br. J. Psychiat.*, News and Notes, January

Sheldon, J. H. (1947). *Social Medicine of Old Age.* Nuffield Foundation, Oxford University Press, London

Sjogren, H. (1956). Neuro-psychiatric studies in presenile and senile diseases, based on a material of 1000 cases. *Acta psychiat scand.*, Suppl. 106, 9

Terry, R. D. and Wiesniwski, H. M. (1970) The ultra structure of the neuro fibrillary tangle and the senile plaque. In *Alzheimer's Disease and Related Conditions* (Ed. G. E. W. Wolstenholme and M. O'Connor), J & A. Churchill, London

Tomlinson, B. E. and Kitchener, D. (1972). Granulovascular degeneration of hippocampal pyramidal cells. *J. Path.*, **106**, 165

Williamson, J., Stokoe, I. H., Gray, S., Fishers, M., Smith, A., McGhee, A. and Stephenson, E. (1964). Old People at home; their unreported needs. *Lancet*, **i**, 1117

Zerbin-Ruedin, E. (1976). Genetics. In *Modern Perspectives in the Psychiatry of Old Age* (Ed. J. Howell), Churchill Livingstone, Edinburgh and London

23 Fasting Girls— Past, Present and Future

H. Gethin Morgan

Severe weight loss due to deliberate reduction of food intake presents many problems to the clinician. Even when organic disease has been excluded, itself not an easy task, there remain a variety of possible psychological causes which are still poorly understood: these include affective disorders such as depressive and phobic anxiety states, certain psychotic conditions with self neglect or specific fears of food contamination, the abdominal hypochondriacal syndromes, psychogenic vomiting and anorexia nervosa.

The last of these is still the subject of many uncertainties regarding its causes and treatment. Although recognition of the paramount importance of psychological factors in its aetiology has rapidly gained momentum in recent years, we still experience many difficulties in achieving an objective attitude to its management, unclouded by our own anxiety, value judgement or indeed hostility towards the patient. This review of the historical development of the concept of anorexia nervosa aims to provide a useful perspective from which to assess our present day approach to the problem of self-induced weight loss.

Attitudes of the Past

Richard Morton (1694) has been credited with the first adequate description of a condition recognisable as anorexia nervosa. He provided details of two cases of what he called 'nervous atrophy', a type of consumption which owed its origin to an 'ill and morbid state of the spirits', characterised by 'want of appetite with a falling away of the flesh'. This condition he distinguished from consumption due to systemic organic disease and he emphasised the total suppression of the monthly menses which might result from 'multitudes of cares and passions of the mind'.

There is an earlier but hitherto unrecognised description by Pedro Mexio (1613) of a young French girl who exhibited a syndrome recognisable as anorexia nervosa. Mexio described a maiden named Jane Balan of Poictu who, for three years or more, was said to have lived without receiving either meat or drink; it was thought by some that her condition was due to some wicked power in an apple which an old woman had given to her two or three months before although Mexio himself dismissed this view and saw the cause as a 'drying up of the liver and of all the parts serving to nourishment due to hurtful humours'. In the 11th year of her age, after an episode of fever and vomiting which began on 15 February, 1599, she became speechless, weak and later fearful, for a short period 'void of good sense', and subsequently no-one could persuade her to eat: 'for both meats and drinkes she altogether loaths, and mightily abhorreth'. She then developed extreme wasting of her abdomen though there was no breast atrophy, 'her pappes prettie and round', her hair remained unchanged and her limbs were 'still fleshy'. No menstrual loss occurred, and it was claimed that no excrement or urine was passed either. Her skin was cold and dry. She remained normally active:

> yet she doth travaile about the house, go to the Market for Victualles, sweep the house, spin on her Wheele, Reele off her Quill; and gives herself to all serviceable Offices in a family and seems as if she were not defective in any part of sense, or motion of her body.

No information is given regarding subsequent outcome. A fasting girl of this kind might at that time have been encouraged by the curiosity of others, perhaps involving financial reward, to malinger and so consciously deceive so that her fasting appeared to be absolute. Although Mexio's account does not permit us to clarify this issue with regard to Jane Balan, from the descriptive point of view her illness may well be the earliest example of a condition recognisable as anorexia nervosa, even though the precise nature of her initial fever and psychological disturbance remains unclear.

Morton's insight into the importance of psychological factors in anorexia nervosa did not at first have much impact on the medical world. Almost two hundred years elapsed before publication of the first two simultaneous yet independent descriptions of the anorexia nervosa syndrome couched in modern scientific terms by William Gull (1868, 1874, 1888) and C. E. Lasegue (1873). Apart from providing lucid clinical details, Gull followed up his patients and was able to strike a note of optimism:

> none of these cases, however exhausted, are really hopeless while life exists; and for the most part the prognosis may be considered favourable.

He placed the cause firmly in the realm of a morbid mental state:

> that mental states may destroy appetite is notorious and it will be admitted that young women at the ages named are specially obnoxious [liable] to mental perversity.

Although Gull noted the difficult relationship which anorexic patients have with their close relatives, Lasegue described this in more detail:

> The family has but two methods at its service which it always exhausts—

entreaties and menaces—and which both serve as a touchstone. The delicacies of the table are multiplied in the hope of stimulating the appetite; but the more the solicitude increases, the more the appetite diminishes.

The family's dilemma is accentuated by the patient's own attitude to the problem, again described by Lasegue:

> . . . the state of quietude – I might almost say a condition of contentment truly pathological. Not only does she not sigh for recovery, but she is not ill-pleased with her condition, notwithstanding all the unpleasantries it is attended with. In comparing this satisfied assurance to the obstinacy of the insane, I do not think I am going too far.

Subsequent to Gull and Lasegue it seems that our understanding became clouded once again, first by anti-feminist attitudes and secondly, to use the words of Ryle (1936) 'by the lure of endocrinology'. The hint of male prejudice in Gull's papers was taken up with relish, and in the early part of the present century the medical literature on anorexia nervosa revealed an undisguised hostility towards the young girl who refused to eat. Thus Allbutt and Rolleston (1911) in their medical textbook described anorexia nervosa under the heading of hysteria in the following way:

> out of such material, when the friends and surroundings supply the element of fraud and credulity, are made the fasting girls who from time to time become notorious and whose exploits have been known to terminate in death.

A further striking example is to be found in Samuel Gee's (1915) discussion of the young woman's repugnance for food:

> a young maiden with small experience of the world expects more from life than life can give: the sympathy desired is not forthcoming; hence dissatisfaction and discontent. In the extreme degree of melancholy the patient suffers from perverse conceit and strange notions. Look at the first wood cut in Sir William Gull's paper for the portrait of a young woman, 13 years old, the very picture of pathetic resignation worthy of a medieval saint.

Such hostility to the young women with eating problems is remarkable and requires an explanation. It may have been related in some degree to the very tragic case of the Welsh Fasting Girl, Sarah Jocobs (Fowler, 1871) who, like Jane Balan in 1599, acquired the reputation of being a miraculous faster, also after an initial serious physical illness of uncertain nature. She died in 1869 after having been placed under close observation for eight days by a committee which included doctors and nurses. Subsequently the parents were sent to prison for the manslaughter of their daughter. Undoubtedly the medical profession felt humiliated for long after this tragedy, which seems to have occurred as a result of an intervention stimulated by public curiosity, and based on an inadequate appreciation of the complex psychological processes involved in such a problem. The confusion of roles on the part of the medical men, when they set out to monitor the girl's eating behaviour without having power to intervene when she began to deteriorate physically, is also a very salutary lesson arising out of this sad story. We need not look far to find reasons for the lack of sympathy subsequently shown by the medical profession at the turn of the century towards anorexic girls.

The second hindrance to full appreciation of the psychological causes of anorexia nervosa at this time makes stranger reading still. Simmonds (1914) published in German a paper entitled 'Fatal hypophyseal atrophy' in which he described a case of atrophy of the pituitary related to previous puerperal sepsis. It so happens that the patient was also generally wasted and there followed a widely held misconception that pituitary atrophy is itself a cause of gross bodily weight loss. As a result, for two or three decades the endocrinological approach to emaciation held precedence and many cases of anorexia nervosa were probably treated with pituitary extracts and implants without attention to psychological issues. In the 1930s, however, certain clinicians protested at the situation. For example, Ryle (1936) stated:

> Physicians subject to the lure of endocrinology have been tempted sometimes to find a basis for the symptoms of anorexia nervosa in a primary deficiency or disharmony of the internal secretions . . . I believe, however, and shall hope to show, some striking physical symptoms notwithstanding, that the origins of the disease are, as Gull maintained, to be sought in a disturbance of the mind and a prolonged insufficiency of food and in nothing more.

Likewise Sheldon (1939) and Richardson (1939) emphasised that any endocrine disturbance in anorexia nervosa was secondary and not the primary cause. Controversy was not finally resolved until Sheehan and Summers (1949) described the post-mortem findings in 95 cases of pituitary gland atrophy unaccompained by hypothalamic involvement, and concluded that emaciation is not regularly associated with this type of lesion. The pre-eminence of psychological factors in anorexia nervosa did not achieve widespread recognition until 50 years after the classic papers of Gull and Lasegue.

The Present Day Approach

Having examined our predecessors' attitudes, we may now turn to our present day difficulties in trying to reach a full and objective understanding of anorexia nervosa. In my discussion particular reference will be made to a follow-up study conducted by the author concerning 41 patients diagnosed as suffering from anorexia nervosa. The series consisted of all patients who had received treatment for anorexia nervosa in the Metabolic Unit of the Maudsley Hospital during the period 1959—66.

Clinical Description

Anorexia nervosa is, of course, a classic example of a psychosomatic condition, one in which psychological and physical factors are closely interwoven. Although one would not wish to quarrel with its name, the point should be made that anorexia is not always strictly appropriate; many of these patients have normal appetites which cause them great distress and against which they struggle relentlessly. Whereas some authors regard anorexia nervosa merely as a nervous malnutrition, secondary to a wide variety of psychological disorders (Bliss and Branch, 1960), the illness is generally seen as something much more specific. Russell (1970) has listed the necessary diagnostic criteria as follows:

(1) The patient's behaviour leads to a marked loss of body weight and malnutrition. The abnormal behaviour consists of a studied and purposive avoidance of foods considered to be of 'fattening nature'. Often, but not invariably, the patient resorts to additional devices which ensure a loss of weight: for example, self-induced vomiting, purgation, or excessive exercise.

(2) There is an endocrine disorder which manifests itself clinically as cessation of menstruation in those patients who are most commonly afflicted by the illness—adolescent girls or women during the reproductive period of life. The amenorrhoea is an early symptom and may precede the onset of weight loss, it is often persistent and may last for several years. In male subjects the equivalent symptom is a loss of sexual interest and lack of potency.

(3) Psychological features such as morbid fear of becoming fat, loss of judgement regarding food requirements and body image, and fears of losing control of eating. Less specific features include depressive, obsessional, hysterical or phobic symptoms.

Others have added more specific criteria: for example, requiring that there should have been amenorrhoea of at least three months duration (Crisp, 1967; Dally and Sargant, 1960; Kay and Leigh, 1954; and Thomä, 1967) or a weight loss of at least 10 per cent (Dally, 1969).

The Maudsley follow-up series consisted of 38 females and 3 males who satisfied these diagnostic criteria. Retrospective analysis of the case notes provided details of the illness at the time of admission to hospital. The series as a whole had the typical clinical features of anorexia nervosa, and a few examples are appropriate here.

The illness had most commonly occurred in adolescence:
Age of onset of food difficulties: Mean 15.5 years, range 11—20 years

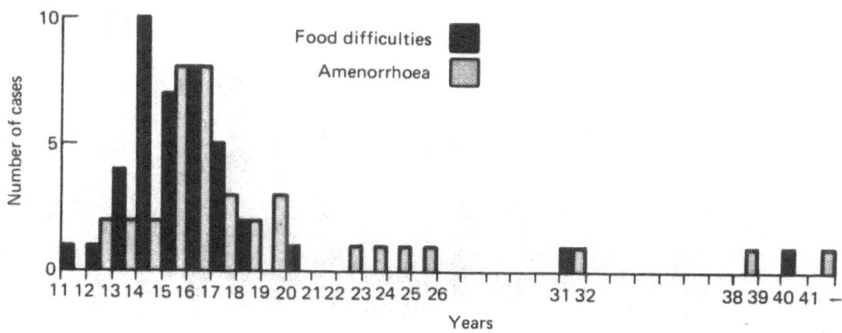

Figure 23.1   **Age onset**

Age of onset of amenorrhoea (figure 23.1): Mean 18.2 years, range 11—41 years.

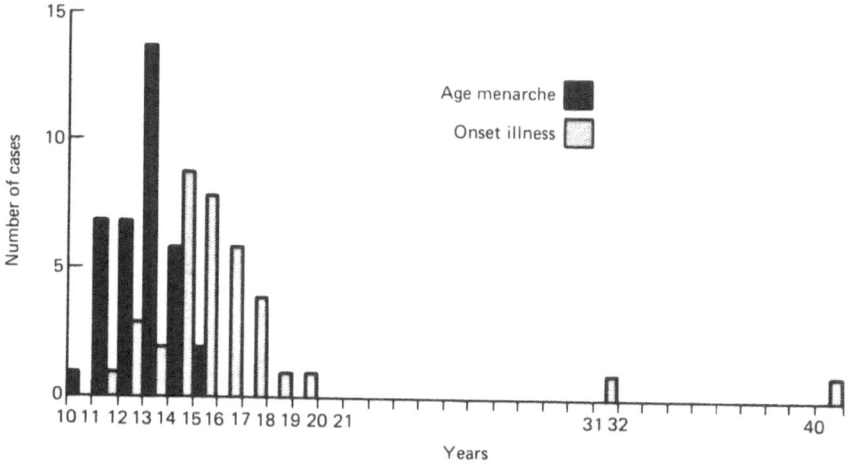

Figure 23.2   Relationship between age of menarche and onset of illness (series analysed as a whole)

Onset of illness in relation to menarche (figure 23.2). In 93 per cent of cases the illness began seven years or less after the menarche.

On the whole the patients had reached a severe degree of weight loss at the time of admission (figure 23.3): body weight on admission (average for series) 63.8 per cent of average body weight.

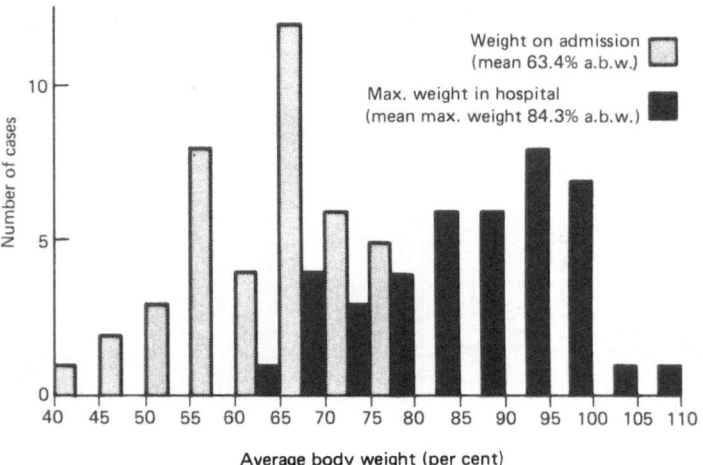

Figure 23.3   Body weight on admission and maximum weight in hospital per cent average for normal population matched for age and sex

Relation between onset of food difficulties and amenorrhoea (figure 23.4): in about half the series (44.7 per cent) food difficulties had preceded the onset of amenorrhoea. Amenorrhoea had preceded food difficulties in 18.4 per cent, and the two had coincided in 34.2 per cent. The remaining patient was pre-menarchal.

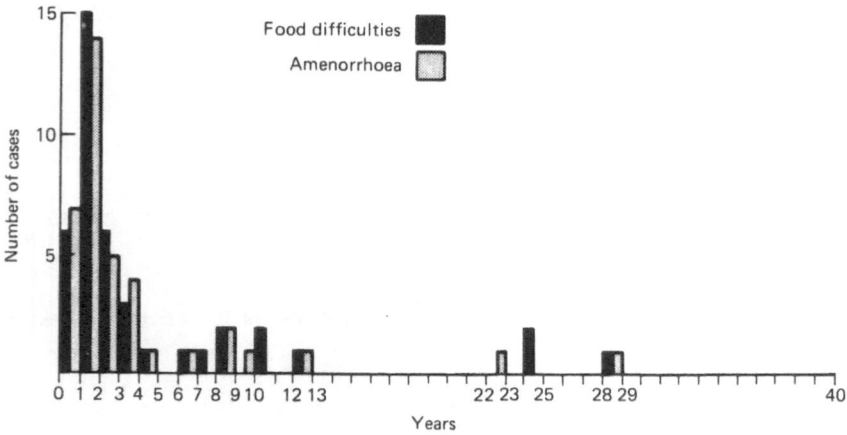

Figure 23.4   Duration of amenorrhoea and food difficulties before admission to hospital

Natural History and Prognosis

Anorexia nervosa, then, may be clearly defined and from the descriptive point of view it appears to be a highly distinctive clinical condition. It is surprising, therefore, to find much difference of opinion concerning its natural history and prognosis. Several studies are optimistic (Beck and Brøchner-Mortensen, 1954; Thoma, 1967, Dally, 1969), a clear majority of cases being regarded as cured or at least significantly improved. Others (Kay and Leigh, 1954; Kay and Schapira, 1965; Crisp, 1965a and b; Meyer, 1961; Warren, 1968; Theander, 1970) are less optimistic and emphasise the high incidence of chronic morbidity.

Detailed examination of these studies suggests that the variable findings are attributable, in some degree at least, to several well recognised sources of bias in patient selection and follow-up methods. Those studies which emphasise the incidence of chronic morbidity may well have included more severe cases and used more direct and complete retrieval methods. Others, the more optimistic ones, may have selected less severe cases, for example, those attending out-patient clinics and not admitted to hospital, and relied upon indirect follow-up assessment methods. Most of the disagreement concerns the proportion which fully recovers; all studies agree that only a small number remain severely ill with chronic, severe weight loss and unremitting amenorrhoea (16–31 per cent in various series). It may well be that much of the variation in findings is more apparent than real, stemming from inadequate definition of terms such as 'recovered', 'improved', or 'relapsed'. It is, of course, very difficult to distinguish between complete recovery and continuing minor illness.

Every effort was made in following up the Maudsley series to avoid these pitfalls. All patients had been admitted to hospital and were suffering from major forms of the illness; the duration of which had ranged from 1 to 28 years (figure 23.4), 27 (65 per cent) had been ill for two years or less, 9 (22 per cent) for seven years or longer. A significant proportion (49 per cent) had received psychiatric treatment previously, 36 per cent for anorexia nervosa. The series therefore includes a substantial proportion of patients with long-standing and refractory anorexia nervosa. The follow-up accounted for all the patients, direct interview was achievecd in 85 per cent and in 70 per cent both the patient and another informant were seen. The duration of follow-up is also, of course, an important variable, and must be sufficiently long to permit a valid estimate of long-term outcome. In this study the minimum duration of follow-up was four years, the maximum ten years after discharge from the unit. Expressed differently, the follow-up period ranged from 4.2 to 32 years after the onset of the illness.

The follow-up interviews provided data concerning body weight, eating habits, menstrual, psychological, and socio-economic status of each patient. Four outcome categories were devised, using the most objective data available, namely, body weight and menstrual function. The *good* outcome category contained those patients who had maintained their weight within 15 per cent of *average body weight* (derived from actuarial tables) and there had been regular menstrual cycles. *Intermediate* outcome included those in whom the body weight had risen to within 15 per cent of average body weight, but this had not been constantly maintained and/or there were continuing menstrual difficulties. *Poor* outcome applied to those patients whose body weight had remained so low that it never approached average body weight minus 15 per cent and it gave rise to concern in the patient or in her attendants. Menstruation had remained absent or very sporadic.

Table 23.1 illustrates the distribution of patients throughout the various outcome categories. Data concerning psychiatric, sexual, and socio-economic adjustment are also shown in this table. *Good* outcome was found in 16 patients (39 per cent), including the three males. The overall mean weight in this group was 97 per cent of average body weight. Psychiatric symptoms were unusual in this group and when present consisted of mild depression or anxiety, although one patient had come to abuse amphetamines and barbiturates. Twelve patients (27 per cent) were found to have *intermediate* outcome, including two who had become obese (119 per cent and 139 per cent average body weight). The former had gained weight after a leucotomy performed in another hospital, two years before the follow-up assessment. The mean weight of the other ten patients was 90 per cent of average body weight. Sporadic or absent menstruation was reported in over half this group. Measures of psychological, sexual and socio-economic adjustment also tended to be less satisfactory in this category. Eleven patients (29 per cent) were found in the *poor* outcome category whose mean weight was only 68 per cent of average body weight. Menstruation was absent or sporadic in all these patients. In eight of them there were continuing and sometimes disabling psychiatric symptoms, usually of a depressive kind. Sexual adjustment was poor, often with aversion from heterosexual contact. Death had occurred in two patients. One had committed suicide soon after leucotomy while in another psychiatric unit. The operation had been followed by obesity which had caused her considerable distress. The second of these patients had died in a hospital from status asthmaticus. She had remained very thin, and shown an erratic life pattern and had become dependent upon alcohol.

It is not possible to consider here the follow-up data in any detail but some of the more striking findings may be mentioned. For example, body weight had frequently returned to normal in spite of persistence of eating difficulties, whether in the form of disturbed attitudes to eating or abnormal pattern of food intake. A further interesting feature is the fact that return of normal menstruation also consistently lagged behind restoration of normal weight (figure 23.5). Exactly half the 36 females had returned to a cyclical pattern of menstruation as measured over the last six months of the follow-up period. The basic psychopathology of anorexia nervosa persisted in some degree in a relatively high proportion of patients: concern about body weight was still present in 65 per cent. However, body weight had returned to near average

Table 23.1
Distribution of 41 patients among the categories of outcome

Category	Patients (No.)	%	Weight as % of 'average' body weight	Menstruation Cyclical	Sporadic	Absent	Rating for adjustment (12 point scales) Mental state	Sexual	Socio-economic
'Good'	16†	39	97	13/13	0	0	10.2	10.9	10.2
Intermediate	12	27	90*	5/12	1/12	6/12	9.0	8.0	7.1
'Poor'	11	29	68	0	2/11	9/11	5.4	6.2	5.7
Death	2	5							
Total	41	100							

* The value for the percentage of 'average' body weight excludes two obese patients.
† The 'good' outcome category includes the three male patients.

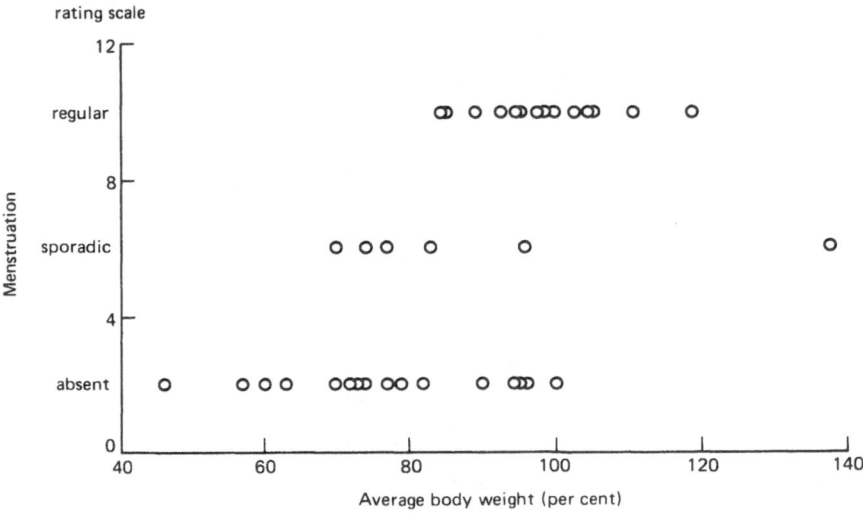

Figure 23.5

levels in over half of the series (55 per cent). While the illness persisted the clinical picture continued to be typical of anorexia nervosa. In only eight patients did food difficulties become partly replaced by other symptoms (one paranoid state, two recurrent self-injury, two affective symptoms, one amphetamine and barbiturate abuse, one predominantly social difficulties).

Prediction of Outcome

By correlating outcome with data concerning family background, childhood development, and clinical features of the anorexic illness (collected at the time of admission to hospital) it was possible to demonstrate certain predictors of poor outcome. Although few in number, they were quite unequivocal, and included long duration of illness, previous admission to psychiatric hospital, onset in late teens or early twenties as opposed to within three years of puberty, a disturbed relationship with the family before the onset of illness, and problems at school. It was perhaps surprising that very few predictors of outcome could be found in the clinical features of the anorexic illness itself: very low body weight on admission may be a valid indicator of poor prognosis, but no significance could be attached to such factors as degree of psychiatric disturbance, vomiting, or age of menarche. Immediate response to treatment again appears to bear no relationship to outcome whether expressed in terms of limited gain in weight, resistance to eating, disturbance of behaviour during re-feeding, or necessity for re-admission. Though these findings are in the main negative, they are of considerable importance in shaping our current attitudes to anorexia nervosa. They suggest that the majority of patients are indeed capable of eventual recovery or considerable improvement no matter how severe the illness, how thin, emotionally upset, or resistant to eating the patient may be, and even though she may relapse on one or more occasion.

Delineation of Anorexia Nervosa from Physical Disease

Knowledge of the highly distinctive clinical features of anorexia nervosa can be most useful in distinguishing it from malnutrition secondary to major organic disease. Such consultative work in medical and surgical hospital wards can as a result be most rewarding. The characteristic symptoms of weight phobia and preferential avoidance of high calorie foods may not have been recognised, and as a result other features of anorexia nervosa such as constipation, vomiting, flatulence, and abdominal discomfort are investigated with excessive zeal, at the same time denying psychiatric help at an early stage of the illness. The diagnosis may have been proposed merely because no other cause for the weight loss can be found, and such an approach by exclusion is of course always highly suspect, particularly in the absence of morbid aversion towards weight increase or calorie avoidance. In uncomplicated nutritional myopathy, muscle power is usually surprisingly good in spite of severe wasting, and tendon reflexes are retained. Localised percussion myotonia is usually marked. While it is important to recognise anorexia nervosa at an early stage, so conversely it is very useful to be able to recognise clinical features which are highly unusual in this illness, if only to encourage the continued search for underlying physical disease. Significant muscle weakness must always be investigated fully: there may, of course, be weakness due to hypokalaemia secondary to persistent vomiting itself, but other organic causes such as thyrotoxicosis must always be high on the diagnostic list, particularly if the muscle weakness is proximal in distribution. Peripheral neuropathy is rare in anorexia nervosa, presumably because the greatly reduced calorie intake means that thiamine requirements are small. Chronic alcoholism is a common cause of peripheral neuropathy in the malnourished individual and it may be difficult to detect because of denial on the part of the patient. Although bradycardia is frequently found in uncomplicated weight loss, a persistently raised pulse rate usually signifies some organic pathology, which, of course, may be secondary to some complication of anorexia nervosa itself: auricular fibrillation in an emaciated young woman indicates in particular that thyroid function should be fully assessed. Vomiting and weight loss also pose diagnostic problems, especially when organic disease has been sought and not found. The vomiting of anorexia nervosa may initially be quite clearly self-induced, although later it may become effortless and apparently involuntary: when it is complicated by secondary hypokalaemia a vicious circle may be created. Vomiting due to oesophageal obstructive lesions should be distinguished relatively easily because there is usually a progressive history of dysphagia for solids more than liquids; when obstruction becomes severe there may be regurgitation of saliva, a symptom which is never found in psychogenic vomiting.

It is not possible to consider here in any detail the interplay of organic and psychological factors in the aetiology of anorexia nervosa. It seems that although the role of endocrinological factors cannot be dismissed outright, psychological causation is paramount. Very probably a great variety of pathogenic factors may occur from childhood onwards, resulting in food avoidance as a maladaptive way of dealing with the various stresses of adolescence. Though clinically distinctive in descriptive terms, its complex aetiology, which may vary from one case to another, means that we should regard anorexia nervosa as a syndrome rather than a disease entity. The latter encourages us to over-simplify and stereotype the illness. The anorexic girl is still, for example, widely regarded as necessarily having a sexual problem, whereas it is probably more accurate to see this merely as one of a wide variety of potential causes. In treatment, individual psychotherapy undoubtedly has an important part to play in order to resolve intra-psychic difficulties, though the patient's denial of psychological problems and her hostility to intervention can make it a very difficult task, and it is still far from clear what form of psychotherapy is best. The outcome in the Maudsley follow-up series compares well with other published series and no more than supportive psychotherapy had been used. 52.5 per cent required subsequent re-admission but in only 7 per cent was more intensive psychotherapy used at a later date. The role of inter-personal factors needs much more systematic study, particularly those concerning the family. The illness usually develops within the family setting and by the quality of its reaction the family as a whole may foster the perpetuation of the illness itself. The high incidence of longstanding parental difficulties in the families of anorexic patients has long been recognised (Kay *et al.*, 1967). The Maudsley follow-up series presented a similar picture: there had been sufficient disharmony between the parents to threaten marital breakdown or even cause separation in 24 per cent of the patients, and the relationship between the family and the patient before the onset of the illness was judged to be disturbed in 22 patients (54 per cent). Further studies of family pathology would be well advised to examine certain themes common to the illness, such as attitudes towards acceptance and avoidance of food, emotional experience and self-control, shared values concerning achievements and ambition, and of course the various influences which parents exert on their children to strive and succeed.

Towards a Better Understanding of the Fasting Girl

The concept of anorexia nervosa as a primarily psychological disorder has emerged after a very chequered developmental career in which fashionable attitudes and prejudices both in society generally as well as within medicine have repeatedly clouded the issues. It is salutary to ask whether we ourselves are any better than our predecessors in understanding and helping these patients. Even when the thin girl is recognised as suffering from anorexia nervosa it is extremely difficult for those in close contact with her, family and others alike, to retain an objective approach to her problem. This may stem from the difficulty of appreciating the very real distress which she experiences when trying to eat, or perhaps it is related to our own anxiety about the dangers and uncertain outcome of this illness. We are all anxious to feed those who clearly need to be fed, but if frustrated our anxiety turns quickly to hostility and a sense of outrage at what seems to be unnecessary self-imposed disease. We still angrily reject the girl who is in so much need of help. As we have learnt more about anorexia nervosa so our optimism has grown and the specialist realises that outcome in general is good, even though the patient is initially extremely thin, resists food intake most strenuously or relapses more than once. Perhaps our most important role in treatment whatever specific approach we may adopt is to maintain a therapeutic optimism, which by preventing despair in the patient and her family and by controlling our own anxiety makes the illness more tolerable and may even hasten its resolution. We may indeed return to Gull's writing once again and remember that in his words:

None of these cases, however exhausted, are really hopeless while life exists: and for the most part the prognosis may be considered favourable.

References

Albutt, C. and Rolleston, H. D. (1911). Hysteria. In *A System of Medicine*, Vol. VIII. Macmillan & Co. Ltd., London, p. 709

Beck, J. C. and Brøchner-Mortensen, K. (1954). Observations on the prognosis in anorexia nervosa. *Acta med. scand.*, **149**, 409–430

Bliss, E. L. and Branch, C. H. H. (1960). *Anorexia Nervosa: Its History, Psychology and Biology*. Hoebner, New York

Crisp, A. H. (1965*a*). Clinical and therapeutic aspects of anorexia nervosa—a study of 30 cases. *J. Psychosom. Res.*, **9**, 67–78

Crisp, A. H. (1965*b*). Some aspects of the evolution, presentation and follow-up of anorexia nervosa. *Proc. R. Soc. Med.*, **58**, 814–820

Crisp, A. H. (1967). *A Psychosomatic Study of Anorexia Nervosa: a Controlled Study of some Aspects of the Constitution and Premorbid Feeding of Patients*. Thesis, University of London

Dally, P. (1969). *Anorexia Nervosa*. Heinemann, London

Dally, P. J. and Sargant, W. (1960). A new treatment of anorexia nervosa. *Br. med. J.*, **1**, 1770

Fowler, R. (1871). *A Complete History of the Case of the Welsh Fasting Girl (Sarah Jacob)*. Henry Renshaw, London

Gee, S. J. (1915). Nervous atrophy (Atrophia nervosa: Anorexia nervosa). In *Medical Lectures and Clinical Aphorisms*, 4th ed. Hodder and Stoughton, London

Gull, W. W. (1868). The Oxford Address in Medicine. *Lancet*, **ii**, 171–176

Gull, W. W. (1874). Anorexia nervosa (Apepsia hysterica, Anorexia hysterica). *Trans. clin. Soc.*, **7**, 22–28

Gull, W. W. (1888). Anorexia Nervosa. *Lancet*, **i**, 516–517

Kay, D. W. K. and Leigh, D. (1954). The natural history, treatment and prognosis of anorexia nervosa, based on a study of 38 patients. *J. ment. Sci.*, **100**, 411–431

Kay, D. W. K. and Schapira, K. (1965). The prognosis in anorexia nervosa. In *Anorexia Nervosa.* Symposium, Göttingen. (Ed. J. N. E. Meyer and H. Feldman), Thieme, Stuttgart

Kay, D. W. K., Schapira, K. and Brandon, S. (1967). Early factors in anorexia nervosa compared with non-anorexic groups. *J. Psychosom. Res.*, **11**, 133–139

Lasegue, C. E. (1873). On Hysterical Anorexia. Archives Generales de Medecine April 1873. In *Evaluation of Psychosomatic Concepts: Anorexia Nervosa a Paradigm.* International Psychoanalytic Library (Ed. M. R. Kaufman and M. Heiman), Hogarth Press, 1965

Mexio, Pedro (1613). Of Wonderfull Fasting. In *The Treasurie of Ancient and Modern Times*, Book VI. W. Jaggard, London, Chapter 8

Meyer, J. V. E. (1961). Das Syndrom der Anorexia Nervosa. Katamnestische Untersuchungen. *Arch. Psychiat. NervKrankh.*, **202**, 31–59

Morgan, H. G. and Russell, G. F. M. (1975). Value of family background and clinical features as predictors of long-term outcome in anorexia nervosa: four-year follow-up study of 41 patients. *Psychol. Med.*, **5**, 355–371

Morton, Richard (1694). Of a Nervous Consumption. In *Phthysiologia or a treatise of consumptions.* Smith and Walford at the Prince's Arms in St. Paul's Churchyard

Richardson, H. B. (1939). Simmonds disease and anorexia nervosa. *Archs Int. Medicine*, **63**, 1–28

Russell, G. F. M. (1970). Anorexia nervosa: its identity as an illness and its treatment. In *Modern Trends in Psychological Medicine*, Vol. **2**, Butterworths, London, pp. 130–164

Ryle, J. A. (1936). Anorexia nervosa. *Lancet*, **ii**, 893–899

Sheehan, H. C. and Summers, V. K. (1949). The syndrome of hypopituitarism. *Q. Jl Med.*, **42**, 319–378

Sheldon, J. H. (1939). In Discussion on Anorexia Nervosa. *Proc. R. Soc. Med.*, **32**, 738–740

Simmonds, M. (1914). Ueber Hypophysisschwund mit todlichem Ausgang. *Deutsche Med. Wochenschrift*, **40**, 322–323

Theander, S. (1970). Anorexia nervosa. A psychiatric investigation of 94 female cases. *Acta psychiat. scand.*, Suppl., 214

Thomä, H. (1967). *Anorexia Nervosa.* International Universities Press, New York

Warren, W. (1968). A study of anorexia nervosa in young girls. *J. Child Psychol. Psychiat.*, **9**, 27–40

SECTION 5
LESS COMMON PROBLEMS

24 Some Rarer Psychiatric Disorders

W. H. Trethowan

Owing to the heterogeneous nature of the disorders to be described, no really adequate classification is possible. For convenience, however, they have been grouped under four main headings: Disorders of Consciousness; Disorders of Ego Functioning; Paranoid States; and Certain Disorders associated with Childbearing.

Disorders of Consciousness

1. Sleep

While early waking is a common and familiar complaint in those who are depressed, of greater interest perhaps, is *hypersomnia*. This too, can be a symptom of depression in which it can be likened to a form of retreat. While most depressed patients sleep poorly, go off their food and lose weight, hypersomnic depressives tend to overeat and to become obese. It would appear that they overeat to stave off on-coming depressive feelings and, by the same token oversleep in order to escape from their problems. Possibly about 5–10 per cent of depressed persons may be placed in this category; although the nosological status of this form of depressive disorder needs to be more clearly defined. It would appear, however, that the condition has more of a neurotic than an endogenous basis; although the possibility that constitutional factors are also operative cannot be entirely discounted.

> Christine M., an obese young university law student started to sleep for about 16 hours daily, a pattern which persisted when she was placed under close observation in hospital and left to her own devices. When, after a few days, she was forcibly woken, well after normal up-and-about hours, and told she was sleeping merely in order to retreat from problems that she was unable to face, her behaviour underwent a dramatic change. She slashed her wrists and began to indulge in other forms of self-threatening behaviour. This 'acting-out' did, however, permit a new and more fruitful approach to her problems, so that finally she worked through these and returned to a more suitable career—it having been discovered during the course of various investigations that law studies were not for her.

A much rarer and more obscure variety of hypersomnia is the *Kleine—Levin syndrome*, defined by Critchley (1962) as 'periodic hypersomnia and megaphagia in adolescent males' a state also accompanied by outbursts of paranoid behaviour when awake. It must be said that neither the aetiology nor the nosological status of this condition has been fully established, so that whether it is or is not an entity cannot yet be determined. Such explanations as have been advanced as to its cause, vary from a frontal-lobe lesion (hyperphagia is, of course a recognised complication of prefrontal leucotomy), a disorder of the hypothalamus, which also may be a source of excessive appetite, to explanations which are basically psychogenic in origin. Pai (1950) who studied 67 patients with somnolence and morbid hunger came to the conclusion that it was not an entity. This, however, was well before Critchley's formulation.

In any event there would appear to be no connection between this condition and *narcolepsy*. While this disorder is also rare, though rather less so, it appears to affect both sexes. Narcolepsy occurs in two forms: symptomatic and idiopathic. A variety of brain lesions may underlie the symptomatic variety although it would appear that it is the hypothalamus which tends mostly to be involved. It is also thought that diabetes mellitus may underlie some cases. The idiopathic variety of narcolepsy was originally considered by Gowers and others to be a variant of epilepsy but this view can no longer be sustained.

There are four principal features of the condition: an undue tendency towards somnolence, often occurring at awkward times such as in the middle of eating a meal; cataplexy—a loss of muscle tone due to sudden emotion, usually surprise; hypnagogic and hypnopompic hallucinations and sleep paralysis. Except for an abnormal feeling of drowsiness all these features are by no means always present in every case. Narcolepsy may also be associated with somnambulism (Brain, 1962). Although, once again even the idiopathic variety of narcolepsy may be regarded as being of neurological rather than primarily of psychiatric origin, this is nevertheless truly a functional disorder and some psychiatrists have therefore construed it as being of psychosomatic origin (Smith, 1958). It may also be regarded as the endpoint of a continuum. Thus narcoleptic drowsiness is apt to occur under conditions in which those persons who could not justifiably be designated as suffering from the disorder to a pathological degree, are also prone to fall asleep: for example, after a meal, in a hot stuffy room, when bored, or when travelling by train, bus or car. Likewise attacks of cataplexy have as their normal equivalent being made 'weak with laughter', as a result, for example, of a comedian on the stage saying something staggeringly funny which, as the saying goes, may have his audience 'rolling in the aisles'; which statement reflects metaphorically the loss of muscle tone which excessive laughter may produce. A sudden unexpected loud noise may have a similar effect in susceptible subjects, occasionally to the point of causing them to fall to the ground.

In established narcolepsy the tendency to cataplexy may be marked:

A patient who worked as a saleslady in a well-known London store had an awkward tendency to fall down behind the counter whenever a customer made her laugh unexpectedly. Another old lady who had been a narcoleptic all her life, rounded a corner and suddenly encountered an old friend she had not seen for 20 years. She was so surprised that she fell and fractured her femur.

Narcoleptic sleep, it should be emphasised, is normal sleep although it is light sleep. Thus the sufferers are easily awakened or often wake spontaneously at intervals, thus passing much of their time 'cat-napping'. The old lady mentioned above was observed while in bed in hospital and, if undisturbed, was found to sleep approximately 20 minutes of every hour of the day. But not only was her sleep lighter by day but also by night. In consequence she, like some other narcoleptic subjects, passed much of the night half-awake, during which she was given to vivid hypnagogic hallucinations, finding some of these highly disturbing. She referred to these as her 'nightmares', although investigation proved that her experiences were much more vivid than dreams and of a hallucinatory nature.

The rarest symptom of narcolepsy is sleep paralysis. This can also occur as an isolated phenomenon and is quite common among nurses on night-duty among whom it is sometimes known as *night-nurses' paralysis*. The cause of this condition is obscure, but it would seem that it is one in which the afferent or sensory nervous system is awake and alert, while the efferent or motor system remains asleep and for a time not under voluntary control.

2. Stupor

Stupor is a state which is difficult to define exactly. In contrast to the comatose patient, the patient in stupor does not appear to be totally unaware of his surroundings, but is more or less unresponsive towards them. The profundity of the condition varies according to its cause.

Depressive stupor, the commonest variety, appears to be the extreme endpoint of psychomotor retardation. Although it may initially be difficult to get the subject to react to an appropriate stimulus he can usually be aroused after a time to the point of making some responses, however slight. This is in contrast to the patient in *catatonic stupor* who exhibits a very much greater degree of frozen immobility and lack of any responsiveness whatsoever. Curiously enough, catatonic stupor of schizophrenic origin appears to have become much rarer in recent years, so that whenever such a condition is seen the possibility of an organic rather than a schizophrenic cause should be considered, particularly encephalitis or epilepsy. Recently a series of cases of ECT-responsive catatonia as a sequel to typhoid fever have been described from Africa (Breakey and Kala, 1977), an event unlikely to be encountered in this country where typhoid is now a rarity.

Much rarer still is *manic stupor*, a very curious mixed affective state described by Kraepelin (1909–13), in which the patient, as in the case of stuporous states of other kinds, is unresponsive and immobile, whose thoughts are inhibited but whose face, at the same time, bears an expression of elation. This condition presents such an odd appearance that the inexperienced are likely to misdiagnose it as being due to schizophrenia. The same diagnostic error is sometimes made in other mixed affective states, such as depression with flight of ideas, again a somewhat rare condition, and usually seen during the transition phase from depression to mania, or vice versa, in those who suffer from cyclothymia without intervening periods of normality.

Other stuporous states include the so-called *epileptic twilight state* which can, in effect, be considered as the psychic equivalent of *epilepsia partialis continuans*; for EEG investigation reveals that the condition is a prolonged psychomotor seizure, characterised clinically by clouding of consciousness and an intense oneiroid or dream-like hallucinatory state. A not altogether dissimilar stuporous state of *'hysterical'* origin can occur as a result of profound emotional withdrawal in which the patient, although apparently conscious, lies speechless and immobile (*akinetic mutism*). In such cases the EEG will show no signs of epileptic activity. A similar type of condition may also occasionally be a complication of treatment with phenothiazines (Behrman, 1973).

Yet another condition which may resemble stupor may follow head injury. Here the patient although appearing unconscious may periodically open his eyes and, as if awake, turn his head from side to side as if inspecting his surroundings. This condition, which is sometimes known as *coma vigil* is probably a type of automatism during which the patient is actually unconscious and behaving in a purely reflex fashion.

Periodic catatonia, a condition originally described by Gjessing (1967), and said to be due to phasic variations in nitrogen balance, has been extensively reinvestigated by Jenner (1970). The catatonic bouts can be controlled by varying the patient's intake of protein and administering thyroxine. Although the condition was regarded by Gjessing as a variety of catatonic schizophrenia accounting, according to most textbooks, for about 2 per cent of cases, the available evidence suggests that it is a type of periodic psychosis which possibly bears a closer relationship to an alternating type of affective disorder rather than to schizophrenia.

Rarest of all is a variety of catatonic delirium associated with fever, which is often fatal in outcome. This, which is known as Stauder's lethal catatonia, was reviewed by Laskowska *et al.* in 1965. The condition carries a high mortality with a death rate of somewhere between a third and half of cases. Females appear to be affected more than males. The origin of the condition is obscure, there being no obvious cause of death to be found.

I have seen two cases which may possibly come into this category although only one was febrile before death, this being due to an intercurrent low-grade bronchopneumonia which was not in itself likely to have been the cause of his death. The other, a known female schizophrenic in a state of remission was afebrile. With the onset of a sudden fresh exacerbation of her condition she developed a state of intense anxiety which caused her pulse rate to rise progressively so that after 10 days it reached a rate of 200 beats per minute or more, at which point she collapsed and died. Her anxiety and rising pulse rate could not be controlled by any measures to hand at that time (although it is tempting to suppose that if beta-blocking agents had been available at the time, these might have had the desired effect). As it was, extensive ante- and post-mortem investigations revealed no cause for these events, so that in the end those who saw her were left wondering if she had not literally 'died from fright'.

3. The Ganser State

It is but a short step from stupor to those disorders in which there may or may not be some degree of clouding of consciousness but which appear primarily to affect cognition, although without having any organic component. In many of these, both depressive and what may be designated as hysterical features are intermingled.

The most striking example is that of the *Ganser syndrome*. Although many textbooks persist in describing this condition as being virtually confined to prisoners, the evidence for this is currently unconvincing. While always uncommon it appears most often to occur as a transient state among those who become depressed as a result of a sudden untoward misfortune of which imprisonment may number as one among many, and in whom the resulting state of depression leads to the mobilisation of certain hysterical features. When fully established the Ganser syndrome is characterised by clouding of consciousness, pseudodementia — as reflected by the giving of approximate answers to questions (*Vorbeireden* or, more correctly *Vorbeigehen*—Enoch *et al.*, 1967), hallucinations and a wide variety of somatic or conversion symptoms, often of a quasi-neurological kind. The most remarkable aspect of the condition is the pseudodementia which manifests itself largely by an appearance of dullness, general unresponsiveness and near-miss answers, such as to give an impression of a series of consistently inconsistent errors, which soon indicate that the subject must really know what the correct answer is. Thus two and two are said to make five; an apple is said to be a pear; a horse a cow, and so on. Pseudodementia may also become evident, in the absence of the other features of the Ganser syndrome, as part of *hysterical puerilism*, when it is usually also accompanied by other forms of childish behaviour, or may occur as part of the so-called *buffoonery state* which is a rather rare manifestation of hebephrenic schizophrenia. It has also been demonstrated experimentally that a considerable proportion of subjects asked to simulate mental disorder will produce similar responses (Anderson *et al.*, 1959).

4. Possession Syndromes

As in the case of catatonic states, gross hysterical manifestations such as *fugues, global amnesia, trance-like* and other *dissociative disorders* all appear to be becoming progressively more uncommon. The most probably reason for this is that casualty officers, psychiatrists and all those who tend to become involved with such patients now tend to adopt a rather more cynical attitude when confronted with patients who exhibit symptoms of this kind. Global amnesia is an excellent case in point, for there can be little doubt that the one-time belief in the reality of the 'lost-memory' man fostered the prolongation of his disorder, helped on, of course, by sensational press reports.

Precisely the same applies to states of supposed *demoniacal possession*, most of which appear to be of hysterical origin, although some present as a pathoplastic feature of a psychosis, usually schizophrenia or an affective disorder. Because, in Western civilisation, only a minority still believe in demoniacal possession as a reality, the occurrence of syndromes suggesting this cause has become rare. There are, however, exceptions, one of which is an outcome of immigration; it having been observed that some West Indians who are intensely religious may, on becoming psychotic, ascribe their symptoms to some diabolical cause. This, however, should be regarded more in the nature of pseudopossession. As suggested 'true' possession both is and was usually either hysterical in origin and allied therefore to trance-states, or alternatively an obsessional phenomenon, in which the 'Devil' is felt by the sufferer to be within, and exerting some effect upon his behaviour, although not, as in the case of hysterical possession, completely controlling all his actions (Oesterreich, 1966). The paradigm of this type of possession can be considered to be Gilles de la Tourette syndrome, the main features of which are convulsive tics and coprolalia, so that the subject commonly barks out obscene four-letter words or alternatively makes explosive utterances in the form of meaningless sounds. Echolalia is also an occasional feature. Although much has been written on Gilles de la Tourette's syndrome, the true origin of this disorder is still in some doubt. While there are those on the one hand who believe it to be a severe form of obsessive-compulsive illness, others have postulated that it may be of organic origin. The truth probably lies somewhere in between, there being both obsessional and organic cases and mixtures of the two.

Recently there seems, in this country, to have been an increase in the number of cases of 'possession' which in turn may have been propagated by an increased interest in exorcism; there being obviously a reciprocal relationship between the one and the other. By this is meant that the availability of an exorcist is likely to foster the notion that certain forms of abnormal behaviour may be due to demoniacal possession and vice versa (Trethowan, 1976). A watchful eye should be kept for such cases for, unchecked, they may sometimes have tragic consequences.

5. Alternating Personality

The so-called *double* or *alternating personality*, while bearing some relationship to some of those conditions already described is probably largely iatrogenic in origin, although, as has been suggested this, too, may also apply to some states of possession. It is indeed often engendered by a belief in its reality or over-zealous attention paid to it by investigators. Perhaps the best example on record is Morton Prince's (1906) case of Sally Beauchamp. The subject was also well treated in a film made a number of years ago entitled 'The Three Faces of Eve', which was said to be based on an actual case. Apart from iatrogenic influences, double personality may arise spontaneously on the basis of attention-seeking, wish-fulfilment and an over-ready tendency to dissociate. I have personally encountered one such subject who clearly demonstrated these aspects of the matter.

A 20-year-old female office worker of no particular attainments who was born and brought up in a suburb of Birmingham, was referred on account of decidedly odd behaviour. During the course of a single psychiatric interview lasting approximately one hour, she 'switched on' a secondary personality on two occasions. Initially she remained herself and gave an apparently fairly truthful account of her life and home circumstances. During her two alternate episodes she assumed a somewhat gutteral accent which could conceivably have been construed as Swedish-English, maintained she had been born and brought up in Gothenberg and recounted a series of other details which she at least seemed to believe might be appropriate to the life of a Swedish girl of somewhat superior social status. Objectively obtained information revealed that she had never left England and knew nothing at first-hand of life in Sweden. When confronted with this she seemed unaffected, but defaulted from the clinic shortly afterwards.

Ego Disorders

1. Disturbances of Ego Identity

These include a number of interesting conditions of which probably the most striking are of schizophrenic origin. They consist for the most part of alterations of self-awareness which are either intrinsic or affect the sufferer's perception of his environment, it being obvious that alterations of self-awareness and of awareness of environment are usually interdependent. Thus the schizophrenic patient is often decidedly unclear as to what constitutes himself, other persons, or even his surroundings, a feature often reflected in the paintings some schizophrenics produce. This loss of sense of personal identity may have bizarre consequences; one of the most remarkable being a disturbance of sexual identity. This is probably much commoner than generally thought, but may have to be closely enquired into before being elicited. Sometimes the patient is led to believe that his sex is actually changing and to behave as if this idea were actually true.

A huge muscular Lithuanian labourer began to suspect that he was changing into a woman and having adorned himself with a necklace and certain articles of female clothing he then examined himself in the mirror as if to find out whether his suspicion was true.

Although this may sound like an example of transvestism or trans-sexualism this was not the case, his behaviour being a direct result of a disturbance of sexual identity. Trans-sexualists, in contrast, are those who feel themselves to have the mentality of the sex opposite to their physical habitus, but are nevertheless not truly deluded, despite their tendency to seek sex-change surgery. Transvestites, who are very much more common are, of course, in quite a different category, being men whose sexual orientation is primarily heterosexual but who obtain autoerotic gratification by dressing in female clothing. The condition is allied to fetishism.

Disturbances of ego identity may lead to other bizarre schizophrenic symptoms, such as, for example, to delusions held by the patient that he is some other person altogether—one perhaps of royal birth or divine descent.

One patient became confused every time he walked along a street behind some other person because he was unsure whether he actually was himself or the person he was following. He also said, in a puzzled way 'Every time I talk to you I feel as if I am you'.

While none of these disorders is really rare they are all of great interest. Probably therefore, a disorder of ego function is the central derangement which in terms of an abnormal psychological process is the source from which all other schizophrenic symptoms flow.

2. Depersonalisation

Depersonalisation although relatively rare, is probably the commonest form of ego disorder other than those which are associated specifically with schizophrenia. Although well-known its origin is still remarkably obscure. The essential feature of the condition is an unpleasant estrangement of the self from the self, so that 'I' becomes separated from 'Me'. It is an *as if* experience, because although the subject feels that this is what has occurred, he knows that this is not actually the case. The condition is commonly, although not invariably, associated with *derealisation*; a circumstance which leads to an extension of the feeling of estrangement from the self to estrangement from the environment. Again this is an *as if* experience. Thus while the subject *knows* that his environment is as it always was, he *feels*, none the less, that it has changed in some strange way so that the trees seem less green, the sky less blue, the birds sing less loudly, and everything around appears to be removed to a greater distance, as if seen, metaphorically speaking, through the wrong end of a telescope.

Depersonalisation may occur as an isolated phenomenon, or as part of an obsessional or other neurotic state. It may occur in states of extreme exhaustion, in febrile conditions or be due to drugs—notoriously lysergic acid. It also occurs as an episodic feature of temporal lobe epilepsy.

3. Cotard's Syndrome

Gross depersonalisation is probably most commonly encountered in the severer forms of depressive illness which occur in late middle life, in which it may contribute to the formation of bizarre nihilistic delusions (*délire de négation*) in which the patient believes that his bowels are rotting away, that his body has turned to stone, that he has no alimentary tract and therefore cannot eat or drink, or even that he is dead. Not only can this be construed as a severe form of hypochondriasis but it also can be interpreted as an internalised paranoid delusional state in which the patient himself is his own accuser. Of very similar quality are those delusional conditions which appertain to size, an oft-quoted example being the patient who refused to pass water because of his fear of flooding the world.

Similarly and possibly related delusional states may occur in association with *microptic* or *Lilliputian hallucinations*. Although these miniscule hallucinations are usually regarded as of organic origin the view has also been advanced that, in psychodynamic terms, they may be interpreted as an effort by the patient to master his environment by, as it were, cutting it down to size. Such an interpretation should however, be given no more than guarded acceptance as microptic or even macroptic hallucinations are usually based on some organic disorder such as cerebral arteriopathy, leading to a disturbance of figure-ground relationships.

4. Disturbances due to Temporal Lobe Disorders

Many queer symptoms including depersonalisation may occur as features of temporal lobe epilepsy. A patient recently seen had a whole series of remarkable symptoms including auditory and visual hallucinations, and feelings of leaving his body. Most of these occurred in the hypnagogic state and only occasionally by day. However there was no doubt from electroencephalographic and other investigations that these phenomena emanated from a temporal lobe lesion. The most familiar kinds of depersonalisation experiences which occur in association with temporal lobe epilepsy are, of course, the *déjà vu* phenomenon and the considerably rarer *jamais vu* phenomenon. However, many other kinds of ego disturbance can occur. Indeed, it is virtually true to say that almost every psychiatric symptom recorded may at times present as a feature of temporal lobe epilepsy so that where there is no other cause for queer subjective sensations to be found, this disorder should always be borne in mind as a likely diagnosis.

5. The Capgras Syndrome

Because this disorder appears to be related to derealisation, although in a somewhat selective way, it is probably best considered here. The *Capgras syndrome* is a rare paranoid disorder which is most commonly a manifestation of schizophrenia although occasionally of affective origin. The essential feature is the *illusion of doubles (sosies)* in which the subject confronted by his spouse or some other family member, while agreeing that the likeness is exact, claims nevertheless that the other person is an imposter (Enoch, 1963). It has even been recorded as extending to include the family dog. Letters also, written to the subject, are believed to be forgeries although he admits that the handwriting appears exact enough. One young female student, during a primary delusional state, looked at her watch, decided it was an exact copy which had been placed on her wrist by the police and, as a consequence of this, took it off and threw it in the river.

6. Ecstacy States

Another much rarer form of ego disorder is the so-called *ecstasy state*. This could well be regarded as a state of 'hyperpersonalisation', a term which I myself have adopted, in view of the fact that in many of its aspects it appears to be a polar opposite to depersonalisation, although it is very much rarer and unlike most cases of depersonalisation tends to be transient. Whereas in the depersonalisation/derealisation syndrome the environment appears flat and dull, changed, removed to a distance and so on, in an ecstasy state the reverse seems to be true; thus trees appear greener than green, the sky bluer than blue, and everything very much more vivid, alive and intense than before, all this being associated with a special feeling of joy. Whereas in derealisation the subject seems in some mysterious way as if removed to a distance from his environment, when, in a state of ecstasy he has the singular experience of 'at oneness' with his environment. Ecstasy, quite understandably, is sometimes associated with a strongly religious content—indeed, it has even been postulated that an attack of temporal lobe epilepsy formed the basis of St Paul's conversion experience on the road to Damascus. In any event epileptics are notorious for their religiosity. Apart from temporal lobe epilepsy, ecstasy states also tend to occur during a sudden upsurge from depression to mania, although as Anderson (1938) has indicated ecstasy is not equivalent to manic elation.

An unmarried patient with long-standing cyclothymia who also had a temporal lobe abnormality underwent an intense ecstatic experience while travelling in the Holy Land. Her surroundings became intensely magnified in beauty and she herself joyous, during which experience she fell suddenly in love with a young Arab guide with whom, it should be added, she had no grounds for affinity whatsoever.

7. Autoscopy

This is another very rare condition which consists, in essence, of a visual hallucination of the self. The notion of a double or a *doppelgänger* has been popular in literature for centuries; reference being found to it in the works of a number of novelists. While sometimes considered as a figment of fancy, it is noteworthy that at least some of those authors who have used this device have themselves suffered from psychiatric disorders in which autoscopic hallucinations have been known to occur. These include Dostoievsky who suffered from epilepsy, de Maupassant who developed General Paralysis and Edgar Allan Poe who was a melancholic given to alcoholism and an epileptic as well. The French psychiatrist Lhermitte (1951) suggested that autoscopic hallucinations might be related to the disturbance of the body image. They can also occur as an epileptic phenomenon. One of my patients who was subject to temporal lobe seizures had as a so-called 'aura' an autoscopic hallucination of herself as seen from above.

Paranoid States

There is a wide variety of these which, although they may vary in content, often bear some relationship to one another and may be seen as psycho-pathological variations on a central theme.

1. Delusions of Jealousy

Many psychiatric textbooks state that *delusions of jealousy* which constitute the core of the so-called 'Othello syndrome', are particularly inclined to occur in chronic alcoholics who have either become impotent as a result of their alcoholism, or who have taken to drink, possibly as a result of sexual inadequacy. Experience clearly indicates, however, that such delusions are more closely related to the occurrence of impotence than to any underlying physical reason; for, indeed, they may occur in association with impotence due to causes other than alcoholism: for example diabetes mellitus, depression, and other disorders giving rise to acquired impotence. It is probable, therefore, that such delusions are essentially related to a feeling of defeat or shame.

2. Sensitivity Reactions

A sense of defeat or shame may also account for so-called *sensitivity reactions*, many of which lead to paranoid ideas, if not actual delusions which surround some part of the body, often the nose; which the subject believes to be misshapen to the point of attracting unfavourable comment both from strangers and others. Plastic surgeons are all too familiar with young men who seek to have the shape of their often quite normally shaped noses altered, on the grounds that some imagined deformity is interfering with their interpersonal relationships, particularly with the opposite sex. Others who are often rather more overtly psychotic believe that they smell (or that others think that they do so), having their beliefs confirmed by seeming to perceive those around them showing signs of aversion: sniffing, coughing, turning away and so on. Psychodynamic theories have it that such subjects have latent homosexual trends which they would strongly disavow. While this may be true of some cases, it is possibly the basic feeling of shame that is more important than what it is that the subject actually feels guilty about. Although often regarded as suffering from schizophrenia, further investigation often reveals that there is a considerable degree of underlying depression in these cases, so that their condition may sometimes respond favourably to adequate antidepressive therapy.

3. Erotomania

This condition takes several forms, ranging from an essentially neurotic disorder which can be regarded as a highly exaggerated 'crush' to a full blown paranoid reaction with or without associated schizophrenic symptoms, in which the principal delusion is one of being loved usually by some seemingly important person who is often a public figure. It is characteristic of all varieties of erotomania that the loved one (or the person whom the subject believes loves him or more usually her) is usually unattainable by reason of differing social status, on account of being already married, being homosexual and thus unmarriageable, or something of the kind. The condition is closely related to delusions of jealousy, it being in a sense the same condition turned, as it were, inside out (Fish, 1967). Where it occurs in pure form, that is unaccompanied by other psychotic manifestations, it is sometimes known as *de Clérambault's syndrome*. Most characteristically it affects middle-aged spinsters (very rarely males) who develop the belief that some exalted person is in love with them but will not admit it. At first the notion of 'confrontation' by the beloved one is apparently eagerly entertained but, with the passage of time, as this anticipated event does not occur, the amorous delusion changes to one of persecution, in the sense that the subject begins to accuse the object of affection, of following her about or otherwise tormenting her; he often knowing nothing of the matter until she takes some action such as informing the police. As has been suggested this form of erotomania which, perhaps a little cruelly, has also been called 'Old Maid's Insanity' (Hart, 1921) has a neurotic equivalent, in which, for example, a young girl may develop a prolonged and more than usually intense passion for her priest, doctor, or some star of stage or screen or some other person to whom she feels strongly attracted, but who is quite out of reach.

4. Delusions of Infestation

These, which are yet another form of paranoid hypochondriasis, sometimes present problems which are extremely difficult to unravel. Those who suffer complain of insects crawling over the skin or in various bodily orifices, about which they may be obsessed or deluded. The difficulty of evaluating such states is well illustrated by a recent example:

> A patient complained, in terms which left little doubt that her notions had a strong delusional basis, that her house was infested with fleas, bed-lice, thrips and other parasites. When confronted with the suggestion that matters might not be all that they seemed to be, she produced a piece of paper which listed no less than five different kinds of insect which she had collected and sent to the Natural History Museum for identification. This understandably produced a therapeutic deadlock as well as providing a ready illustration of the fact that it is possible for a patient to have obsessions or even paranoid delusions about matters of fact, a paradox with which it can be extremely difficult, if not impossible, to deal.

5. Folie à Deux

One of the most remarkable forms of paranoid state is *folie à deux*. Here one person who develops a paranoid psychosis, who is thought to be the more intelligent or dominant of the two, gradually imposes it upon his or her partner. Although some have considered that the partners should not be blood-relatives for, in this event, hereditary factors may be operative, none the less about 90 per cent of the reported cases have a common heredity. Sometimes more than two persons may develop a similar psychosis, thus one may speak of *folie à trois, à quatre, à cinq*, or where a whole family is involved, *folie à famille*. While the initial description of *folie à deux* has been attributed to Lasègue and Falret (1877) the condition was in actual fact described well before then by Baillarger (1860), who gave the first really comprehensive account. A number of varieties of the condition have been described. These include *folie imposée*, in which the more forceful individual imposes his delusion on the partner; *folie simultanée*, in which the same delusion arises spontaneously in both partners; *folie communiquée*, where the person developing a secondary psychosis shares the delusions of the first person in the beginning but, in the course of time, his own psychosis expands and assumes an autonomy of its own; and *folie induite*— the rarest form of all—where two unrelated patients confined in a psychiatric hospital influence one another and come to share the same delusions. These sub-divisions, it must be admitted, are not only somewhat academic but, in practice it is often difficult if not impossible to distinguish in any particular case which is which.

The principal criteria which give birth to a *folie à deux* relationship are first the occurrence of a paranoid psychosis in the inducer; secondly a prolonged and intimate association of both partners; thirdly, the relative isolation of both from the community and, lastly, a personality disorder or latent psychotic tendency in the recipient which, after an initial period of resistance, leads him to accept the inducer's delusions. Separation of the two affected partners does not necessarily bring about a resolution of the condition of either, although this is said to be more likely in the recipient or passive partner in cases of *folie imposée*.

Disorders Associated with Childbearing

Not much need be said of post-partum mental illnesses since these are common and usually differ in no essential respect from other mental disorders which occur without any relationship whatsoever to pregnancy. A possible exception, however, is *oneirophrenia*, a form of acute schizophrenia which may occasionally be encountered. As clouded consciousness may be a prominent and presenting feature it may bear, at first sight, a close resemblance to a toxic confusional state for which it may be mistaken.

1. Pseudocyesis

False pregnancy or *pseudocyesis* is an extremely uncommon condition which has also been observed in animals. In humans it takes two forms: a hysterical variety which occurs in younger women and may be accompanied by amenorrhoea and tumescence of the abdomen and sometimes by signs of 'quickening' brought about apparently by flickering movements of the abdominal musculature. The abdominal swelling which occasionally deceives even experienced obstetricians, at least for a time, is not due, as is sometimes thought, to aerophagy but to downward pressure of the diaphragm and lordosis of the lumbar spine (Simpson, 1872). Thus if the swelling is reduced by pressure or under anaesthesia, there is no escape of flatus.

The second variety of pseudocyesis occurs in older usually childless and often unmarried women around the time of the menopause. This variety is not accompanied by abdominal swelling or other physical manifestations of false pregnancy but is more akin to paranoid hypochondriasis. In both types however, there is clearly an underlying element of wish-fulfilment.

2. The Couvade Syndrome

Abdominal swelling resembling pregnancy can occur as a very rare manifestation of the otherwise fairly common *Couvade syndrome* (Trethowan, 1968, 1972). Although when it does occur, its basis appears to be identical with the false tumescence of female pseudocyesis, the subject does not entertain the notion that he is pregnant, this despite the fact that delusions of pregnancy although rare are not unknown in psychotic male patients. The Couvade syndrome is a psychosomatic disorder more usually expressed by the occurrence of digestive or other abdominal symptoms which appear for the most part to be an outcome of anxiety over the pregnancy or labour of the spouse. In the earlier months of pregnancy loss of appetite, nausea and morning sickness and toothache are the commonest symptoms. These may persist during the wife's pregnancy or disappear for a few months, only to be replaced at the time the wife starts labour, by abdominal cramp-like pains. All these symptoms tend to disappear spontaneously as soon as labour is complete (Trethowan and Conlon, 1965). Often their origin passes unrecognised; although in some cases an interpretation of their likely cause may bring about a resolution of all symptoms.

Various theories have been advanced to account for the occurrence of this strange disorder. These include jealousy over a woman's ability to bear children (dubious); anxiety on the part of the husband at having placed his wife in jeopardy (more feasible); and a strong sense of empathy and identification together with a willingness to share in her experience (possibly the most reasonable hypothesis of all). It should be noted, however, that none of these explanations is mutually exclusive.

Acknowledgement

Although much new material has been added, this chapter is based considerably on a paper entitled 'Obscure Psychiatric Disorders' first published as part of a 'Symposium on Practical Psychiatry', published in *The Practitioner* in January 1973, **210**, 96–104. The author is grateful for permission to use some of the material originally presented in this paper.

References

Anderson, E. W. (1938). *J. Neurol. Psychiat.*, **1**, 1–20
Anderson, E. W., Trethowan, W. H. and Kenna, J. C. (1959). *Acta psychiat. scand.*, **34**, Suppl., 132
Baillarger, J. G. F. (1860). *Gaz. Hôp., Paris*, **33**, 149
Behrman, S. (1973). *Br. J. Psychiat.*, **121**, 599–604
Brain, Lord (1962). *Diseases of the Nervous System*, 6th ed. Oxford University Press, London
Breakey, W. R. and Kala, A. K. (1977). *Br. med. J.*, **2**, 357–59
Critchley, M. (1962). *Brain*, **85**, 627–56
Enoch, M. D. (1963). *Acta psychiat. scand.*, **39**, 437–62
Enoch, M. D., Trethowan, W. H. and Barker, J. C. (1967). *Some Uncommon Psychiatric Syndromes*, John Wright, Bristol
Fish, F. (1967). *Clinical Psychopathology*. John Wright, Bristol

Gjessing, R. (1967). *Somatology of Periodic Catatonia*, Pergamon Press, Oxford

Hart, B. (1921). *The Psychology of Insanity*, Cambridge University Press, Cambridge

Jenner, F. A. (1970). The physiology and biochemistry of periodic psychoses including periodic catatonia. In *Biochemistry, Schizophrenia and Affective Illnesses* (Ed. H. Himwich), Williams & Wilkins, Baltimore

Kraepelin, E. (1909–13). *Psychiatry*, 8th edn. Thieme, Leipzig

Lasègue, C. and Falret, J. (1877). *Arch. gén. Méd., Paris*, **30**, 257–97

Laskowska, D., Urbaniak, K. and Jus, A. (1965). *Br. J. Psychiat.*, **111**, 254–57

Lhermitte, J. (1951). *Br. med. J.*, **1**, 431–34

Oesterreich, T. K. (1966). *Possession, Demoniacal and Other, among Primitive Races, in Antiquity, the Middle Ages, and Modern Times*. University Books, New York

Pai, M. N. (1950). *Br. med. J.*, **1**, 522–24

Prince, M. (1906). *The Dissociation of a Personality*. Longmans, New York

Simpson, Sir J. (1872). *Clinical Lectures on Diseases of Women*, Black, Edinburgh

Smith, C. M. (1958). *J. ment. Sci.*, **104**, 593–607

Trethowan, W. H. (1968). *J. psychosom. Res.*, **12**, 107–15

Trethowan, W. H. (1972). In *Modern Perspectives in Psycho-obstetrics* (Ed. J. G. Howells), Oliver & Boyd, Edinburgh

Trethowan, W. H. (1976). *J. med. Ethics*, **2**, 127–37

Trethowan, W. H. and Conlon, M. F. (1965). *Br. J. Psychiat.*, **111**, 57–66

25 Arsonists and the Psychiatrist

M. Faulk

Historical Background

Esquirol in 1835 in his *Text Book of Mental Disorder* showed that arson could be due to mental illness. He had borrowed his case histories from Dr Marc's essay of 1833. The descriptions indicate that although firesetting might be due to jealousy or revenge as well as attempts by criminals to cover other offences, there were certainly cases which were associated with hallucinations and delusions, dementia, subnormality and epilepsy. At that time a diagnosis of monomania was in fashion. This diagnosis was made where the patient demonstrated an abnormal preoccupation and thus the term 'pyromania' for recurrent arsonists came about. Several threads about the psychopathology of firesetting run through the literature. Some workers believe that 'pyromania' was a real illness characterised by the presence of an irresistible impulse. This clearly would have, and indeed did have in Germany, substantial legal consequences in terms of responsibility and insanity of the offender. Antagonists of this view held there was no such entity as 'pyromania' and generally insisted that a motive could always be found. The development of this argument, which seems to have persisted into the second half of the nineteenth century, was described in detail by Lewis and Yarnell (1951).

The second area of discussion was the sex and age of arsonists. Early German writers (from clinical experience) believed that the bulk of firesetters were adolescent female domestic servants. A number believed that this reflected disorders of pubertal development, while others pointed to the difficulties and loneliness experienced by such people away from their own homes. A third group of workers were concerned to explain firesetting as the outcome of many different conditions, sometimes psychiatric (illness, etc.) or non-psychiatric (jealousy, criminal causes, etc.) The psychiatric conditions included, of course, concepts now considered archaic, for example the influence of genital development on the brain or bloodstream and the theories of pathological inheritance and moral degeneration.

There seems to have been, throughout the latter half of the nineteenth century, a recurrent theme connecting either sexual development or sexual fantasy with firesetting. Early hypotheses were very organic, for example, Lewis and Yarnell refer to Osiander (1813) who appears to have believed that during puberty arterial blood was diverted to the genitals depriving the organs of sight of such blood, which made these organs irritable and requiring light. This need 'caused the individual to make fires'. Later writers began to draw attention to the psychological associations between firesetting and sexual activity. Firesetting was seen sometimes as an outlet for sadistic impulses and sometimes as an outlet for frustrated sexual desires. Attention was drawn to the use of language in the descriptions of the passions—'aflame with desire'. In 1914 Schmidt gave the first description of a man who had masturbated while watching a fire he had set. This association of fires and disturbed sexual feelings was discussed a great deal in the first quarter of this century, culminating in Stekel's work in 1924. He had observed sexual difficulties in some firesetters, particularly impotence and frigidity, and postulated three possible relationships with masturbation and firesetting. First, masturbation may occur during the fire with sadistic, destructive fantasies, the fire being a sort of fetish. Secondly, masturbation may be a defence against the arson impulse, that is to say, during an enforced abstinence from masturbation, arson would occur as a relief of tension. Thirdly, arson may free the masturbator from the habit which was producing marked guilt and anxiety and tension. The field was now set for formal surveys.

Surveys

The classical study and biggest survey in this field was done in the United States by Lewis and Yarnell and published in 1951. They reviewed two thousand case records of Fire Underwriters which gave accounts of incendiary fires, that is those which were not accidental. They then made an intensive study of those cases in which there was information and they hoped that this was a representative sample. The study also incorporated additional cases from Fire Marshalls, Psychiatric Clinics and Institutions, and in addition thoroughly reviewed current arrests. A follow-up study was attempted but this was not completed. Although their sampling was uneven and statistically unsophisticated, they ended up with the records of 1145 men over the age of 16, 238 below 16 and 201 females. Arson constituted only 0.1 per cent of all major crimes (murder constituting 1 per cent and rape 0.9 per cent), and tended to occur in waves, perhaps due to imitation of notorious cases.

The peak incidence occurred at 17 years with minor peaks in the 40s and 60s. Lewis and Yarnell classified the arsonists into two major groups. The first group consisted of those who had lit only a few fires and had little interest in the ritual of firemen or in assisting firemen, or in watching the fire. These included psychotic persons, those motivated by anger, revenge and jealousy, and those who were covering up a crime, committing an insurance fraud or driven by political motives. The use of firesetting for such clear motives is well described by D.F. Scott (1974).

The second big group consisted of those who were associated with a number of fires, whose interest was primarily in the fire, not in the object destroyed and whose interest was, perhaps, in watching the fire or the associated activities and enjoying the excitement or attempting to be seen as heroes. Tramps and migrant workers were described, who, although claiming revenge on society as a reason for the fire, were really using the fire to dispel feelings of depression and oppression. Also included were a few men who were sexually aroused by fire. However, much the biggest group of all in terms of numbers were those who were impelled to make fires for no reason that they could articulate—the real so-called irresistible impulse groups or 'pyromaniacs'.

Psychiatric classification of all the males showed that 10 per cent were schizophrenic, 10 per cent were otherwise psychotic and 50 per cent were of subnormal intelligence. A psychopathic personality with or without one of these aforementioned was the commonest diagnosis. Lewis and Yarnell found that 10 per cent or 20 per cent of firesetters, regardless of age, had some recorded sexual delinquency, and 4 per cent admitted to some definite sexual satisfaction from setting the fires. Half their cases had a previous offence, ranging from petty offences to manslaughter, and up to 30 per cent had been in an institution. They paint a picture of a very handicapped group of people. One third were found to repeat fire raising incidents after arrest but there may be a delay of years between incidents. The incendiaries who were potential recidivists seemed to be those whose fires centred upon a struggle for masculine ascendancy in the community; this group included all the pyromaniacs, some revenge firesetters and some paranoid firesetters. The impulsive firesetter does not lose his impulse easily; the revenge firesetter may repeat if he has a basically immature paranoid personality; and the fire fetishist is a very dangerous person and must be confined for long periods.

Studies in Institutions

Surveys from institutions must necessarily be biased because their population has been specially selected. Conclusions from such surveys should be generalised with great care. In the Broadmoor Hospital (a Secure Hospital catering for dangerous mentally abnormal offenders) Fry and Le Couteur found that arsonists accounted for 1 per cent of the intake, with males outnumbering females 10 to 1. A high percentage came from broken homes, institutions and orphanages and, the sample was heavily weighted with psychotic patients (75 per cent suffered from schizophrenia). Yarnell's classification was found to be useful but many people fell into several categories. A further group was added—'the cry for help' group—whose behaviour is likened to a suicidal gesture, in a depressive state or in difficult and deteriorating social circumstances. It was very difficult to estimate the dangerousness of patients and gauge the time for discharge. Some patients unexpectedly did well and others failed having been discharged as no longer appearing disturbed. The value of the restriction order is emphasised, even a brief recall to Broadmoor had a very chastening effect on unwanted or potentially dangerous behaviour.

McKerracher and Dacre (1966) studied patients referred for tests of conditioning to the Psychology Department at Rampton Hospital (a Special Hospital for dangerous mentally abnormal offenders, particularly the sub-normal). Earlier observations, that arsonists seem to have a more normal GSR response than other offenders, were not confirmed although their results were in the same direction. Arsonists committed fewer sexual offences and were less aggressive than the other patients in the Rampton control group but were more suicidal and more psychotic. This was interpreted as indicating that the arsonist is unable to express aggression directly, and displaces it to fire-raising instead. The lower sexual offending rate may also mean a sublimation of this energy into arson due to severe inhibition of normal behaviour. Hurley and Monahan (1969) compared 50 arsonists who have been through Grendon Prison (a prison specialising in the treatment of mentally disturbed offenders, particularly those with psychopathic disorders) with 100 non-arson offenders at Grendon. These arsonists (who mainly suffered from personality disorder) had committed fewer previous offences than the other Grendon inmates though the pattern of these offences was similar. Ten per cent of the arsonists had previous offences of arson but 40 per cent of the arsonists had no previous offence. The range of motivations was as described by Lewis and Yarnell. Although 3 of the 50 had sexual excitation at the fire itself the incidence of sexual maladjustment among the arsonists did not differ from that in the control group. They were unable to find criteria to distinguish those with repeated firesetting from those with only one arson offence.

Tennent et al. (1971) compared 56 female patients from English Special Hospitals who had a history of arson, with a control group. In this particular study, the arsonists had more symptoms relating to sexual disturbance than the controls, that is more dysmenorrhea, promiscuity and prostitution associated with negative feelings about sex. Psychiatric symptomatology was similar in the two groups but personality disorder as a secondary diagnosis was more common in the arsonist. The over-all impression, however, is of similarity between the female arsonist and her non-arson counterpart in Rampton. Although there was a high incidence of sexual disability, only in very few cases could the firesetting be related to a specific sexual anxiety. They discussed their findings in the light of two main explanations of arson

(1) that there is a disturbed sexual development which leads to a sublimation of energy into arson, or
(2) that arsonists are inhibited aggressive people.

Either hypothesis fits the findings, though the Grendon findings do not support the sexual hypothesis. They make a third suggestion; that the early separation and environmental experience leads to poor tolerance of frustration, though it is still puzzling why patients choose arson to deal with their tension.

Dangerousness

From these studies, a picture is built up of the arsonist as a severely handicapped person, committing grave offences, causing considerable anxiety among those who have to estimate his dangerousness, and likely to have a substantial recidivism rate. Soothill and Pope (1973) studied the documentary evidence on 67 offenders convicted of arson in a Higher Court in England and Wales in 1951, and then checked for recidivism by consulting the Records Office for the next 20 years. The offenders received all grades of sentences for the arson varying from fines through probation to imprisonment up to 14 years and including hospital orders. Over the follow-up period only three were reconvicted of arson and one was found guilty of malicious damage due to firesetting, whilst 52 per cent were reconvicted for a standard list offence. Thus whereas almost half did not re-offend, 4 per cent set fires, 3 per cent committed a sexual offence, 7 per cent a violent offence, 13 per cent property damage and 25 per cent committed property or motoring offences. Where the arson was the first conviction, 66 per cent did not re-offend and only one repeated the firesetting. Where there had been previous offences 10 per cent repeated the arson, that is, 3 out of the 38. Although undiscovered arsonists would be missed, arson, from these figures, does not have a high repeat rate, especially when it is a first offence. This conclusion, until confirmed, must remain *sub judice*, particularly as it does not, at first sight, match clinical experience or the findings of Lewis and Yarnell. The assessment of dangerousness in individual cases has been discussed by Scott (1977) who draws attention to understanding the act both in terms of the individual's history as well as the current situation. From clinical experience, factors which may be taken to increase the suspicion of dangerousness in fire-raising unless treatment is provided, include:

(1) history of previous fires;
(2) firesetting associated with psychosis;
(3) firesetting associated with severe subnormality or dementia;
(4) marked pleasure in the firesetting as such, for example sexual excitement;
(5) an awareness expressed by the patient of associations with sadistic activity;
(6) an awareness by the patient of a recurrent overwhelming urge to set fires, often as a relief for tension, anxiety or depression.

Case Histories, Treatment and Management

A classification of arsonists is outlined in table 25.1. This classification is based on that by Lewis and Yarnell (1951) with modifications derived from other studies. Unfortunately for investigators, patients frequently fall into several classifications at the same time and there can be no perfect classification scheme. The following are examples of the type of problem seen in clinical practice and illustrate the sub-groups in the above classifications, with discussion of management to illustrate the wide variety of causes and disposals.

Table 25.1
Classification of Arsonists

Group I. The fire as a means to an end

Relatively Few Fires
1. Deluded, psychotic patients
(the fire is directed by the delusion or disturbed emotion)
2. Revenge/anger/jealousy states
(aimed at a specific target)
3. Cry for help states
(the act draws attention to their plight)
4. Covering up evidence of a crime
5. Insurance fraud
6. Political motives
7. Gang activity for excitement
(adolescents)

Relatively More Fires
1. Desire to be seen as a hero
(may act bravely at the scene of the fire)
2. Desire to feel powerful
(enjoys the feeling of having caused all the commotion)
3. Desire to earn money
(part-time firemen who are paid for their trips)

Group II. The fire as the focus of interest

1. Irresistible impulse group
(inarticulate but aware of a repeated urge)
2. Sexual excitement group
(sexually aroused by fires)
3. Anti-depressive or anxiety reducing group
(impulse firesetting in disturbed emotional states, often associated with inadequate personality)

Group I. The Fire as a Means to an End

Relatively Few Fires

1. Psychotic Patient
Case A
A middle-aged seaman recently increased his intake of alcohol substantially. He became abstinent and within a week developed a schizophreniform

psychosis as a consequence of alcohol withdrawal. He thought people on the ship were trying to kill him. He saw no way out except to kill himself by setting fire to his cabin to escape his 'persecutors'. He was arrested and charged with arson on the high seas. Assessment by a psychiatrist on his return to England showed that his psychosis was much improved and the prognosis was thought to be good. There was no previous history of offences and especially no history of fire-raising. He had a good marriage and his wife was prepared to have him back. From a psychiatric point of view, therefore, it seemed that if his psychosis could be relieved, the chance of his re-offending would be minimal. He was prepared to accept treatment. In the Report to Court it was stated that he had been mentally ill at the time of the offence and that his offending was largely a result of his mental illness. Even though it was associated with alcohol he could not have anticipated that stopping drinking would have produced such a severe mental reaction. It was recommended that his sentence should ensure continued treatment initially in hospital, and later as an out-patient; and that the treatment be a condition of probation, so that if he then required further treatment it would be possible to insist on his return to hospital. A disposal under Section 60 of the Mental Health Act of 1959 would have been possible, but this has the disadvantage that the longer treatment follow-up possible under probation supervision is not so easy to organise.

2. The Revenge/Anger Group
Case B
An immature, isolated man of 20, superficially plausible but without deep emotional relationships, mistrustful and hypersensitive, was employed in a large store. He had an altercation with his manager at the store and that evening in a state of anger and resentment he set fire to a pile of cardboard cases in the storeroom. At interview he was found to be superficially pleasant almost to the point of unctuousness. In view of his youth and the extent of the damage, the Court requested a Psychiatric Report. During examination it become clear that he suffered from neither mental illness nor subnormality, but the history of his emotional development and relationships revealed the difficulties in his personality. Where there is no associated history of persistent firesetting or other destructive or dangerous activities, and the motivation is simply anger, the law usually takes its course and the offender can expect a prison sentence, despite the personality difficulties. If, as in this case, the patient had previously set fires of a similar nature, and had also shown dangerous, aggressive behaviour in other spheres (such as sexual assaults or even rape), then the case falls within the Mental Health Act definition of psychopathic disorder. Under the present legislation such patients may well have to be considered for Special Hospital because their history suggests they may be an immediate danger to others. Should this be the case, then an application to the Department of Health and Social Security would have to be made by two doctors, agreeing on the diagnosis and the disposal for admission to a Special Hospital under Section 60 of the Mental Health Act.

Alternatively where there has been persistent dangerous behaviour the Court may take the view that a life sentence or a very long sentence would be the more appropriate disposal. Once the patient is in prison or Special Hospital, attempts should be made to offer treatment—generally psychotherapy to increase the man's self-perception and improve his social functioning, where necessary (for example in cases of persistent high tension) with appropriate medication.

3. Cry for Help State

Case C

A patient with chronic schizophrenia in his mid-30s was discharged after several years in hospital. After an argument in his lodgings he left in a state of indignation and wandered around the countryside becoming increasingly despondent. He slept rough and one night set fire to a barn. He was arrested, charged with arson, and remanded in custody as he had by then lost his lodgings and his behaviour was not understood. Psychiatric assessment was requested by the Court in view of his psychiatric history and it was clear that at the time of the offence he was not floridly psychotic. His act of firesetting could be understood as an attempt to draw attention to his plight, for there was no evidence of it being directly due to a delusion or hallucination. He was very willing to accept further hospital care and treatment and was admitted to a local hospital under Section 60 of the Mental Health Act.

The Judge, believing that the man was still very potentially dangerous to the public, placed restrictions on his discharge, unlimited in time, under Section 65 of the Mental Health Act. The patient rapidly settled into the hospital routine and his mood and mental state soon became normal. After some months, application was made to the Home Office for permission for him to obtain work in the community. If this is successful then application will be made for him to become an out-patient. The decision to take him into an ordinary hospital was based on the lack of a history of firesetting or other dangerous behaviour and the presence of an understandable precipitating cause.

Case D

A very conscientious married man in his late 20s had run into occupational and domestic difficulties. He had been made redundant and he was unable to meet his financial responsibilities. His wife had put a certain amount of pressure on him not realising how earnestly he would treat her demands. Under these various stresses he became more depressed and tearful and, following yet another rejection for a job, he set fire to his house. At first it was thought he had set the fire to obtain the insurance money, but later this explanation was discarded. He was, nevertheless, charged with setting a fire which might endanger the lives of other people in the building. A Psychiatric Report was requested in view of the bizarreness of his behaviour. Considering his previous ability, the history of the recent depressive episode, his despondency at his predicament and his inability to see his way out of it, his firesetting could be understood as a cry for help. The incident brought his difficulties out into the open, and his family rushed to his aid. From the psychiatric point of view the chance of his setting further fires seemed remote and this explanation of his behaviour and the offer of out-patient treatment was put to the Court.

4. Covering up Evidence of a Crime

Such cases are unlikely to come a psychiatrist's way but may do so if the whole situation seems bizarre enough. What is required is that the psychiatrist makes sure that he has seen, as in all cases, all the relevant statements (depositions) which are made to the Court. The depositions can be supplied either by solicitors or the Court itself. A study of the depositions often throws light on what appears to be a perplexing event, especially if the patient is attempting to mislead the psychiatrist about the nature of the act. A psychiatrist may be involved where a serious crime such as murder has been committed and the accused has attempted to hide the body or evidence of the crime by setting fire to the building in which the body or crime rests. The assessment of the patient should follow the usual psychiatric routine and this, taken in conjunction with the evidence from the statements, will allow the psychiatrist to make a judgement about the man's mental state. The crime itself will not guide the psychiatrist to the patient's mental state; one may find psychotic patients, subnormal or just very angry patients setting fires for this purpose.

5. Insurance Fraud

It is unlikely that a psychiatrist will be asked to see such a case except where the accused has a history of mental illness, or there is a suspicion of mental illness. Descriptions of insurance frauds for gain are given by Scott (1974). The treatment, if required, will depend on the underlying disorder.

6. Political Motives

It is unlikely that a psychiatrist will be asked to see a person who has set a fire for this purpose unless someone has been killed, in which case the accused may well be charged with murder, and psychiatric reports are generally provided in all such cases of homicide. Most politically motivated firesetting will be committed by people who do not suffer from mental illness or subnormality, and such people are often at great pains to point out that their action is that of a sane and reasonable man. Some may have a history of personality instability but generally a hospital disposal in such cases would be found to be inappropriate, and the law will take its course.

7. Gang Activities for Excitement

This group contains young, often immature, people who work themselves up into a state of excitement during which they may commit various offences, including arson, for which there seems to be a very good prognosis from the re-offending point of view. They are unlikely to be seen by a psychiatrist as on the whole they are not seriously disturbed. One sometimes sees, however, cases where there is one very disturbed member influencing a group of relatively normal boys to indulge in wild behaviour, or cases where a disturbed youth attempts to gain attention or status with other youths by behaving in a dangerous way. The important point is that the relatively normal youths are unlikely to set further fires once the dominating leader or disturbed youth is separated from them.

Group I. Relatively more Fires

1. Desire to be Seen as a Hero
Cases have been described of men with rather inadequate personalities with low self-esteem, who construct a situation in which they may appear to be a hero. They will set a fire, call the fire brigade and rush to the rescue of the people caught in the blaze in the hope of capturing the admiration of others and of seeing themselves the hero of the day, reported in the newspapers, etc. The long-term follow-up studies do not clarify whether this motivation in itself necessarily means a bad prognosis. One might expect that supportive therapy might be very helpful to some such men.

2. Desire to Feel Powerful
Cases are described of inadequate men of low status who obtain considerable satisfaction in setting a fire, and standing back and watching all the commotion, reading about it the next day.

Case E
A middle-aged man with a history of numerous offences of theft and one of firesetting had spent most of his adult life in prison and had no roots or friends in the community. He was charged with a further case of firesetting. It appeared that he had been feeling despondent and knew from his previous experience that he would feel better if he were to set a fire. His pattern was as described above. In the absence of any formal mental illness or hope that a hospital approach would influence his behaviour, he received a prison sentence. This case overlaps in motivation with the tension reducing group.

3. Desire to Earn Money
Cases have been described where part-time firemen have deliberately created work for themselves by setting fires. Such cases are unlikely to come the way of a psychiatrist and usually receive prison or other penal sentences.

Group II. The Fire as the Focus of Interest

1. Irresistible Impulse Group

People in this group are aware of a repeated urge to set fires which they do not appear fully to understand, and when questioned about it are very inarticulate. They usually have a history of setting several fires before being caught, and the fires often seem to escalate in severity. It appears as if the offender has an increasing feeling of tension which the firesetting releases.

Case F

A man of 50 who had spent most his adult life in prison for violent behaviour, mainly aggressive sexual assaults, was taken into hospital and received anti-libidinal treatment. After 2 or 3 years of apparently settling down well, it was discovered that he had set a fire which had led to considerable destruction. It then became clear on questioning him that in fact he had been setting fires intermittently for several months. He had seemed through this period to be quite well and he was quite unable to explain his motivation. The nearest he could come to it was to talk of a feeling of anger or tension which was relieved by setting the fire. He also was aware that the urge was likely to persist and stated that he could not say that he would now stop setting fires. In this man's case, in view of the fact that he was also subnormal and had a long history of violence, an application was made, on the grounds of his subnormality and psychopathic disorder, for his admission to a Special Hospital. He was transferred under Section 60 of the Mental Health Act. The Judge placed a restriction order on his discharge unlimited in time, under Section 65 of the Mental Health Act. One could speculate whether the suppression of his sexual feelings had led to the firesetting or whether his sexual attacks were really expressions of anger or resentment stemming from the frustrations in his childhood, and that this anger or resentment became diverted to other activity. It is expected that, with time, his tension and urge to set fires will die down; it will then be appropriate to transfer him back to an open hospital.

Case G

A subnormal man, aged 30, was charged with breaking and entering. He had broken into a garage and then set fire to it. At first he said he had set the fire because he was angry that he had been unable to find anything to steal. Information from his Probation Officer, however, made it clear that the man was in fact much more disturbed than this, and that he had set other fires. On further interview, the man admitted that he had the recurrent urge to set fires which he could not explain. He feared that the firesetting would continue. In view of his subnormality and his dangerousness, an application was made to a Special Hospital where he was transferred under Section 60 of the Mental Health Act with a restriction order under Section 60/65.

2. Sexual Excitement Group

Although fire as a fetish was once thought to be a common cause of firesetting, men who are directly sexually stimulated by fires seem to be rare. Cases are described in the literature of people being sexually aroused by the fire they have set, but surveys, as already discussed, indicate that these are a very small proportion of the firesetters. There is no clear management of such men. Some receive prison sentences and receive psychotherapy at prisons such as Grendon. Others may, depending on how dangerous they are, find themselves with very long prison sentences, or be admitted to Special Hospitals. The motivation seems so bizarre in these cases that a psychiatric approach would seem desirable and necessary and the treatment would be that of fetishism or sexual deviation, though it is usually believed that the prognosis must be very guarded.

3. Anti-Depressive or Anxiety Reducing Group

In this group the principal motivation for setting a fire is the discovery by the patient that the act will make him feel better during periods of extreme despondency or tension. This group overlaps with the 'irresistible impulse' group and with the 'cry for help' states. Their management depends on how easily one feels one can reduce the depression or anxiety, either by offering asylum in hospital, supportive therapy as an out-patient, with or without medication, or whether it is necessary to contain the man in a more secure establishment until, through time and treatment, he has matured and gained greater self-control.

Case H

An isolated 19-year-old boy from an apparently stable family was arrested for setting fire to a shed and it became apparent on interview that he had been setting fires to various objects for a number of years. He described in a rather inarticulate way periods of increasing despondency at which time he would set a fire with a relief of his inner tension. He had great difficulty in relating to others, particularly girls, and had developed a fetish for female underclothes. He was of borderline, subnormal intelligence, and loneliness and frustration were his common emotional states. He was remanded for reports because of his behaviour. It was felt that the combination of his personality difficulties and dull intelligence was such that he required treatment. It seemed unlikely that out-patient supervision or simple measures would suffice. Application was successfully made to a Special Hospital in view of his dangerousness. This case illustrates how firesetting might be related to tension states arising from both social and sexual difficulties, but also it is an interesting example of the associations sometimes seen in individual cases between sexual difficulties and firesetting.

Summary of Management

The important theme which runs through the study of firesetting is that the causes are numerous. People will set fires for many reasons and in many different psychological states. Management is equally variable and can vary from out-patient supervision to containment in high security conditions. Points which would guide the doctor would be the persistence of the firesetting, underlying mental disturbance and historical background as described in the preceding section on dangerousness.

References

Esquirol, J. E. D. (1965). *Mental Maladies. Treatise on Insanity*, Hafner, London

Fry, J. F. and Le Couteur, B. (1966). Arson. *Medico-Legal J.*, **XXXIV**, 108–121

Hurley, W. and Monahan, T. M. (1969). Arson: the criminal and the crime. *Br. J. Crimin.*, **9**, 4–21

Lewis, N. D. C. and Yarnell, H. (1951). Pathological firesetting. *Nervous and Mental Disease Monographs*, No. 82. New York

Marc, M. (1833). Considérations medico-légales sur la monomanie et particulièrement sur la monomanie incendiaire. *Annls Hygs. publ. Méd. lég.*, **10**, 367–484

McKerracher, D. W. and Dacre, A. J. I. (1966). A study of arsonists in a special security hospital. *Br. J. Psychiat.*, **112**, 1151–1154

Osiander, F. B. (1813). Ueber den Selbstmord, seine Uraschen Arten, medicinischgerichtliche Untersuchung und die Mittel gegen denselben. *Eine Schrift sowohl für Policei-und Justiz-Beamte, als für gerichtliche Aerzte und Wundärzte für Psychologen und Volkslehrer*, **XII**, Hannover

Schmid, Hans (1914). Zur Psychologie der Brandstifter. *Psychologische Abhandlungen*, Bd. 1, 80–179

Scott, D. F. (1974). *Fire and Fire-Raisers*. Duckworth, London

Scott, P. D. S. (1977). Assessing dangerousness in criminals. *Br. J. Psychiat.*, **131**, 127–142

Soothill, K. L. and Pope, P. J. (1973). Arson. A twenty year cohort study. *Med., Sci. Law*, **13**, 127–138

Stekel, Wilhelm (1924). *Pyromania*, Vol. II, *Peculiarities of Behaviour*. Boni-Liverwright Co., pp. 124–232

Tennent, T. G., McQuaid, A., Loughnane, T. and Hands, A. J. (1971). Female arsonists. *Br. J. Psychiat.*, **119**, 497–502

Topp, D. O. (1973). Fire as a symbol and as a weapon of death. *Med., Sci. Law*, **13**, 79–86

26 Trans-sexualism

J. Christie-Brown

Trans-sexualism is a rare disorder which is difficult to manage or treat. It is of great theoretical interest and its study may eventually throw light on normal psychosexual development.

Historical and Transcultural Aspects

In 1949 Cauldwell, writing in the journal *Sexology*, described a girl who 'obsessively wanted to be a boy' and coined the term Psychopathia Transsexualis. In 1953 Benjamin first used the term trans-sexualism in an address to the New York Academy of Medicine to describe anatomical males of apparently normal physique who felt themselves to be female and often wanted to become more so, and anatomical females with the converse problem. Benjamin then published an article using the term, and comments rather darkly that the majority of the very large number of requests for reprints came from Army doctors.

This relatively new term, trans-sexualism, refers of course to a very old problem. But a considerable impetus was given to the study of it when at about the time of Benjamin's paper, Hamburger (1953) published in the medical literature his account of a so-called 'sex conversion' operation on an American soldier called George Jorgensen who subsequently became Christine Jorgensen. Until then, trans-sexualism had had to lurk in obscure corners of medical practice, and surgical procedures did not see the light of day in respectable journals. Perhaps Hamburger was responding to changes in public acceptance of these problems that were already occurring, but the publication of his article was followed by hundreds of letters from people asking for help and by an alteration in medical attitudes. Since then, so-called Gender Identity Clinics have been opened at many Centres, mostly in the States but also in other parts of the world. Discussion of 'sex change' and trans-sexualism often appears in the popular press and there has been a sharp increase in medical articles on the subject, although to put it in perspective, Trans-sexualism follows Transposition of the Great Vessels in the Index Medicus and usually only occupies about one third as much space. The study of trans-sexualism then, and its management, has now become fairly acceptable and public rather than reprehensible and private.

This is probably all to the good, but even now the problem of making sense of the findings is considerable. The fact that trans-sexualism is of unknown aetiology and prevalence is less serious than the fact that there is no generally agreed definition. This difficulty is compounded by the very large effect of selection. Even today, to be a trans-sexual is very different from having measles or schizophrenia in terms of public and medical acceptance. Trans-sexual patients who reach doctors have to show great determination to do so and are more often than not well armed with knowledge of the literature and the advice of other trans-sexuals. Therefore, every conclusion about this problem, however limited or tentative, must be qualified by the fact that the patients are highly selected and often single-minded in the pursuit of a particular treatment.

As has been said, trans-sexualism is a new word for an old problem. No doubt changing social mores play a major part in influencing the readiness of patients to present the problem and may have pathoplastic and perhaps even pathogenic effects. But a brief survey can show that trans-sexualism is not simply a product of the decline of the West, permissiveness or bourgeois capitalist repression. There are, of course, many ancient myths in which some sort of change of sex plays a central part. It was said, for example, that among the Phrygians the male priests were supposed to castrate themselves and live as women. Juvenal, referring to presumed trans-sexuals of his day wrote:

But why are they waiting?
Isn't it now high time for them to try
The Phrygian fashion to make the job complete
Take a knife and lop off that
Superfluous piece of meat

Philo of Alexandria wrote of men who 'expending every care on outward adornment, are not ashamed even to employ every device to change artificially their nature as men into women . . . Some of them, craving a completed transformation into women . . . have amputated their generative member'. There are many other possible examples, including King Henry III of France who used to wear a low cut dress and pearls, and Lord Cornbury who showed the stuff of which the Empire was made by arriving in New York to take up his post as the first Colonial Governor dressed as a woman and continued to dress that way throughout his term of office. Several first hand and quite extensive descriptions of nineteenth century cases are given by Krafft-Ebbing.

Examples from history are useful but often the descriptions that are available are very sketchy. It is also important to know that probable trans-sexuals occur in cultures very different from our own where they may well have an important place in the society. In several tribes of American Indians there is recognition and acceptance of boys who show marked feminity when small and who grow up to live as women, and for similarly masculine girls. Among the Mohave Indians, boys with feminine traits were chosen to become priests and their feminity was cultivated by the women of the tribe. In some cases when grown up, such young men would 'marry' other men and would imitate menstruation by scratching themselves with sticks. After a time this menstruation would stop and later a stool would be passed which would be designated a stillbirth and ceremoniously buried with a period of mourning to follow. There are similar findings among Siberian tribes, Eskimos, and peoples from Africa, India, South America, Borneo and elsewhere.

This compression of a vast body of evidence is put forward simply to show that trans-sexualism is not confined to our society or our time.

Clinical Aspects

In turning to clinical aspects of the problem, one immediately comes up against the difficulty of the lack of a generally agreed definition (Meyer *et al.*, 1971; Finney, 1975). To call trans-sexual all those people who come to doctors asking for an operation to 'change sex' is clearly unsatisfactory. It is loosely analogous with calling any patient who asked for chlorpromazine a schizophrenic. The best that can be offered is a description of those patients who would almost certainly be diagnosed as trans-sexual to illustrate what clinical attributes belong to the term.

These attributes can be grouped under five headings (table 26.1).

Table 26.1
Clinical Features of Trans-sexualism

1. Subjective sense of Gender Discordance
2. Distaste for the evidence of anatomical sex
3. Behaviour more appropriate to psychological gender
4. Other abnormalities of psychosexual development
5. Other psychiatric and social problems

The first attribute is deviance of psychological gender, or of primary psychological sex-differentiation. In normal people psychological gender can usefully be broken down into two components: the first can be called *gender identity*, which refers to the subjective sense of maleness or femaleness, together with associated attitudes, interests and so on. The second is *gender role behaviour* which refers to the repertoire of behaviours that are sex specific to some degree: habits of dress, speech, gesture, activity and so on. Unfortunately, some of these theoretically obvious notions turn out to be remarkably elusive in practice. Clearly, the most reliable indicator of gender as a whole is anatomy, followed at some distance by dress, adornment and hair style. Where psychological gender is concerned, one is dealing with much less clear-cut indicators. If one puts aside behaviour related to sexual interaction itself, there is a great deal of evidence to show that the everyday behaviour of men and women is less gender dimorphic than we often think and that the differences that exist are hard to specify or measure. The overlap is so great where attitudes are concerned, that the difference almost disappears. Nevertheless, there remains a strong and irreducible subjective sense of gender identity.

In trans-sexuals, gender deviance is often apparent from an early age. To simplify matters, this and subsequent descriptions will be confined to anatomical males, although most applies *mutatis mutandis* to females. As a young boy the patient experiences a puzzling sense of being female, of wanting to be a girl, and of hoping to grow up to be one. He may prefer girls' games and their companionship, but one is always left with the irreducible sense of gender discordance. As Jan Maris says

> Trans-sexualism is something different . . . it is not an act of sex at all . . . (but) a lifelong ineradicable conviction . . . I equate it with the idea of soul, or self . . . it will be harder to systematize gender . . . it is a more nebulous entity.

The second major attribute of trans-sexualism is the distaste for the evidence of anatomical sex, which is sharply intensified at the time of puberty. The external genitalia, secondary sex hair, and the need to shave are all sources of great distress. In a few cases the penis may be mutilated or amputated by the patient.

The third attribute is that of behaviour appropriate to psychological gender. The adult male trans-sexual is usually feminine in gesture and in intonation of voice, and often this behaviour has an exaggerated 'camp' quality. Female trans-sexuals make better men than male ones do women.

A particular aspect of this behaviour is cross dressing, which occurs persistently in about 40 per cent of adult male patients. Usually, they dress up completely in women's clothes, with great attention to grooming and make-up, and without deriving sexual excitement from doing so but rather a general sense of well-being.

From cross dressing they go on to demands for hormones and surgical treatment, all aimed at crushing anatomy to fit psychological gender. This process can become a crusade in which the mildest suggestion of back tracking is brusquely dismissed as ridiculous.

Fourthly, there are often abnormalities of other aspects of psychosexual development. In general, the level of interest in sexual relationships is low, and patients stress the importance of being cared for or loved. Puberty is often reported as being late, but this has to be set against the fact that the changes of puberty are bitterly resented and evidence of anatomical sex denied.

Many trans-sexuals have experienced heterosexual relationships but often need a fantasy of having intercourse with a man to arouse them. Most of their sexual relations are homosexual where they play a passive role and avoid as far as possible the penis being touched. They will, of course, point out that in terms of their true nature, such relationships are heterosexual.

Finally, there is a fairly high incidence of other deviance. Histrionic personality, depressive episodes, overdose taking, alcohol abuse, instability of employment, and convictions for sexual and other offences have all been recorded. It is impossible to draw a precise dividing line between problems which are secondary to the trans-sexual state and those which are evidence of primary disorders of development of other aspects of personality. Nevertheless some trans-sexuals are of exemplary character, and much of what is known about these people is distorted by the highly selected sample we see in psychiatric clinics.

This description applies to what can be called the 'nuclear' group. But if the net is thrown wider, we can catch many variants (Meyer, 1974). First, there are undoubtedly a number of patients who show the basic syndrome, but to a milder degree. In this group could be placed a 23-year-old male patient who for as long as he can remember has felt uneasy in the male role, and conscious of a feminine aspect to his nature, but who does not accord it supremacy. He is a passive homosexual with a low level of sexual interest and looks for relationships in which he is cared for. He dislikes his penis and particularly resents having to shave but emphatically does not wish for any surgical treatment. He occasionally cross dresses.

Then there are those who report no early awareness of gender discordance, but rather one which arises at or after puberty. They may pass through a phase of fetishistic cross dressing or common-or-garden homosexuality and gradually shift into the trans-sexual syndrome.

Beyond these two variants, there are other types of patient described in the literature who may turn up asking for 'change of sex operations'.

Table 26.2
'Differential diagnosis' of Trans-sexualism

1. Fetishistic transvestism
2. Effeminate homosexuality
3. Gross personality disorder
4. Schizophrenia

First, there are those who obtain sexual satisfaction from cross dressing, and who have had more extensive heterosexual experience: the fetishistic transvestites. Then there are the passive homosexuals, occasional cross dressers with a strong streak of femininity but who do not show low sex drive or distaste for their genitalia. Then there are patients with severe personality disorders for whom a brief excursion into the trans-sexual scene seems to be just another adventure. Finally, and in a very different category, are occasional schizophrenic patients with delusions of sex change.

A great deal of ink has been spilled in arguments about these differential diagnoses. There are those who argue that it is of vital importance to identify the true trans-sexual and that the other types fall into clearly defined and distinct categories. Then there are the surgical pragmatists who speak of a general 'gender dysphoria syndrome' and say that anyone who can live successfully for one or two years in his chosen gender role qualifies for surgery and that diagnostic minutiae are of little importance—one imagines that they leave out the schizophrenics.

I would like to propose a view which falls somewhere between these two extremes. There is no convincing evidence that 'nuclear' trans-sexualism is a discrete entity, although it is referred to as a syndrome for convenience, but there is some evidence of varying degrees of gender discordance perhaps distributed along a continuum. It is then a kind of personality deviance in the statistical sense. There can then be severe and mild gender anomalies with or without other forms of personality deviance. Another dimension, to some degree independent, is that of sex object choice. Thus, there may be many homosexuals with little or no gender discordance, and some trans-sexuals who are not entirely homosexuals. This view hardly deserves the name of hypothesis because it describes rather than explains, but perhaps it is a model from which to derive hypotheses. It can encompass those occasional and perplexing patients who ask for 'sex change operations' in order to be homosexual: for example, men who wish to become women in order to live as lesbians. One would then say that their psychological gender is strongly discordant but their object choice heterosexual.

The prevalence of trans-sexualism can only be guessed at from surveys of patients known to doctors or from counting the number of replies to well publicised requests for information from Gender Clinics (Walinder, 1968). These guesses are that from 1:40 000 to 1:100 000 males are trans-sexual and about half to one-third as many women. One can never be sure what degree of gender discordance is included.

Aetiology

The question of aetiology is best introduced with a very brief account of normal sexual differentiation, anatomical and psychological. There are many factors in this process, but among these there are certainly variables in a chain, each of which sets the scene as it were for the operation of the next. Each one of these can be influenced by other factors which can deflect the process from its central course (Money and Ehrhardt, 1972).

First, the chromosomal constitution XX or XY almost invariably determines the differentiation of the gonad into ovary or testis. Then, secretion of androgen promotes male anatomical development. In the absence of androgen, female differentiation occurs. In the testicular feminisation syndrome, for example, there is a failure of tissue response to androgen and an XY child with undescended testes is born with female external genitalia. The anomaly is usually discovered when primary amenorrhoea is being investigated.

Of great interest are the discoveries over the past twenty years of the organising effects of androgen on brain mechanisms, particularly in the hypothalamus. Most of this work has been done with rats, but the findings also apply to some extent to other species including guinea pigs and the rhesus monkey. There is a critical period of a few days only in late foetal or early neonatal life according to species in which the presence or absence of androgen has permanent effects on hypothalamic organisation and determines whether gonadotrophic hormones are produced in a steady, characteristically male fashion or a cyclical characteristically female fashion when sexual maturity is reached. For example, a female rat exposed to androgen during the critical period will at maturity be anovulatory with steady gonadotropin production. In contrast, male rats treated with anti-androgen and later castrated can evoke the changes of oestrus in implanted ovaries.

There are also behavioural consequences of the action of this critical-period androgen, although the findings are complicated by variation from species to species and are influenced by the hormonal changes at sexual maturity and the setting in which the observations are made. Broadly speaking, the anatomical female rat that has been exposed to androgen is more likely than other females to mount females, and the male deprived of androgen to be receptive to the mounts of other males. In the rhesus monkey the androgen-ised female plays in a characteristically 'rough and tumble' male way.

There is a little evidence about the importance of these mechanisms in humans. Girls with the adrenogenital syndrome have a metabolic block, preventing the normal production of adrenal steroids and produce large quantities of androgenic hormones instead. They may be born with a large clitoris and fused labia and require surgery as well as treatment with steroids to suppress the androgen production. Money has shown that compared with controls they show more masculine tomboyish behaviour during development even when the abnormality is treated immediately after birth, but they grow up with female gender identity and ovulate. In fact, studies of a wide variety of children who are pseudo-hermaphrodites, that is to say who have some ambiguity of anatomical differentiation, have shown that gender identity is mainly determined by sex of assignment whatever the chromosomal or gonadal sex. If a mistake is made, reassignment becomes increasingly difficult after the age of 18 months and almost impossible after 5 years although there are reports of cases that do not follow this rule. Of course, these are not true experiments because the gender identity of pseudo-hermaphrodites may be more easily moulded by other influences than that of normal children. But Money quotes one case of a normal male child who suffered a severe burn to his external genitalia and for whom female genitalia were constructed. He is being fairly successfully reared as a girl, being now 7.

So, in humans it seems that it is psychological and social influences which are of prime importance in psychological gender development. Anatomy is the crucial focus in mobilising these influences, but there may be certain innate psychological differences as well between the sexes. In a vast review, Maccoby and Jacklin (1975) came up with four such differences which they believe to be to some degree independent of environment. Boys are more aggressive than girls, and have greater mathematical and visuo-spatial ability and less verbal ability but there is considerable overlap, and the differences are small. Subsequent gender differentiation depends partly on imitation or identification and partly on differential reinforcement of behaviour and attitudes by parents and peers. There is, however, an important and obvious cognitive principle which is a second focus after anatomy in organising these influences, which is the development of a stable concept of being a boy or a girl, this being usually fixed by the age of 18 months.

In summary, post-natal social and psychological influences seem to be the most important factors in human psychological gender development. However, there are innate psychological differences between boys and girls, and foetal endocrine or other organic factors cannot be ruled out on present evidence.

Returning now to trans-sexualism, if there is indeed a continuum of severity of the abnormality, a multifactorial aetiology is likely. The possible factors that have been investigated so far can be grouped under five headings (Money and Ehrhardt, 1972).

(1) Chromosomal.
(2) Genetic.
(3) Temporal lobe dysfunction.
(4) Endocrine.
(5) Environmental.

To take the first, there is no evidence of any chromosomal abnormality in the vast majority of trans-sexuals. There is a doubtful excess of gender discordance in Klinefelter's syndrome and one case of trans-sexualism in an XX/XO mosaic has been reported.

As far as a possible genetic aetiology goes, two monozygotic twin pairs have been reported both discordant for trans-sexualism, showing at least that other factors are important. There have been four reports of sibships in which more than one member is affected, but none where earlier generations have been. This is taken to support an environmental aetiology, but would also be consistent with recessive genetic inheritance. However, much more often than not the siblings of trans-sexuals are unaffected and a recent study found no excess of cousin marriages in the parents of trans-sexuals (Walinder and Thuwe, 1977).

Reports of rare associations between temporal lobe abnormalities and fetishism occur: for example the case of the safety-pin fetishist cured by temporal lobectomy. There has therefore been a thorough search of the EEGs of trans-sexuals and in up to 28 per cent some temporal lobe dysrhythmia has been claimed but these abnormalities disappear when the EEGs are assessed blind against those of a control group (Blumer, 1969).

In a number of endocrine studies which have measured plasma and urine levels of gonadotropins, androgens and oestrogens, the only abnormalities found have turned out to be due to the patients surreptitiously taking hormone pills. However, if there is an endocrine abnormality, it might be the result of some failure of the foetal critical period development mentioned earlier. An abnormality of this kind would probably not be detected by cross-sectional studies, but only by investigating the dynamics of the system. Dorner has recently reported on six trans-sexual men and four trans-sexual women. The basis of his work is that in normal females oestrogen has a positive feedback effect on luteinising hormone (LH) production: that is to say, giving oestrogen produces a surge of LH. In males the effect is to suppress LH production. In two of the six trans-sexual men a positive feedback effect occurred and in two of the four women the feedback effect was only weakly positive. Results like these need careful replication but they are of great interest (Dorner *et al.*, 1976).

It is, of course, environmental factors that have received greatest attention. Stoller (1974), a psychoanalyst, has made extensive studies on very feminine boys who in some cases become trans-sexual as adults. He has described a very specific family constellation which he believes to be the rule. The mother has been a tomboyish girl, ambivalent about her femininity. She spends an inordinate amount of time in close physical contact with the infant, carrying him everywhere and lying for hours with him. The father is present in the family but totally committed to his work. He appears briefly at breakfast and in the evening after a few noncommital grunts, shuts himself in a room by himself. In this way the child forms an intense identification with his mother. Perhaps there is one glimmer of hope for these children, in that psychotherapy with a man who takes a rather directive and involved role seems to deflect a few of them from their trans-sexual path.

Table 26.3
22 cases (18 male, 4 female)

	Early onset $n = 11$	Late onset $n = 11$
Mild gender discordance	1	6
Family 'Stoller' type	4	2
Other family abnormality	2	4
Possible endocrine disorder	0	4
Severe personality disorder	1	4

Table 26.3 shows the first 22 cases in my own series. There are 18 men and 4 women. The patients have been divided into 11 in whom there was clear evidence of gender disturbance in early childhood and a second group of 11 in whom the disorder did not emerge until after puberty. Seven cases were thought to show the trans-sexual syndrome to a mild degree, and six of these

were in the late onset group. Only six cases had been exposed to the sort of family influences described by Stoller, with four of the six in the early onset group. In six cases there was definite evidence of other family disturbance, but of a non-specific kind, with disorganisation of the family by parental death, violence and alcoholism; four of these six were in the late onset group. In three of this same group there was convincing evidence of late puberty and in a fourth case a strong clinical suggestion of Cushing's syndrome for which the patient refused investigation. Lastly, there were five cases of severe general personality disorder, four of these being in the late onset group. Although not shown in the table, there were no EEG abnormalities at all.

It would be reckless to try to draw firm conclusions from this small and certainly distorted sample. It can be said that EEG abnormalities are not an essential finding in trans-sexualism and that the 'Stoller family' is not the rule. A hypothesis to be tested is that the early onset cases are less severe and show more features and background factors to suggest that their trans-sexualism is part of a more general disorder of personality development.

Management

Trans-sexual patients who reach doctors are almost always determined to obtain hormone treatment; in males, electrolysis for the removal of body hair; and surgery. Psychotherapy and aversion therapy are virtually useless in changing the patient's mind, although there has been a single case report of success with behavioural methods.

The usual procedure is as follows. First, there must be careful assessment to exclude the mentally ill and the sensation seekers, or those with severe personality disorders. The first at least are very rare, although I have seen one patient whose trans-sexual urge only emerged fully when he was depressed. The critical step is to insist that the patient must live publicly in his chosen role for at least one year, because no medical treatment can lessen the impact of this adjustment. In this country there is no problem in obtaining suitable employment documents and a passport. A male patient will then be given oestrogen which will produce some breast development and slight reduction in hair growth, but electrolysis will usually be necessary. In the female, testosterone suppresses menstruation. In some centres, classes are provided to educate patients in deportment, dress, makeup and so on. Finally, comes the surgery. For men this involves mammaplasty, castration, penectomy and the construction of an artifical vagina. Some patients also ask for plastic surgery to the nose, the eyelids, the ears and the larynx. In women, mastectomy, hysterectomy and occasionally attempts to construct a penis are carried out.

No doctor can embark on this process without considerable misgivings. For one thing the operation in males has a high rate of complications, around 40 per cent. These include recto-vaginal fistula, urethral stenosis and an unsatisfactory short and narrow vagina.

Technical considerations apart, there is an ethical dilemma. The first, and least important, part of this is that doctors dislike giving treatment prescribed by the patient. This problem applies to much of plastic surgery. Secondly, it seems that the doctor is colluding with the bizarre and morbid ideas of the patient: the patient will reply that it is equally grotesque to insist that anatomy must have supremacy over mental life. Perhaps the most crucial question is, does this treatment help the patient to a more contented life?

Unfortunately, there is no satisfactory answer to this question. The few follow up studies that have been done are short, small, and there is a large dropout rate.

Assessment is by those who were responsible for the treatment and is usually highly subjective and must be distorted by enormous pressure from the patient as well to justify what has happened. In general, it is said that few are worse and 60–70 per cent are better. However, there are two series in which the assessment of results has been more careful than most (Randell, 1971; Money, 1971).

Table 26.4
Postoperative follow up (Randell), $n = 37$

	Preoperative adjustment	Postoperative adjustment
Excellent		15
Good	4	14
Fair	21	3
Poor	12	1
Very poor		4

Table 26.4 shows Randell's series which gives data on 37 out of 52 cases who had surgery. Adjustment was assessed in a global way, but in general there was an improvement after surgery except in four cases, two of whom committed suicide. In fact, it is not possible from the data to trace the improvement of individual cases. The duration of follow up is not given.

Table 26.5 shows Money's series in which patients were assessed on four variables before and after surgery. In only one instance, on the first variable,

Table 26.5
Postoperative follow up (Money), $n = 24$

	Better	No change	Worse
Patient satisfaction	23		1
Employment record	12	12	
Police record	4	20	
Psychiatric disability	10	14	

was a patient adjudged to have got worse. The median follow up time was four years.

Compared with the way in which other treatments are assessed, even the better follow-up studies of operated trans-sexuals are unsatisfactory, and clearly there is an urgent need for better designed studies. Nevertheless, the practising psychiatrist will see some trans-sexuals who are entirely convincing in their new role so that they will be automatically referred to by the pronoun of their choice. Their lives are stable and any difficulties they have seem to be secondary to the gender disorder and its social consequences. It is easy to say that prevention would be preferable and that surgery should be avoided, but I believe that surgery can be justified in some of these cases although the decision is never easy and is best shared with an experienced colleague.

References

Benjamin, H. (1953). Transvestism and transsexualism. *Int. J. Sexol.*, **7**, 12–14

Blumer, Dietrich (1969). Transsexualism, sexual dysfunction and temporal lobe disorder. In *Transsexualism and Sex Reassignment* (Ed. R. Green and J.Money), Johns Hopkins University Press, Baltimore, pp. 213–219

Cauldwell, D. C. (1949). Psychopathia transsexualis. *Sexology*, **16**, 274–280

Dorner, G., Rhoda, W., Seidel, K., Hass, Willi and Schott, G. (1976). On the evocability of a positive oestrogen feedback action on LH secretion in transsexual men and women. *Endokrinologie*, Band 67, Fest 1, pp. 20–25

Finney, Joseph C. (1975). A study of transsexuals seeking gender reassignment. *Am. J. Psychiat.* **132**(9), 962–964

Hamburger, C. (1953). Desire for change of sex as shown by personal letters from 465 men and women. *Acta endocr.*, **14**, 361–375

Maccoby, E. E. and Jacklin, C. N. (1975). *The Psychology of Sex Difference*. Oxford University Press, London

Meyer, Jon K., Knorr, Norman J. and Blumer, Dietrich (1971). Characterisation of a self-designated transsexual population. *Archs Sexual Behav.*, **1**(3), 219–230

Meyer, Jon K. (1974). Clinical variants among applicants for sex reassignment. *Archs Sexual Behav.*, **3**(6), 527–537

Money, John (1971). Prefatory remarks on the outcome of sex reassignment in 24 cases of transsexualism. *Archs Sexual Behav.*, **1**(2), 163–165

Money, John and Ehrhardt, Anke A. (1972). *Man and Woman, Boy and Girl: the Differentiation and Dimorphism of Gender Identity from Conception to Maturity*. Johns Hopkins University Press, Baltimore and London

Randell, John (1971). Indications for sex reassignment surgery. *Archs Sexual Behav.*, **1**(2), 153–161

Stoller, Robert J. (1974). *Sex and Gender*, Vol. 1, *The Development of Masculinity and Femininity*. Jason Aronson, New York

Walinder, J. (1968). Transsexualism: definition, prevalence and sex distribution. *Acta psychiat. scand.*, Suppl. 203, 255–257

Walinder, J. and Thuwe, I. (1977). A study of consanguinity between the parents of transsexuals. *Br. J. Psychiat.*, **131**, 73–4

Author Index

Subject Index

Numbers in brackets refer to chapters in *Current Themes in Psychiatry* Vol. 1.
Numbers in italic refer to complete chapters.